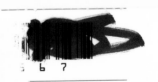
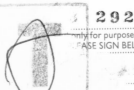

CANCER CHEMOTHERAPY AND
SELECTIVE DRUG DEVELOPMENT

DEVELOPMENTS IN ONCOLOGY

3

CANCER CHEMOTHERAPY AND SELECTIVE DRUG DEVELOPMENT

Proceedings of the 10th Anniversary Meeting of the
Coordinating Committee for Human Tumour Investigations,
Brighton, England, October 24–28, 1983

edited by

K.R. Harrap
W. Davis
A.H. Calvert

Technical Editor: A.S. Robinson

Martinus Nijhoff Publishing
a member of the Kluwer Academic Publishers Group
Boston/The Hague/Dordrecht/Lancaster

Distributors for North America:
Kluwer Academic Publishers
190 Old Derby Street
Hingham, MA 02043

Distributors for all other countries:
Kluwer Academic Publishers Group
Distribution Centre
P.O. Box 322
3300 AH Dordrecht
The Netherlands

Library of Congress Cataloging in Publication Data
Main entry under title:

Cancer chemotherapy and selective drug development.

   (Developments in onology)
   Includes bibliographies and indexes.
   1. Cancer--Chemotherapy--Congresses. 2. Anti-
neoplastic agents--Testing--Congresses. I. Harrap,
K. R. II. Davis, Walter. III. Calvert, A. Hilary.
IV. Co-ordinating Committee for Human Tumour
Investigations. V. Series. [DNLM: 1. Antineoplastic
Agents--therapeutic use--congresses. 2. Neoplasms--
drug therapy--congresses. W1 DE998N / QZ 267 C21o5 1983]
RC271.C5C3135   1984   616.99'4061   84-14677
ISBN 0-89838-673-X

PREFACE

Over the past 30 years many significant advances have been made in the management of a number of disseminated malignant diseases. The prognosis for diseases such as childhood leukaemia, choriocarcinoma and Hodgkin's disease has gradually been transformed as better antitumour agents have become available and their clinical use has been refined. During the past 10 years the advent of new agents, particularly cisplatin, bleomycin and the podophyllotoxins, has allowed the cure of disseminated testicular tumours. This degree of success has not, however, been achieved in the case of a number of other common cancers. Ovarian carcinoma is tantalisingly chemo-sensitive and although there are long term survivors from disseminated disease, these are only a small proportion of the total. Breast cancer, although "sensitive" to a multitude of drugs appears to have yielded neither survival benefit, nor cure to the efforts of therapists, while tumours such as those of the colon remain stubbornly unresponsive.

Against this backcloth it is apparent that additional more selective treatments are needed if further impact is to be made on the problem of cancer. The development of such agents requires the integration of a multidisciplinary effort encompassing the fields of chemistry, biology and medicine.

This symposium provided a forum for clinical and preclinical scientists, where current aspects of cancer treatment were reviewed and approaches to the development of a new generation of more selective anticancer drugs discussed.

THE EDITORS

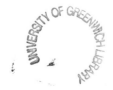

CONTENTS

CHAPTER I: ADVANCES IN CANCER TREATMENT

1. NEW APPROACHES TO OLD PROBLEMS

2. CURRENT CLINICAL PROGRESS WITH NEW AGENTS

CHAPTER IV: DESIGN AND DEVELOPMENT OF NEW DRUGS

CHAPTER V: CHROMATIN AS A TARGET IN CANCER CHEMOTHERAPY

CHAPTER VI: ENDOCRINE THERAPY

ABSTRACTS OF PROFFERED PAPERS AND POSTERS

1. NEW AGENTS: EXPERIMENTAL STUDIES

2. NEW AGENTS/COMBINATIONS: CLINICAL STUDIES

3. NEW AGENTS: CYTOTOXIC MECHANISMS

4. NEW AGENTS: METABOLISM AND PHARMACOKINETICS

CONTRIBUTORS

G.E. ADAMS, MRC Radiobiology Unit, Harwell, Didcot, Oxon OX11 ORD, England.

P. ALEXANDER, Department of Medical Oncology, Southampton General Hospital, Southampton SO9 4XY, England.

J.M. ALLEN, Hammersmith Hospital, DuCane Road, London W12, England.

M.J. BAINES, St. Christopher's Hospice, Lawrie Park Road, London SE26, England.

M.H. BAKER, Institute of Cancer Research, Belmont, Sutton, Surrey, England.

P. BEDFORD, Christie Hospital and Holt Radium Institute, Manchester M20 9BX, England.

A. BELANGER, MRC Unit Mol Biol,Le Centre Hospitalier de l'Universite Laval, Quebec G1V 4G2, Canada.

J. BESSERER, Warner Lambert/Parke Davis Pharmaceutical Research Division, Ann Arbor, Michigan, U.S.A.

P. BILLIAERT, Department of Oncology, Glasgow University, Scotland.

L.J. BLACK, The Lilly Research Laboratories, Indianapolis, Indiana, U.S.A.

A. BLOCH, Roswell Park Memorial Institute, 666 Elm Street, Buffalo, New York 14263, U.S.A.

S.R. BLOOM, Hammersmith Hospital, DuCane Road, London W12, England.

A. BOGDEN, EG & G Mason Research Institute, 57 Union Street, Worcester, Mass 01608, U.S.A.

W.A. BOGGUST, Cancer Research Unit, Department of Experimental Medicine, Trinity College & St. Luke's Hospital, Dublin, Ireland.

P. BONDY, Veterans Administration Medical Center, West Spring Street, West Haven, CT 06516, U.S.A.

R.J. BOOTH, Department of Pathology, Auckland University, Private Bag, Auckland, New Zealand.

T.J. BORITZKI, Warner Lambert/Parke Davis Pharmaceutical Research Division, Ann Arbor, Michigan, U.S.A.

A. BRODIE, University of Maryland, Baltimore, U.S.A.

W. BRUNNER, Institut of Medical Oncology, University of Bern, Inselspital, CH-3010 Bern, Switzerland.

K.C. CALMAN, Department of Oncology, Glasgow University, Scotland.

Z.N. CANELLAKIS, Veterans Administration Medical Center, West Spring Street, West Haven, CT 06516, U.S.A.

S.K. CARTER, Bristol-Myers Company, 345 Park Avenue, New York, NY 10022, U.S.A.

A.M. CASAZZA, Farmitalia C. Erba, Via imbonati 24, 20159 Milano, ITALY.

F. CAVALLI, Department of Medical Oncology, Ospedale san Giovanni, CH 6500 Bellinzona, Switzerland.

S. CHRAPUSTA, Institute of Oncology, Warsaw, Poland.

M.J. CLEARE, Johnson Matthey Research Centre, Blount's Court, Sonning Common, Reading RG4 9NH, England.

J.A. CLEMENS, The Lilly Research Laboratories, Indianapolis, Indiana, U.S.A.

H. CLINK, Royal Marsden Hospital, Belmont, Sutton, Surrey, England.

W.R. COBB,EG & G Mason Research Institute, 57 Union Street, Worcester, Mass 01608, U.S.A.

V.M. COLE, Tenovus Building, Southampton General Hospital, Tremona Road, SouthamptOn SO9 4XY.

P.D. COOK, Warner Lambert/Parke Davis Pharmaceutical Research Division, Ann Arbor, Michigan, U.S.A.

R.C. COOMBES, Ludwig Institute for Cancer Research, Belmont, Sutton, Surrey, England.

V.D. COURTENAY, Institute of Cancer Research, Belmont, Sutton, Surrey, England.

M. CROFTS, Royal Marsden Hospital, Belmont, Sutton, Surrey, England.

H.A. DE HAAN, Medical Department, ICI Pharmaceuticals Division, Alderley Park, Macclesfield, Cheshire SK10 4TG, England.

N. DEVLEESCHOUWER,Lab. de Cancerologie Mammaire, Institut Jules Bordet, 1 rue Heger Bordet, B-1000 Brussels, Belgium.

H.S. DHALIWAL, ICRF Dept. Medical Oncology, St. Bartholomew's Hospital, London EC1A, England.

A. DI MARCO, Farmitalia C. Erba, Via imbonati 24, 20159 Milano, Italy.

W. DIETRICH, Central Institute for Cancer Research, 1115 Berlin-Buch, G.D.R.

J. DIVER, Medical Department, ICI Pharmaceuticals Division, Alderley Park, Macclesfield, Cheshire SK10 4TG, England.

A. DRUMM, Cancer Research Unit, Department of Experimental Medicine, Trinity College & St. Luke's Hospital, Dublin, Ireland.

D.S. DUCH, Dept. Medicinal Biochemistry, Wellcome Research Labs, 3030 Cornwallis Road, Research Triangle Park, NC 27709, U.S.A.

D.C. DUMONDE, St. Thomas' Hospital, Lambeth Palace Road, London SE1, England.

A. DUPONT, MRC Unit Mol Biol, Le Centre Hospitalier de l'Universite Laval, Quebec G1V 4G2, Canada.

S. ECKHARDT, National Institute of Oncology, 1525 Budapest PF. 21. XII, Rath Gu. U. 7/9, Hungary.

L.H. EINHORN, Section of Medical Oncology, University of Indiana Medical Centre, Indianapolis, Indiana 46207, U.S.A.

G. EISENBRAND, Department of Food Chemistry and Environmental Toxicology, University of Kaiserslautern, 6750 Kaiserslautern, F.R.G.

U. EPPENBERGER, Laboratory of Biochemistry-Endocrinology, Research Department and Department of Gynecology, Kantonsspital Basel, CH-4031 Basel, Switzerland.

L.C. ERICKSON, Section of Oncology, Department of Medicine, Loyola University Medical Center, Maywood, Illinois 60153, U.S.A.

B.D. EVANS, Institute of Cancer Research, Belmont, Sutton, Surrey, England.

T. FACCHINETTI, Farmitalia C. Erba, Via imbonati 24, 20159 Milano, Italy.

A.B. FOSTER, Institute of Cancer Research, Belmont, Sutton, Surrey, England.

B. FOX, Christie Hospital and Holt Radium Institute, Manchester M20 9BX, England.

K.R. FOX, Department of Pharmacology, Medical School, Hills Road, Cambridge, England.

F. FRIEDLOS, Institute of Cancer Research, Belmont, Sutton, Surrey, England.

D.W. FRY, Warner Lambert/Parke Davis Pharmaceutical Research Division, Ann Arbor, Michigan, U.S.A.

N.W. GIBSON, Laboratory of Molecular Pharmacology, National Cancer Institute, Bethesda, Maryland, U.S.A.

U. GLAS, The Stockholm-Gotland Oncologic Center, Stockholm, Sweden.

M.J. GLENNIE, Tenovus Building, Southampton General Hospital, Tremona Road, Southampton SO9 4XY, England.

A. GOLDHIRSCH, Ludwig Institut for Cancer Research (Bern-Branch), Inselspital, CH-3010 Bern, Switzerland.

A. GOLDIN, Vincent T. Lombardi Cancer Research Center, Georgetown University School of Medicine, Washington, DC 20007, U.S.A.

G.H. GOODWIN, Chester Beatty Laboratories, Institute of Cancer Research, Fulham Road, London, England.

G. GOSS, Royal Marsden Hospital, Belmont, Sutton, Surrey, England.

P.E. GOSS, Institute of Cancer Research, Belmont, Sutton, Surrey, England.

H. GRUNICKE, Institute of Medicinal Chemistry and Biochemistry, University of Innsbruck, A-6020 Innsbruck, Austria.

T. HABESHAW, Institute of Radiotherapy, Western Infirmary, Glasgow, Scotland.

G.W. HANKS, Royal Marsden Hospital, Fulham Road, London.

H.H. HANSEN, Finseninstitute, Strandboulevarden 49, Copenhagen O, Denmark.

K.R. HARRAP, Institute of Cancer Research, Belmont, Sutton, Surrey, England.

A.L. HARRIS, Regional Radiotherapy Centre, Newcastle General Hospital, Newcastle upon Tyne NE4 6BE, England.

J. HARTLEY, Christie Hospital and Holt Radium Institute, Manchester M20 9BX, England.

B. HARTLEY-ASP, Leo Research Laboratories, S-251 00 Helsingborg, Sweden.

S. HAYLOCK, Department of Pharmacology, Medical School, Hills Road, Cambridge, England.

E. HEISE, Central Institute for Cancer Research, 1115 Berlin-Buch, G.D.R.

W. HELLIGER, Institute of Medicinal Chemistry and Biochemistry, University of Innsbruck, A-6020 Innsbruck, Austria.

J.C. HEUSON, Lab. de Cancerologie Mammaire, Institut Jules Bordet, 1 rue Heger Bordet, B-1000 Brussels, Belgium.

J.A. HICKMAN, CRC Experimental Chemotherapy Group, University of Aston, Birmingham B4 7ET, England.

K. IDESTROM, The Stockholm-Gotland Oncologic Center, Stockholm, Sweden.

B.F. ISSEL, Bristol Laboratories, PO Box 657, Syracuse, New York 13201, U.S.A.

D. JACKSON, Lederle Laboratories, Division of American Cyanamid Co, Middletown Road, Pearl River, NY 10965, U.S.A.

I.M. JACKSON, Ciba-Geigy Pharmaceuticals Divison, Wimblehurst Road, Horsham, West Sussex RH12 4AB, England.

R.C. JACKSON, Warner Lambert/Parke Davis Pharmaceutical Research Division, Ann Arbor, Michigan, U.S.A.

M. JARMAN, Institute of Cancer Research, Belmont, Sutton, Surrey, England.

A. JENEY, I. Institute of Pathology, Semmelweis Medical University, 1085 Budapest, Ulloi ut 26, Hungary.

R. JOSS, Institut of Medical Oncology, University of Bern, Inselspital, CH-3010 Bern, Switzerland.

B. KAHN, Royal Marsden Hospital, Belmont, Sutton, Surrey, England.

M. KAIGAS, The Stockholm-Gotland Oncologic Center, Stockholm, Sweden.

L. KARNSTROM, The Stockholm-Gotland Oncologic Center, Stockholm, Sweden.

D.J. KERLE, Hammersmith Hospital, DuCane Road, London W12, England.

J. KLASTERSKY, Institut Jules Bordet, rue Heger Bordet 1, 1000 Brussels, Belgium.

B. KONOPKA, Institute of Oncology, Warsaw, Poland.

W. KUNG, Laboratory of Biochemistry-Endocrinology, Research Department and Department of Gynecology, Kantonsspital Basel, CH-4031 Basel, Switzerland.

F. LABRIE, MRC Unit Mol Biol, Le Centre Hospitalier de l'Universite Laval, Quebec G1V 4G2, Canada.

H. LAGAST, Institut Jules Bordet, rue Heger Bordet 1, 1000 Brussels, Belgium.

G. LECLERCQ, Lab. de Cancerologie Mammaire, Institut Jules Bordet, 1 rue Heger Bordet, B-1000 Brussels, Belgium.

C-S. LEUNG, Institute of Cancer Research, Belmont, Sutton, Surrey, England.

O-T. LEUNG, Institute of Cancer Research, Belmont, Sutton, Surrey, England.

B. LEYLAND-JONES, Memorial Sloan Kettering Cancer Centre, 1275 York Avenue, New York, NY 10021, U.S.A.

T.A. LISTER, ICRF Dept. Medical Oncology, St. Bartholomew's Hospital, London EC1A, England.

A. LOIDL, Institute of Medicinal Chemistry and Biochemistry, University of Innsbruck, A-6020 Innsbruck, Austria.

S. LONN, Department of Histology, Karolinska Institute and Radiumhemmet Karolinska Hospital, 104 01 Stockholm, Sweden.

U. LONN, Department of Histology, Karolinska Institute and Radiumhemmet Karolinska Hospital, 104 01 Stockholm, Sweden.

R. LOSER, Klinge Pharma GmbH & Co., 8000 Munich 40, F.R.G.

R. McCAGUE, Institute of Cancer Research, Belmont, Sutton, Surrey, England.

J.G. McVIE, Department of Medicine, Netherlands Cancer Institute, Plesman Laan 121, 1066 CX Amsterdam, The Netherlands.

B.C. MILLAR, Institute of Cancer Research, Belmont, Sutton, Surrey, England.

J.L. MILLAR, Institute of Cancer Research, Belmont, Sutton, Surrey, England.

M.G. MOTT, Dept. Pediatrics, Royal Hospital for Sick Children, Bristol, England.

V.L. NARAYANAN, Drug Synthesis and Chemistry Branch, DTP, DCT, NCI, Blair Building, Room 4A-07, Silver Spring, Maryland 20910, U.S.A.

R.L. NELSON, Division of Oncology, Eli Lilly & Co., McCarthy Street, Indianapolis, Indiana, U.S.A.

A.M. NEVILLE, Ludwig Institute for Cancer Research, Belmont, Sutton, Surrey, England.

C.A. NICHOL, Dept. Medicinal Biochemistry, Wellcome Research Labs, 3030 Cornwallis Road, Research Triangle Park, NC 27709, U.S.A.

B. NORDENSKJOLD, The Stockholm-Gotland Oncologic Center, Stockholm, Sweden.

S. O'CONNELL, Cancer Research Unit, Department of Experimental Medicine, Trinity College & St. Luke's Hospital, Dublin, Ireland.

R.K. OLDHAM, Biological Development Branch, National Cancer Institute, Bethesda, Maryland 20014, U.S.A.

R.M. ORR, Institute of Cancer Research, Belmont, Sutton, Surrey, England.

H. PADZIK, Institute of Oncology, Warsaw, Poland.

Z. PASZKO, Institute of Oncology, Warsaw, Poland.

A. PEDRAZZINI, Royal Marsden Hospital, Belmont, Sutton, Surrey, England.

D. PEREZ, Royal Marsden Hospital, Belmont, Sutton, Surrey, England.

R.L. POWLES, Royal Marsden Hospital, Belmont, Sutton, Surrey, England.

T.J. POWLES, Royal Marsden Hospital, Belmont, Sutton, Surrey, England.

R.L. PRESTIDGE, Department of Pathology, Auckland University, Private Bag, Auckland, New Zealand.

B. PUSCHENDORF, Institute of Medicinal Chemistry and Biochemistry, University of Innsbruck, A-6020 Innsbruck, Austria.

F. RANDALL, Macmillan Unit, Christchurch Hospital, Christchurch, Dorset, England.

C.J. RAWLINGS, Institute of Cancer Research, Belmont, Sutton, Surrey, England.

J.J. ROBERTS, Institute of Cancer Research, Belmont, Sutton, Surrey, England.

W. ROOS,Laboratory of Biochemistry-Endocrinology, Research Department and Department of Gynecology, Kantonsspital Basel, CH-4031 Basel, Switzerland.

M.G. ROWLANDS, Institute of Cancer Research, Belmont, Sutton, Surrey, England.

G.J.S. RUSTIN, Dept. of Medical Oncology, Charing Cross Hospital, London W6, England.

J.L. RYAN, Veterans Administration Medical Center, West Spring Street, West Haven, CT 06516, U.S.A.

R.R. SANDHU, Institute of Cancer Research, Belmont, Sutton, Surrey, England.

P.S. SCHEIN, Division of Medical Oncology, Lombardi Cancer Research Center, Georgetown University, Washington, DC 20007, U.S.A.

S. SHALL, The University of Sussex, Biology Building, Falmer, Brighton, Sussex, England.

P.W. SHELDON, MRC Radiobiology Unit, Harwell, Didcot, Oxon OX11 ORD, England.

C.W. SIGEL, Dept. Medicinal Biochemistry, Wellcome Research Labs, 3030 Cornwallis Road, Research Triangle Park, NC 27709, U.S.A.

W.E. SIMON, Universitats Fraenklinik, Hamburg-Eppendorf, 2000 Hamburg, F.R.G.

L. SKOOG, The Stockholm-Gotland Oncologic Center, Stockholm, Sweden.

C.L. SMITH, Professorial Medical Unit, Southampton General Hospital, Southampton SO9 4XY, England.

I.E. SMITH, Royal Marsden Hospital, Fulham Road, London, England.

G.G. STEEL, Institute of Cancer Research, Belmont, Sutton, Surrey, England.

M.F.G. STEVENS, CRC Experimental Chemotherapy Group, University of Aston, Birmingham B4 7ET, England.

G.T. STEVENSON, Tenovus Building, Southampton General Hospital, Tremona Road, Southampton SO9 4XY, England.

I.J. STRATFORD, MRC Radiobiology Unit, Harwell, Didcot, Oxon OX11 ORD, England.

J.F.B. STUART, Department of Pharmacy, University of Strathclyde, Glasgow, Scotland.

M.H.N. TATTERSALL, Ludwig Institute for Cancer Research, Sydney Cancer Therapy Unit, Syndey, N.S.W. 2006, Australia.

K.D. TEW, Division of Medical Oncology, Lombardi Cancer Research Center, Georgetown University, Washington, DC 20007, U.S.A.

N-O. THEVE, The Stockholm-Gotland Oncologic Center, Stockholm, Sweden.

P.E. THORPE, Imperial Cancer Research Fund, Lincoln's Inn Fields, London, England.

M. TILBY, Institute of Cancer Research, Belmont, Sutton, Surrey, England.

J.L. TOY, Wellcome Research Labs, Langley Court, Beckenham, Kent BR3 3BS, England,.

G. TRAMS, Universitats Fraenklinik, Hamburg-Eppendorf, 2000 Hamburg, F.R.G.

C.P. TURNBULL, American Cyanamid Company, One Cyanamid Plaza, Wayne, N.J. 07470, U.S.A.

R.G. TWYCROSS, Sir Michael Sobell House, The Churchill Hospital, Headington, Oxford OX3 7LJ, England.

J.M. VENDITTI, Division of Cancer Treatment, National Cancer Institute, National Institutes of Health, Bethesda, Maryland 20014, U.S.A.

A. WALLGREN, The Stockholm-Gotland Oncologic Center, Stockholm, Sweden.

A.L. WANG, Division of Medical Oncology, Lombardi Cancer Research Center, Georgetown University, Washington, DC 20007, U.S.A.

M.J. WARING, Department of Pharmacology, Medical School, Hills Road, Cambridge, England.

J.D. WATSON, Department of Pathology, Auckland University, Private Bag, Auckland, New Zealand.

H.F. WATTS, Tenovus Building, Southampton General Hospital, Tremona Road, Southampton SO9 4XY, England.

J. WELSH, Department of Oncology, Glasgow University, Scotland.

J.M.A. WHITEHOUSE, CRC Medical Oncology Unit, Centre Block CF 93, Southampton General Hospital, Southampton SO9 4XY, England.

N. WILKING, The Stockholm-Gotland Oncologic Center, Stockholm, Sweden.

C.J. WILLIAMS, Medical Oncology Unit, Royal South Hants Hospital, Southampton, England.

G. WILLIAMS, Hammersmith Hospital, DuCane Road, London W12, England.

J. WILLIAMS, Ludwig Institute for Cancer Research, Belmont, Sutton, Surrey, England.

E. WILTSHAW, Royal Marsden Hospital, Fulham Road, London, England.

R.E. WITTES, Memorial Sloan-Kettering Cancer Center, 1275 York Avenue, New York, NY 10021, U.S.A.

R.L. ZERBE, The Lilly Research Laboratories, Indianapolis, Indiana, U.S.A.

C. ZLOTOGORSKI, Laboratory of Molecular Pharmacology, National Cancer Institute, Bethesda, Maryland, U.S.A.

H. ZWIERZINA, Institute of Medicinal Chemistry and Biochemistry, University of Innsbruck, A-6020 Innsbruck, Austria.

CHAPTER I

ADVANCES IN CANCER TREATMENT

1. NEW APPROACHES TO OLD PROBLEMS

awogbeif at f.fraßoun-sbn.ac.uk.

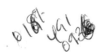

CLINICAL DRUG RESISTANCE

J. M. A. Whitehouse

Clinical characteristics of resistance

If it were possible to assume adequate exposure to an active agent, anything less than complete regression must indicate a degree of resistance.   In practice, varying degrees of resistance may be seen at initial presentation or subsequently.   These range from no response at all, initial tumour regression followed by stabilisation, to stabilisation without regression.   Between patients with identical tumours there may be profound differences in the time taken to respond to identical therapies.   To attribute either incomplete response or delay to inherent tumour resistance makes many assumptions.   Pharmaco- logical explanations, are frequently quoted as possible mechanisms contributing to reduced effectiveness of cancer treatment.   In practice none of these factors can be implicated with certainty, and the activity of a drug regimen is assessed on the basis of a reduction in tumour volume.   Clinical evidence of response, therefore, is virtually the sole means by which resistance may be assessed with any applicability to the individual tumour within the environment of the particular host.   In vitro assays using the influence of drugs on the growth of tumour stem cells or the influence upon xenografts, may give some indication, but in practice while resistance can be predicted with 90% certainty, the selection of definitely potent agents within the host is much less successful (1).

Many criteria of response exist, but only total disease eradication and complete response appear to have real survival significance (2). The former cannot be predicted, and is a diagnosis by default.   The direct impact of therapy can only be assessed in the crudest terms, but since it is the change in tumour burden which gives some guide to the interpretation of drug activity and by doing so influences management, it is a measurement of some importance (Fig. 1).

Fig. 1.   CATEGORIES OF RESPONSE

ERADICATION (= 'CURE')	[	TYPE I	TOTAL
	[	TYPE II	COMPLETE (No detectable disease but subsequent relapse)
	[	TYPE III	MAJOR (Microscopic detectable disease only)
NO ERADICATION	[	TYPE IV	MINOR (Measurable reduction)
	[	TYPE V	SYMPTOMATIC (+ stabilisation)
	[	TYPE VI	NIL

Complete Response

While total and complete responses bring substantial improvements
in quality of life, lesser responses while implying a degree of resistance
to therapy, may bring temporary benefits. The list of Type II responses
is substantial and includes some common cancers (Fig. 2). Why such a
fundamental difference should exist between Type I and II responses is
ill understood. The activity of drugs as single agents in the latter,
is well established and although dose escalation appears to increase
the percentage of complete remission in some conditions (Fig. 3), this
is not associated with a conversion to Type I responses.

Fig. 2   CONDITIONS IN WHICH COMPLETE RESPONSE IS REPORTED

TYPE I
HODGKIN'S DISEASE
GERM CELL TUMOURS
SEMINOMA
CHORIOCARCINOMA
HISTIOCYTIC LYMPHOMA
CHILDHOOD –
  ACUTE LYMPHOBLASTIC LEUKAEMIA
  RHABDOMYOSARCOMA
  EWING'S TUMOUR

TYPE II
ACUTE LEUKAEMIAS
LYMPHOMAS
NEUROBLASTOMA
SOFT TISSUE SARCOMAS
MYELOMA
PLASMA CELL LEUKAEMIA
MELANOMA

SQUAMOUS CELL CARCINOMA OF
  HEAD AND NECK
OSTEOSARCOMA
CHILDHOOD BRAIN TUMOUR
CARCINOMAS OF LUNG
                OVARY
                BREAST

Fig. 3   CONDITIONS IN WHICH HIGH DOSE
        CHEMOTHERAPY SUBSTANTIALLY INCREASES
                RESPONSE RATE

MELANOMA	Methotrexate	Fisher et al, 1979 (3)
	Melphalan	Lazarus et al, 1983 (4)
MYELOMA)	Melphalan	McElwain et al, 1983 (5)
PLASMA CELL LEUKAEMIA)		
SMALL CELL LUNG CANCER	Cyclophosphamide	Souhami et al, 1982 (6)

BREAST CANCER	Methotrexate	Yap et al, 1979	(7)
OSTEOSARCOMA?	Methotrexate	Jaffe et al, 1977	(8)
OVARIAN CANCER	Cis DDP	Bruckner et al, 1981	(9)
NEUROBLASTOMA	Melphalan	Lazarus et al, 1983	(4)

This shortfall of achievement is emphasised by the fact that while
complete remission rates of 70% occur in adult acute lymphoblastic
leukaemia, 80% in acute myelogenous leukaemia, 50% in small cell
bronchial carcinoma, 33% in carcinoma of the ovary and 10% in carcinoma
of the breast, eventual relapse approaches 100% in each. A striking
feature of these relapses is that while initially the tumour may appear
responsive to chemotherapy with a variety of different agents, eventually
the tumour becomes unresponsive, not only to all previously used
agents, but also to compounds to which there has been no exposure.
Such 'resistance' is well documented and poorly explained although
recent studies suggest that gene amplification may be implicated (10,
11). Even in tumours for which Type I responses are recorded, there
is a significant proportion of patients whose tumours are largely
unresponsive 'de novo'. These patients identify themselves by their
ultimate course which may sometimes be predicted only on clinical or
pathological grounds, but without any more objective discriminant.
Those patients who achieve a Type II response, but in whom a Type I
response is not seen, may well share biological characteristics similar
to tumours such as AML, adult ALL and carcinoma of the lung, ovary and
breast. This is particularly so if their disease is uninfluenced by
dose escalation, implying a dissociated relationship between drug
dosage and response.

Although complete response is an identifiable state, the rate at
which this may be achieved varies with the tumour type, so that complete
remission virtually never occurs with maximal treatment after 15 weeks
in testicular teratomas, but may occur as late as 72 weeks in AML and
breast cancer. Earlier assessment might be interpreted as a failure
of therapy, and thus of 'resistance'. Nonetheless, there is clearly a
difference in responsiveness of tumours having the same histology
implying diminished sensitivity to the drugs used, and thus a degree of
resistance. If the end result is the same, such semantic discrimination
does not have clinical relevance, although it may eventually be shown
to be of pharmacological significance. Even within one patient,
response of metastases may vary considerably from tissue to tissue.

In breast cancer, the median time to resolution of skin lesions is 7 weeks, whereas that of lesions in the liver and bone is 32 weeks (12). In bone, this may well reflect the natural rate of healing, while in liver more complex interpretations are possible. Complete response depends for its definition on available methods for disease detection. This imposes a severe limitation since with the exception of choriocarcinoma and some cases of germinal tumours where residual tumour can be identified from raised beta HCG or alphafoetal protein levels, a considerable volume of tumour must remain unidentified using current techniques. As techniques of detection improve, it is likely that in patients with Type II responses, residual disease will be found. Immunological techniques have already established that in poorly differentiated nodular lymphomas patients with Stage I disease often have a monotypic population of lymphocytes in blood or bone marrow implying that this is truly Stage IV disease (13). Years may pass before this becomes clinically apparent. Complete remission in this condition is not uncommon, but intensification does not improve survival (14) implying that the neoplastic nidus either remains resistant, or that neoplastic transformation is a continuing process.

Clinical features contributing to resistance

While the existence of sanctuary sites has been found to be a feature of ALL, and the introduction of appropriate prophylactic therapy has substantially altered the natural history of this condition, in no other tumour has this been found to be of equal importance. However, CNS prophylaxis in histiocytic lymphoma and small cell lung cancer may substantially reduce the frequency with which disease appears in this site. Much debate has surrounded the significance of tumour mass as a contributing factor to resistance. In Burkitt's lymphoma, ovarian cancer and some childhood malignancies unrandomised studies suggest a benefit from debulking procedures. Some suggestion has also been made that phenotypic variation within some bulky tumours develops because of a greater mutation rate and may contribute to the risk of resistant lines developing (15). Others, such as histiocytic lymphoma and testicular teratoma may respond overwhelmingly to chemo-therapy, despite considerable bulk implying genetic stability and a low mutation rate. Further experimental evidence is required to substantiate the importance of tumour bulk reduction as a therapeutic procedure. Advantages in survival and response seen in patients with resectable disease may be a reflection of real differences in intrinsic behaviour of individual tumours. The concept of giving chemotherapy to reduce tumour volume yet further once minimal disease is present is a seductive one. If chemotherapy has been the primary treatment, then only in one condition, acute lymphoblastic leukaemia, is 'maintenance' chemotherapy still considered to extend survival. In other 'adjuvant' situations involving childhood tumours, i.e. Wilm's and Ewing's tumour where prior therapy has been surgery, radiotherapy or both, chemotherapy undoubtedly contributes to improved survival. However, the role of adjuvant chemotherapy for the majority of tumours remains to be clearly defined, for even in breast cancer, overall survival is only marginally improved in some studies and the principal effect appears to be on disease free survival in certain patient sub-groups.

It is a remarkable fact that 'resistance' of normal tissues is a clinical rarity - possibly because 'resistance' of the tumour develops more readily. The induction of tolerance by normal tissues is a feature of the priming phenomenon reported to occur with cyclophosphamide and melphalan (16, 17). Unlike tumours where induced resistance persists, this phenomenon appears temporary and of short duration. The limitations imposed by normal tissue tolerance may prevent adequate therapeutic doses of drugs being given, i.e. cisplatinum with extensive renal damage, or when concurrent therapy with an aminoglycoside antibiotic is essential; any bone marrow suppressive drug when the bone marrow is heavily infiltrated; adriamycin where the myocardium is profoundly compromised etc. Resistance in these situations is compounded by inadequate therapy. These problems may also be accentuated in situations where drug metabolism or excretion is affected by primary organ failure.

A characteristic of second malignancies is their refractoriness to therapies which are normally active in tumours appearing as a first malignancy. Why this should be so is a matter of conjecture, and is not yet understood. Other features which may possibly be of importance in relationship to clinical drug resistance include interference with metabolism by non anti-cancer drugs administered concurrently, and the mode of administration (i.e. bolus, infusion or oral). Any element of malabsorption whatever the cause reduces available drug levels. Although much has been written concerning the vulnerability to drugs at different times in the cell cycle, no logically derived schedule has been shown to have any advantage over drugs administered synchronously.

Problems for the future

Many unresolved questions remain – perhaps the most important of which is not how to eradicate disease which cannot be identified, located or quantified, but rather how best to achieve knowledge of these characteristics. Only then can mechanisms contributing to resistance be defined for each situation. Exploitation of this knowledge would be a certain route to improved management, and would greatly facilitate logical drug design. Until this can be achieved, the meticulous documentation of disease extent, coupled with improved assessments of response, may aid a greater understanding of resistance.

The role of chemotherapy in the treatment of tumours which are partially resistant needs to be more clearly defined. Methods for documenting palliation require standardisation, and some quantification is required for clinical situations of the contribution chemotherapy may make to tumour response when integrated with other treatment modalities.

It may be that certain tumours may actually be made more sensitive to chemotherapy by the provision of factors which facilitate growth (i.e. oestrogen in the presence of oestrogen receptor breast carcinoma). So far this has been incompletely explored. The significance of variations in resistance associated with different histological types also merits attention. In planning chemotherapy metastases should be regarded as potential 'sanctuary sites' for which new approaches are required.

To avoid surmise, and the dependance on assumption when planning therapy 'resistance' must be more precisely defined and given specific interpretations of clinical significance.

REFERENCES
1. Alberts DS, Salmon SE, Chen H-SG, Surwit EA, Soehnlen B, Young L, Moon TE. In vitro clonogenic assay for predicting response of ovarian cancer to chemotherapy. Lancet(2):340-342,1980.
2. Carter SK. Cancer chemotherapy: new developments and changing concepts. Drugs(20):375-397,1980.
3. Fisher RI, Chabner BA, Myers CE. Phase II study of high dose methotrexate in patients with advanced malignant melanoma. Cancer Treat Rep(63):147-148,1979.
4. Lazarus HM, Herzig RH, Graham-Pole J, Wolff SN, Phillips GL, Strandjord S, Hurd D, Forman W, Gordon EM, Coccia P, Gross S,

Herzig GP.   Intensive melphalan chemotherapy and cryopreserved autologous bone marrow transplantation for the treatment of refractory cancer. Jnl Clin Oncol(1):359-367,1983.

5. McElwain TJ, Powles RL. High-dose intravenous melphalan for plasma-cell leukaemia and myeloma. Lancet(2):822-824,1983.

6. Souhami RL, Harper PG, Linch DC, Goldstone AH, Richards JDM, Trask C, Tobias JS, Spiro SG, Geddes DM. Single agent high dose cyclophosphamide with autologous bone marrow transfusion (ABMT) as initial treatment for small cell carcinoma of the bronchus (SCCB) (Abstract). The III World Conference on Lung Cancer(235):169,1982.

7. Yap HY, Blumenschein GR, Yap BS, Hortobagyi GN, Tashima CK, Wang AY, Benjamin RS, Bodey GP. High dose methotrexate for advanced breast cancer. Cancer Treat Rep(63):757-761,1979.

8. Jaffe N. American Journal of Surgery(133):405,1977.

9. Bruckner HW, Wallach R, Cohen CJ, Deppe G, Kabakow B, Ratner L and Holland JF. High-dose platinum for the treatment of refractory ovarian cancer. Gynecologic Oncology(12):64-67,1981.

10. Ling V. Genetic aspects of drug resistance in somatic cells. In: Schabel FM (ed) Antibiotics and chemotherapy. S. Karger, Basel, 1978, pp 191-200.

11. Biedler JL et al. J. Cell Biochem. Suppl 6 (30),1982.

12. Henderson TC, Gelman R, Canellos GP, Frei E. III. Prolonged disease-free survival in advanced breast cancer treatment with "super-CMF" adriamycin: An alternating regimen employing high-dose methotrexate with citrovorum factor rescue. Cancer Treat Rep(65): 67-75,1981.

13. Smith J. Personal communication.

14. Longo DL, Young RC, DeVita VT. What is so good about the "good prognosis" lymphoma. In: Williams CJ, Whitehouse JMA (eds) Recent Advances in Clinical Oncology. Churchill Livingstone, Edinburgh, 1982, pp 223-231.

15. DeVita VT. The relationship between tumor mass and resistance to chemotherapy. Cancer(51):1209-1220,1983.

16. Hedley DW, Millar JL, McElwain TJ, Gordon MY. Acceleration of bone-marrow recovery by pre-treatment with cyclophosphamide in patients receiving high-dose melphalan. Lancet(2):966-967,1978.

17. Millar JL, Phelps TA, Carter RL, et al. Cyclophosphamide pretreatment reduces the toxic effect of high dose melphalan on intestinal epithelium in sheep. Eur J Cancer(14)1283-1285,1978.

NEW THERAPIES WITH OLD DRUGS

I.E. SMITH

INTRODUCTION

There are around 30 non-investigational cytotoxic drugs currently available for cancer treatment. It is commonly and correctly stated that not all of these have yet been assessed against common cancers and that several hundred possible combinations of these drugs have likewise not been fully assessed. This argument is not supported by clinical experience: most tumours are either generally chemo-sensitive or chemo-resistant and while there are a few exceptional tumour types dramatically sensitive only to one or two agents (e.g. AML or testicular teratoma) it is nevertheless unlikely that the common solid tumours which are already relatively resistant to most forms of chemotherapy so far tried should prove to be uniquely sensitive to an as yet untried agent. This means that better treatment must depend either on new drugs or on better ways of using currently available drugs.

METHOTREXATE-5FU INTERACTIONS

Studies with experimental tumours have suggested that methotrexate given before 5-FU has synergistic activity, whereas the two drugs are antagonistic if methotrexate is given after 5-FU (I). The biochemical rationale for this is uncertain but may be based on the anti-purine effect of methotrexate, resulting in increased phosphoribosylpyro-phosphate levels which increase the rate of metabolic conversion of 5-FU to all its nucleotides. Clinical studies in breast cancer have reported response rates of I4-53% with sequential methotrexate followed by 5-FU, and in colo-rectal cancer response rates of 0-80% (2). Control randomised trials are required to establish whether this combination has benefit; preliminary results from such trials have so far shown no added efficacy.

13

5 FU AND FOLINIC ACID

5-FU as a single agent in the treatment of advanced gastrointestinal carcinomas has been disappointing and the drug has recently
been given in combination with high dose folinic acid on the basis that
an excess of intra-cellular reduced folate is necessary for optimal
inhibition of thymidylate synthetase and for an increased cytotoxic
effect of 5-FU. Preliminary results have shown a 56% complete and
partial response rate in the 30 patients with advanced colo-rectal
carcinoma, with responses seen in patients previously resistant to
5-FU alone (reference 3). In the same study 3 out of 5 patients with
gastric carcinoma also achieved response. These promising early
results require confirmation.

HIGH DOSE METHOTREXATE

The rationale for high dose methotrexate with folinic acid
rescue and early clinical experience have already been widely
described. At present the best randomised trial comparing doses of
50 mg, 500 mg. and 5 G. in patients with head and neck carcinoma have
shown only a modest increase in response rate with increasing dose;
no survival benefit was achieved and toxicity was very much more severe
with higher doses (reference 4). Results with high dose methotrexate
in other tumours including poor risk lymphomas and osteosarcoma are
encouraging, but the need for a high dose methotrexate component in
the overall treatment here has yet to be fully established.

AMINOGLUTETHIMIDE IN ADVANCED BREAST CANCER

Aminoglutethimide was first developed in the 1950s as an anticonvulsant but was withdrawn from clinical use after the reporting of
endocrine side-effects including adrenal corticoid insufficiency. The
drug was subsequently demonstrated to inhibit the desmolase enzyme
series responsible for the conversion of cholesterol to pregnenolone.
Several groups have subsequently shown that aminoglutethimide in
combination with hydrocortisone is effective in the treatment of
advanced breast carcinoma and the term "medical adrenalectomy" has been
coined. As with other forms of endocrine therapy, an overall response

rate of around 30% has been consistently achieved and randomised trials have found aminoglutethimide to be as effective as surgical adrenalectomy or tamoxifen. Aminoglutethimide is particularly useful in the treatment of bone metastases and in the control of associated bone pain. Side-effects however are common and include lethargy, drowsiness, ataxia and a transient erythematous rash in some patients. Most of the side-effects (except the rash) are dose-related.

Recently, aminoglutethimide has been further investigated in our own Unit as an inhibitor of aromatase, an enzyme responsible for the conversion of androstenedione to oestrogens in peripheral tissues. Invitro studies have demonstrated that this can be achieved at a much lower drug concentration than those required for desmolase inhibition. We are currently investigating aminoglutethimide in a very low dose (I25 mg. twice daily) without hydrocortisone. We have demonstrated that at this low dosage plasma oestrone levels in post-menopausal patients are suppressed to the same degree as that achieved with high dosage and hydrocortisone, but without the associated adrenal corticoid suppression of the higher dose, as measured by plasma DHA-S and cortisol. At this low dosage the drug is clinically active and responses have already been seen in patients currently being entered into a phase II study. These preliminary results tend to support the hypothesis that advanced breast cancer might be controlled by aromatase inhibition. Whether low dose aminoglutethimide has any clinical advantage over conventional dosage awaits the outcome of future trials.

LONG TERM INFUSIONS

The use of long term infusions of chemotherapy in the treatment of solid tumours is currently being investigated using two slightly different approaches.

First, the development of totally implantable subcutaneous pumps (e.g. Infusaid) has led to the use of 5-FUdR given by prolonged hepatic arterial infusion in the treatment of liver metastases predominantly arising from colo-rectal carcinoma. Initial studies suggested very high response rates of up to 80%, but a more recent detailed study from the Sydney Farber Institute found responses in only 29% of patients (5).

No evidence of survival benefit was seen and toxicity including epigastric pain and toxic hepatitis was significant.

An alternative approach has been the use of an external portable pump allowing long term venous drug delivery through a subclavian catheter. A 30 day infusion of adriamycin to a total dose of 90 mg/m^2 has been investigated in a phase II study. Some tumour responses have been seen, and interestingly this treatment has been associated with very minimal toxicity and with the absence of alopecia.

At present these approaches remain experimental but merit further study.

HIGH DOSE CYCLOPHOSPHAMIDE

In general, dose escalation studies in the treatment of small cell carcinoma of lung have shown that moderate increases in drug dosage (e.g. 2-fold increases) are not associated with any significant survival benefit, but are associated with increased toxicity. In contrast very high dose cyclophosphamide with autologous bone marrow rescue has recently been shown to achieve an 80% response rate with around 50% complete remissions in selected patients with small cell lung cancer (6). Again however no obvious survival benefit has been demonstrated.

We have therefore investigated very high dose cyclophosphamide (7 G/m^2) in patients who have already achieved a complete remission or good partial response to conventional chemotherapy for small cell lung cancer (adriamycin, vincristine and VPI6).

Thirty-five patients have so far been treated in a phase II study. Overall results are disappointing and no long term remissions have been seen in any patients who have achieved only a partial response to conventional chemotherapy, or in any patient initially presenting with extensive disease (whether or not achieving a complete or partial response). However 6 out of I4 patients originally presenting with limited disease who achieved a complete remission to conventional chemotherapy so far remain in remission from 8-22 months from diagnosis and the median survival in this group is I8 months.

The initial I7 patients in this study received autologous bone marrow rescue and the remaining patients did not. Autologous bone marrow rescue did not improve duration of neutropenia or enhance peripheral white blood count or platelet recovery and we have concluded that this procedure is unnecessary with high dose cyclophosphamide.

If this intensive chemotherapeutic approach has any long term value, then it would appear to be limited only to those patients who have already achieved a good complete remission to conventional chemotherapy and real benefit could only be demonstrated in a randomised trial.

REFERENCES

1. Mulder, J.H., Smink, T. and Van Putten, L.M.
    5-FU and methotrexate combination chemotherapy: the effect of drug scheduling. Eur. J. Cancer Clin. Oncol. (17) (7):831-837, 1981.

2. Bertino, J. Clinical application of the scheduled combination of methotrexate and 5-FU. Pharmanual Ed. Bertino, J.R. published Pharmalibri, page 109-120, 1983.

3. Machover, D., Schwarzenberg, L., Goldschmidt, E. et al.
    Treatment of advanced colo-rectal and gastric adenocarcinoma with 5-FU combined with high dose folinic acid: a pilot study.
    Cancer Treat. Rep. (66):1083-1087, 1982.

4. Woods, R.L., Fox, R.M. and Tattersall, M. Methotrexate treatment of head and neck cancer: a dose response evaluation.
    Cancer Treat. Rep. (65) (1):155-159, 1981.

5. Weiss, G.R., Garnick, M.E., Osteen, R.T. et al.
    Long-term hepatic arterial infusion of 5-FUdR for liver metastases using an implantable infusion pump. J. Clin. Oncol. (1)337-344, 1983.

6. Souhami, R.L., Harper, P.G., Linch, D. et al.
    High dose cyclophosphamide with autologous marrow transplantation as initial treatment of small cell carcinoma of the bronchus.
    Canc. Chemother. Pharmacol. (8):31-34, 1982.

ANTIMETABOLITE COMBINATIONS POSSESSING ENHANCED EFFICACY

M.H.N. TATTERSALL

Goldin et al were the first to document the important modulating effects of citrovorum factor rescue in the treatment of murine leukaemia by methotrexate (1). The notion of "methotrexate rescue" programmes was pioneered clinically by Djerassi et al in the late 1960s (2). The scientific basis for the prevention of methotrexate toxicity by citrovorum factor rescue, without major reduction of antitumour effects, has been the subject of several clinical and laboratory studies during the last few years (3,4).

The metabolic perturbations caused by methotrexate treatment were first studied in the early 1970s and the potential for antagonistic interactions was recognised at that time (5,6). The remarkable therapeutic synergy of combinations of methotrexate and asparaginase was first reported experimentally in the mid-1970s (7), and the clinical efficacy of these programmes has been confirmed in recent years. Animal studies reporting enhancement of the therapeutic index of methotrexate treatment using thymidine $\pm$ purine nucleosides as modulators was first reported in the mid-1970s (8,9), and the biochemical bases for these effects have only recently begun to be understood. However the clinical role of purine or thymidine modulation of methotrexate treatment is still uncertain (10-12). In the last five years, several groups have studied in detail the biochemical and therapeutic interaction of methotrexate with either fluorouracil or cytosine arabinoside (13-15). While these studies have led to greater understanding of the molecular basis of antimetabolite drug action, it is not yet clear what is the clinical role of variations in the schedule of administration of these agents in clinical cancer management. In this manuscript, some of our own results investigating the modulation of methotrexate action by nucleosides and fluorouracil will be presented together with the preliminary results of a randomised clinical trial comparing two sequences of administration of methotrexate and fluorouracil therapy.

MODULATION OF METHOTREXATE ACTIVITY BY NUCLEOSIDES

The acute effects of methotrexate treatment on deoxyribonucleoside triphosphate levels was documented during the 1970s and the majority of studies reported a fall in the thymidine triphosphate pool with varying changes in purine deoxyribonucleoside triphosphate pools (6,9). It was noted that thymidine and purines had differing effects on the reversal of methotrexate growth inhibition among different cell lines, and this observation led to the evaluation of thymidine and purines as modulators of methotrexate activity in vivo. The majority of studies confirmed the initial report that thymidine improved the therapeutic index of methotrexate treatment of murine L1210 leukaemia allowing substantially higher doses of methotrexate treatment to be administered with improved antitumour effects and reduction in normal tissue toxicity (8,9). Several groups subsequently studied the modulating effects of thymidine in patients receiving methotrexate treatment (10,11). These showed that thymidine could be used as a methotrexate rescue agent and might also when given simultaneously with methotrexate, enhance the therapeutic ratio in some cancers. The precise role of thymidine modulation of methotrexate treatment in vivo has been the subject of a recent review article (18). Further studies of the biochemical and cell kinetic perturbations caused by methotrexate treatment in vivo may identify tumour types in which methotrexate + thymidine may have improved antitumour activity compared to methotrexate alone.

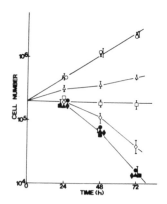

FIGURE 1. Effects of MTX on the growth of CCRF-CEM cells in culture. x, Untreated controls; 0, 10^{-9}M; △, 10^{-8}M; □, 2×10^{-8}M; ◇, 6×10^{-8}M; ●, 10^{-7}M; ▲, 10^{-6}M; ■, 10^{-5}M; ◆, 10^{-4}M. Error bars represent $\pm$ 2 SE from the mean obtained from four individual experiments. Counts are of live cells only as measured by phase-contrast microscopy.

21

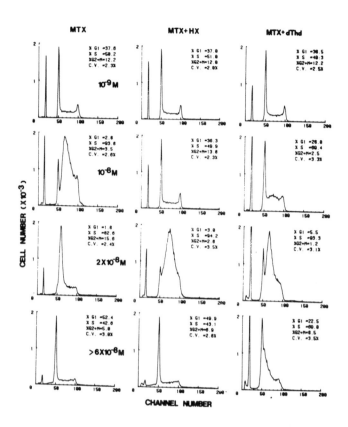

FIGURE 2. Changes in the DNA distribution of CCRF-CEM cells treated with MTX for 24hr in the presence or absence of dThd (10^{-5}M) or Hx (10^{-4}M). The DNA distribution of untreated CCRF-CEM cells (not shown) was identical with that found for 10^{-9}M MTX. Channel number represents relative fluorescence intensity, which is directly proportional to cellular DNA content. Numbers of cells are shown on the ordinate. The peak between channels 10 and 20 represents chicken red blood cells, which act as an internal biological standard and thus allow correct placement of the G_1 DNA peak which appears in channel 50. The ratio of the G_1 DNA peak channel number to that of untreated controls was 3.3. The DNA peak of cells treated with 2×10^{-8}M MTX represents cells accumulated in early S-phase as judged from the peak/chicken red blood cell ratio of 3.8 C.V., coefficient of various of G_1 DNA peak.

In recent years we have undertaken detailed studies of the biochemical and cell kinetic perturbations caused by methotrexate treatment (19-21). Figure 1 shows the effect of methotrexate on the growth of CCRF-CEM cells over a 72 hour period. With methotrexate concentrations between 10^{-9}M and 10^{-7}M, a concentration-dependent inhibition of cell growth was observed but methotrexate concentrations >10⁻⁷M had no further effect on cell growth. An increasing inhibition of cell cycle progression shown by an increase in the proportion of cells with an S-phase content was observed at 24 hours for methotrexate concentrations ⩽2x10⁻⁸M (Fig. 2). At methotrexate concentrations ⩾6x10⁻⁸M only minor changes in DNA content distribution were seen when compared with controls. Correlated 2-parameter analysis of acridine orange stained cells was used to study the relative effects of methotrexate treatment on DNA (green fluorescence) and RNA content (red fluorescence) (Fig. 3). It can be seen from the increases in red fluorescence that methotrexate (2x10⁻⁸M – 10⁻⁶M) resulted in classical unbalanced growth. No unbalanced cell growth was seen with either 10⁻⁸M or 10⁻⁴M methotrexate, although perturbations of DNA synthesis were seen.

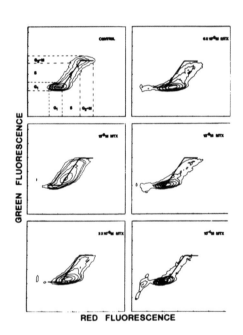

FIGURE 3. Correlated two-parameter analysis of acridine orange-stained CCRF-CEM cells. Red and green fluorescence represents RNA and DNA, respectively. Each contour plot was generated by using six contour levels of 50, 100, 150, 300, 600 and 1000 cells. To facilitate comparisons between individual plots, a heavy solid line, representative of control values, has been superimposed on each contour plot. The drug exposure time in each case was 24hr.

The effect of exogenous thymidine and/or hypoxanthine in methotrexate treated cells was also studied. Thymidine reduced cytotoxicity at all dose levels of methotrexate examined, and flow cytometric studies showed a decreased inhibition of DNA synthesis (Fig. 2). At the lower methotrexate concentrations hypoxanthine also reduced cytotoxicity (Table 1) and inhibition of DNA synthesis (Fig. 2) to an extent similar to that caused by thymidine. However hypoxanthine significantly potentiated the cytotoxicity of 10^{-4}M methotrexate and had no rescuing effect on DNA synthesis.

Table 1. Modification of the growth inhibitory effects of MTX in CCRF-CEM cells by dThd (10^{-5}M) and/or Hx (10^{-4}M). All values represent the mean of four individual experiments $\pm$ 2 SE. Counts are of live cells, as judged from phase-contrast microscopy, at 72hr after treatment. Drug treatment commenced 24hr after initial seeding of culture flasks with 10^5cells/ml. Cell cycle time is approximately 22hr.

MTX	Cell Count			
	Control	+dThd	+Hx	+dThd+Hx
M	$x10^5$/ml			
0	24.0 ± 2.0	23.0 ± 2.8	22.5 ± 3.1	10.0 ± 1.5
10^{-8}	4.9 ± 0.5	11.5 ± 1.0	20.3 ± 2.7	9.8 ± 1.3
$2x10^{-8}$	1.8 ± 0.4	3.5 ± 0.4	4.5 ± 0.5	2.5 ± 0.5
10^{-4}	0.15 ± 0.04	1.5 ± 0.2	0.05 ± 0.02	10.0 ± 1.1[a]

[a]Additional dThd (10^{-5}M) at 48hr

The combination of thymidine and hypoxanthine completely prevented methotrexate cytotoxicity, but with 10^{-4}M methotrexate, this "rescue" failed between 48-72hrs. The potentiation of methotrexate cytotoxicity ($>10^{-7}$M) by hypoxanthine has been studied further. The effects of a 48 hour exposure to methotrexate on the growth of CCRF-CEM cells in the presence or absence of added hypoxanthine (10^{-4}M) is shown in Fig. 4. A similar series of experiments using drug exposures equivalent to two cell-doubling times with PMC-22 or L1210 cells is shown in Fig. 5. In both sets of data exogenous hypoxanthine reduced methotrexate toxicity at low methotrexate concentrations but potentiated toxicity greatly at higher methotrexate concentration ($>6x10^{-8}$M MTX).

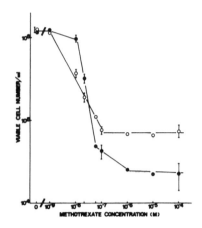

FIGURE 4. Modulation of MTX cytotoxicity by Hx in CCRF-CEM cells. O , MTX alone (5x10^{-6}mM Hx present in the growth medium); ●, MTX + 10^{-4}M Hx. All cell counts were made 48hr after drug addition. Initial cell numbers at time of drug addition was 2x10^{-5}/ml. Points, at least 2 individual experiments; bars, S.D. of the mean obtained from at least 4 individual experiments.

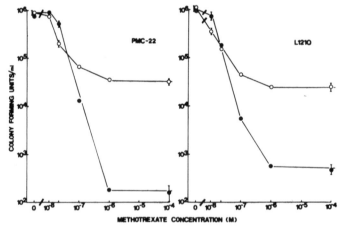

FIGURE 5. Modulation of MTX cytotoxicity by Hx in PMC-22 and L1210 cells. O , MTX alone (5x10^{-6}M Hx present in the growth medium); ●, MTX + 10^{-4}M Hx. Drug exposure times were 48 and 24hr for PMC-22 and L1210, respectively. Points, at least 2 individual experiments; bars, S.D. of the mean obtained from at least 4 individual experiments.

The effects of these drug treatments on cellular deoxyribonucleoside triphosphate levels were studied. Methotrexate-induced changes in dATP, dTTP and dGTP were almost identical in all three cell lines. The effects of exogenous hypoxanthine on these pool changes varied with methotrexate concentration. At low methotrexate concentrations (10^{-8} - 2×10^{-8}M) where hypoxanthine reduced cytotoxicity, hypoxanthine prevented the fall in dATP and reduced the fall in dTTP and dGTP. At higher methotrexate concentrations (10^{-7}M-10^{-4}M) where hypoxanthine potentiated toxicity, hypoxanthine caused a considerable dATP elevation and had no significant effects on dTTP or dGTP. Further studies of these interactions showed that other purines can modulate methotrexate toxicity, and that there is a striking relationship between the extent of purine potentiation of methotrexate toxicity and their effects on dATP which strongly supports the hypothesis that dATP levels are critical determinants of toxicity (21).

These data call into question the relevance of purine and thymidine concentrations in vivo as modulators of methotrexate activity. Thymidine levels in human plasma range between 0.5 and 5µM (22) and would be expected to have some modulating effect on methotrexate growth inhibition particularly at lower methotrexate dosages. We have recently measured plasma purine levels in man and documented major regional variations with purine levels in bone marrow supernatants being 10 to 50-fold higher than those in the peripheral plasma (23) (Table 2). Presumably the high concentrations of purines in the bone marrow supernatant is caused by breakdown of cell nuclei in the bone marrow associated with nuclei being lost from maturing red cells, and ineffective myelopoiesis.

Table 2. Extracellular purine levels

Source	Hx/X	IR	AR
Normal Plasma (18)	1.32 $\pm$ 1.07	0.37 $\pm$ 0.36	1.03 $\pm$ 0.71
Bone Marrow*			
Amyloid (N)	16.2 (0.7)**	0.4 (n.d.)	5.3 (1.9)
Osteoporosis (N)	15.0 (1.5)	7.7 (0.7)	6.9 (1.6)
Thrombocythaemia (A)	18 (3.0)	10 (0.1)	54 (8.8)
Myeloma (A)	4.5 (0.7)	2.0 (0.3)	10.8 (2.5)
Cryoglobulin (A)	36 (1.1)	11 (0.4)	60 (6.6)

* Diagnosis - A = abnormal marrow morphology
              N = normal marrow morphology

**Results in parenthesis are simultaneous. Peripheral venous plasma levels.

These data also may go some way to providing an explanation for the modulating effects of thymidine on methotrexate action in vivo. The majority of investigators have documented that thymidine infusions prevent the myelotoxicity of methotrexate treatment but are less effective in reducing the mucosal toxicity (10-12). It now seems likely that raised plasma thymidine levels caused by thymidine infusion and the high regional concentrations of purines in the bone marrow are sufficient in bone marrow to prevent methotrexate growth inhibitory effects. However in the gut the absence of high physiological concentrations of purines means that thymidine alone may be insufficient to prevent the growth inhibitory effects of methotrexate.

METHOTREXATE-FLUOROURACIL

The interaction of methotrexate and fluorouracil has been the subject of investigation for a number of years. Our initial studies in vitro and in vivo suggested that the interaction might be antagonistic under some circumstances (6). Subsequently Bertino reported synergistic antitumour activity of sequential methotrexate-fluorouracil in Sarcoma 180 bearing mice (24). A number of detailed animal studies of methotrexate-fluorouracil have been undertaken subsequently, and it is clear that the combination of methotrexate and fluorouracil rarely influences the therapeutic index although it has varying effects depending upon the sequence of administration (25).

The series of studies from Cadman's group and also from Bertino have investigated the interaction of methotrexate and fluorouracil treatment in cell culture (13,14). Cadman's group have documented that under some circumstances methotrexate treatment increases cellular phosphoribosyl pyrophosphate levels leading to enhanced anabolism of fluorouracil to nucleotides and incorporation into RNA. Bertino's group have demonstrated that accumulation of dihydropteroyl polyglutamates in methotrexate treated cells enhances the binding of fluorodeoxyuridine monophosphate to thymidylate synthetase and that this may be the basis for the enhanced sensitivity to fluorouracil of methotrexate pre-treated cells. We have undertaken a series of studies investigating the modulating effects of TdR and Hx on the interaction of sequential methotrexate-fluorouracil treatment (26), and we have also initiated a randomised prospective clinical trial in which sequential methotrexate followed by fluorouracil treatment is compared to the same drugs given in the opposite order (27).

MODULATION OF SEQUENTIAL METHOTREXATE-FLUOROURACIL SYNERGY BY NUCLEOSIDES

Our studies have investigated the growth inhibitory effects of sequential methotrexate for three hours followed by fluorouracil one hour on the growth of murine L1210 cells cultured in media supplemented with varying types of serum. Pretreatment with methotrexate (three hours 10μM) markedly potentiated

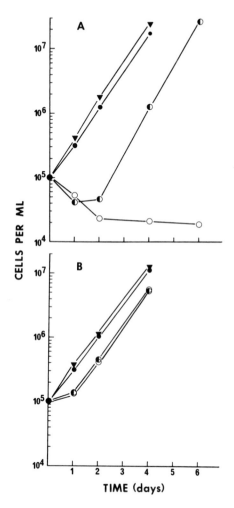

FIGURE 6. Effect of serum source on sequential MTX-FUra cytotoxicity. L1210 cells were exposed to either FUra (30μ M, 1hr) (●); MTX (1μM, 4hr) (■); MTX (10μM, 4hr) (◐); MTX (1μM, 3hr) followed by FUra (30μ M, 1hr) (□); or MTX (10μM, 3hr) followed by FUra (30μM, 1hr) (○); in medium containing either 10% horse serum (A) or 10% FCS (B). Cells were then washed and suspended in appropriate drug-free medium, and subsequent growth was compared to that of non-drug-treated cells (▼).

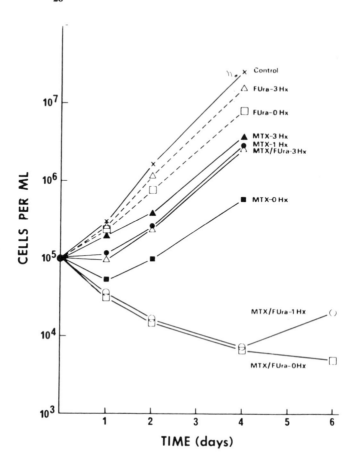

FIGURE 7. Prevention by hypoxanthine or synergistic MTX-FUra cytotoxicity in medium containing 10% dialysed FCS. L120 cells cultured in medium containing 10% dialysed FCS were supplemented with either 0, 1 or 3μM hypoxanthine (0 Hx, 1 Hx, 3 Hx) and then exposed to either FUra (30μM, 1hr), MTX (10μM, 4hr), or MTX (3hr) followed by FUra (1hr). Growth in the appropriate hypoxanthine-containing drug-free medium was then determined. Controls are similar at all 3 hypoxanthine concentrations. Growth of FUra-1μM hypoxanthine was between that of FUra-0μM hypoxanthine and FUra-3μM hypoxanthine; data not shown.

the growth inhibitory effects of a one hour exposure to 30μM fluorouracil in medium containing 10% horse serum but had no such effect on cells growing in medium containing 10% foetal calf serum (Fig. 6).

The growth inhibitory effects of a one hour exposure to 30μM fluorouracil alone was similar in both horse serum and foetal calf serum containing media but the growth inhibition caused by a four hour exposure to methotrexate (10μM) was slightly less in foetal calf serum than horse serum - media. Synergistic cytotoxicity produced by sequential methotrexate-fluorouracil could however by demonstrated with foetal calf serum if the serum was dialysed before use. Undialysed foetal calf serum contains approximately 100 μM hypoxanthine compared to less than 1μM in horse serum. We have investigated the effect of hypoxanthine on the synergy produced by sequential methotrexate-fluorouracil in dialysed foetal calf serum containing media. In the experiment shown in Figure 7, the addition of 1μM hypoxanthine during and after methotrexate-fluorouracil exposure did not reduce the cytotoxicity seen during the first four days after drug exposure. However 3μM hypoxanthine almost completely abolished the sequential methotrexate-fluorouracil synergy. These data call into question the significance of the experimental results obtained in media supplemented with horse serum or dialysed foetal calf serum to the clinical situation where hypoxanthine concentrations in peripheral plasma are usually in the range 1-3μM or greater.

CLINICAL TRIAL OF SEQUENTIAL METHOTREXATE-FLUOROURACIL IN PATIENTS WITH SQUAMOUS CELL CARCINOMA OF THE HEAD AND NECK AND GASTROINESTINAL TRACT NEOPLASMS

During the past 18 months, we have been conducting a randomised prospective controlled trial comparing the outcome of treatment in patients with measurable squamous carcinoma of the head and neck, or gastrointestinal tract cancer, treated with methotrexate one hour - fluorouracil or the opposite sequence. To date 90 patients have been entered on this study which is continuing to accrue patients. No differences in response rate or survival duration have been observed and the toxic effects (Table 3) are similar in the two treatment arms. The overall response rate (complete plus partial response) in head and neck cancer is 52%, and 58% in previously untreated patients. In colorectal cancer the response rate is 38% but the median survival from start of chemotherapy is only 4.7 months.

Table 3.   Toxicity of sequential methotrexate-fluorouracil

	Treatment Sequence	
	M – F	F – M
No evaluable	34	34
Toxicity grades	3	
WBC $\geqslant$2	3	7
Mucositis $\geqslant$2	8	8
Nausea & vomiting $\geqslant$2	8	9
Diarrhoea $\geqslant$ 2	6	4
Treatment related death	2	2

The trial is still relatively small, and the type II error remains considerable. The trial is continuing, and has been widened to include patients with advanced gastric adenocarcinoma. This interim analysis shows no suggestion that the theoretically "antagonistic" fluorouracil-methotrexate sequence is inferior to the opposite sequence. Such antagonism could have provided a therapeutic advantage if it were more marked in normal tissues than in tumour, as higher doses could then have been used in the fluorouracil-methotrexate arm. Such a differential effect was conceivable in view of the widely differing purine concentrations in bone marrow and peripheral blood.

CONCLUSION

Improved understanding of the modulating effects of natural metabolites and other drugs on the activity of antimetabolites will increase the rational scheduling of these agents. New factors to be considered are regional variations in purine nucleoside concentrations, and the critical modulating effects of these compounds on methotrexate and fluorouracil toxicity.

ACKNOWLEDGEMENT

I am grateful to my colleagues Dr. I.W. Taylor, Dr. A.A. Piper and Dr. A.S. Coates for their help and collaboration undertaking these studies.

REFERENCES

1. Goldin A, Venditti JM, Kline I, Mantel N: Eradication of leukaemic cells (L1210) by methotrexate and methotrexate plue citrovorum factor. Nature: 1548-1550, 1966.

2. Djerassi I, Abir E, Roger GL: Long term remission in childhood acute leukaemia: use of infrequent infusion of methotrexate; supportive rate of platelet transfusions and citrovorum factor. Clin Pediats (5): 502-509, 1966.
3. Pinedo HM, Zaharko DS, Ball JM, Chabner BA: The reversal of methotrexate cytotoxicity to bone marrow cells by leucovorin and nucleosides. Cancer Res (36): 4418-4424, 1976.
4. Sirotnak FM, Donsbach RC, Moccio DM, Dorick DM: Biochemical and pharmacokinetic effects of leucovorin after high dose methotrexate in a murine leukaemia model. Cancer Res (36): 4679-4686, 1976.
5. Tattersall MHN, Harrap KR: Combination chemotherapy: the antagonism of methotrexate and cytosine arabinoside. Europ J Cancer (9): 229-232, 1973.
6. Tattersall MHN, Jackson RC, Connors TA, Harrap KR: Combination chemotherapy: the interaction of methotrexate and 5-fluorouracil. Europ J Cancer (9): 733-739, 1973.
7. Capizzi RL, Nichols R, Mullins J: Long term survival of leukemic mice by therapeutic synergism between asparaginase and methotrexate. Fed Proc (31): 553, 1972.
8. Tattersall MHN, Brown B, Frei E: The reversal of methotrexate toxicity by thymidine with maintenance of antitumour effects. Nature (253): 198-200, 1975.
9. Grindey GB, Seman JH, Pavelic ZP: Modulation versus rescue of antimetabolite toxicity by salvage metabolites administered by continuous infusion. Antibiot Chemother (23): 295-304, 1978.
10. Howell SB, Herbst K, Boss GR, Frei E: Thymidine requirements for the rescue of patients treated with high dose methotrexate. Cancer Res (40): 1824-1829, 1980.
11. Ensminger WD, Frei E: The prevention of methotrexate toxicity by thymidine infusions in humans. Cancer Res (37): 1857-1863, 1977.
12. Howell SB, Mansfield SJ, Taetle R: Thymidine and hypoxanthine requirements of normal and malignant human cells for protection against methotrexate cytotoxicity. Cancer Res (40): 1824-1829, 1980.
13. Cadman Ed, Heimer R, Benz C: The influence of methotrexate pretreatment on 5-fluorouracil metabolism in L1210 cells. J Biol Chem (256): 1695-1704, 1980.
14. Fernandes DJ, Bertino JR: 5-Fluorouracil-methotrexate synergy. Enhancement of 5-fluorodeoxyuridylate binding to thymidylate synthase by dihydropteroylpolyglutamates. Proc Natl Acad Sci (77): 5663-5667, 1980.
15. Cadman ED, Eiferman F: Mechanism of synergistic cell killing when methotrexate precedes cytosine arabinoside. Study of L1210 and human leukemic cells. J Clin Invest (64): 788-798, 1979.
16. Tattersall MHN, Jackson RC, Jackson STM, Harrap KR: Factors determining cell sensitivity to methotrexate: sudies of folate and deoxyribonucleoside triphosphate pools in 5 mammalian cell lines. Europ J Cancer (10): 818-826, 1974.
17. Harrap KR, Taylor GA, Browman GP: Enhancement of the therapeutic effectiveness of methotrexate and protection of normal tissues with purines and pyrimidines. Chem-Biol Interactions (18): 119-128, 1977.
18. Schornagel JH, Leyva A, Pinedo HM: Is there a role for thymidine in cancer chemotherapy. Cancer Treat Rev (9): 331-352, 1982.
19. Taylor IW, Tattersall MHN: Methotrexate cytotoxicity in cultured human leukemic cells studied by flow cytometry. Cancer Res (41): 1549-1558, 1981.
20. Taylor IW, Slowiaczek P, Francis PR, Tattersall MHN: Biochemical and cell cycle perturbations in methotrexate-treated cells. Mol Pharmacol (21): 201-210, 1982.

21. Taylor IW, Slowiaczek P, Francis PR, Tattersall MHN: Purine modulation of methotrexate cytotoxicity in mammalian cells. Cancer Res (42): 5159-5164, 1982.
22. Holden L, Hoffbrand AV, Tattersall MHN: Thymidine concentrations in human sera: variations in patients with leukaemia and megalaoblastic anaemia. Europ J Cancer (16): 115-120, 1980.
23. Tattersall MHN, Slowiazczek P, De Fazio A: Regional variation on human extracellular purine levels. J Lab Clin Med (102): 411-420, 1983.
24. Bertino JR, Sawicki WL, Lindquist CA, Gupa VS: Schedule dependent antitumour effects of methotrexate and 5-fluorouracil. Cancer Res (37): 327-328, 1977.
25. Mulder JH, Smink T, Van Putten LM: 5-Fluorouracil and methotrexate combination chemotherapy: the effects of drug scheduling. Europ J Cancer (17): 831-838, 1981.
26. Piper AA, Nott SE, MacKinnon WB, Tattersall MHN: Critical modulation by thymidine and hypoxanthine of the sequential methotrexate-5-fluorouracil synergism in murine L1210 cells. Cancer Res (43): 5701-5705, 1983.
27. Coates AS, Tattersall MHN, Slowiaczek P, Swanson C, Hedley D, Fox RM, Raghavan D: Sequential versus reversed methotrexate and 5-fluorouracil. A prospective randomized clinical trial of order of administration. J Clin Oncolol, 1983 (in press).

MISMATCHED BONE MARROW TRANSPLANTATION

R. POWLES, G. GOSS, A. PEDRAZZINI, M. CROFTS, H. CLINK, J. MILLAR, B. KHAN AND
D. PEREZ

In the United Kingdom, based on family size, the probability of a patient
having a histocompatible sibling as a donor is only about 0.3 (1). Moreover,
matched transplants are rarely successful for recipients over the age of 45
years. Thus for bone marrow transplantation to make any impact on the
management of bone marrow disorders, particularly acute leukaemia, the
availability of donors must be extended outside of those with complete
identical inheritence of chromosome no. 6. HLA matched unrelated donors are
being used to a limited extent to determine the feasibility of their use, but
even with very large panels of normal donors the number of such transplants
that have been undertaken is so small that no statement can be made on the
efficacy of such a treatment. Seattle have previously reported a study in
which donors were matched for one haplotype of chromosome no. 6, the other
haplotype having antigenic similarities (2). These patients were given
methotrexate as prophylaxis to prevent graft versus host disease (GvHD); many
of them had active disease at the time of transplantation and in consequence
there were many failures, but there were also some long term survivors.
However, selecting patients whose donors are more than half identical at the
MHC can only slightly extend the proportion of patients eligible for grafting.

Following encouraging results using Cyclosporin A (CyA) in matched grafts
(3) we embarked upon a study of unselected patients who did not have MHC
matched donors, choosing the most suitable non-matched member of the family as
the donor. This study was therefore a report on a procedure that could be
applicable to most young patients with acute leukaemia who were in remission
and probably could be applied to other diseases also. In the original series
(June 1979 to July 1982) 35 patients between the ages of 3 and 45 years were
studied (4). There is now a minimum follow-up of 18 months of all patients.
Thirty three patients had AML, 2 had ALL, and all received allogeneic
mismatched transplants from family members. At the time of grafting 14
patients were in first remission, 15 were in later remission and 6 were in
relapse. In 16 cases the donor was a sibling, in 16 a parent and in 4 a

33

child. This included one patient who received marrow first from her father and then from her child. All patients except one shared one HLA haplotype with the donor, and of the 34 one haplotype mismatched patients, 19 shared one or more antigens of the non-identical haplotype with the donor. All the MLC tests that could be evaluated were at least weakly positive in one direction in the one way test. Of this original series of 35 patients, 31 were conditioned with cyclophosphamide and total body irradiation as for matched transplants (4) and in 4 a single dose of melphalan 240mg/m^2 (5) was given 7 days after a priming dose of cyclophosphamide (300mg/m^2). Patients were given intramuscular or oral Cyclosporin A (CyA) at 12.5 - 37.5mg/kg per day (in two 12 hourly doses) starting 24 hours before the infusion of marrow and continuing for 5 days. From the sixth day the drug was administered orally at a dose of 12.5mg/kg per day (in two 12 hourly doses) for six months. The dose of Cyclosporin A was reduced as renal function deteriorated. The first 8 patients received this protocol and 3 of them died of a previously unseen problem of massive pulmonary oedema of which the immediate cause of death appeared to be occurring 12-48 days after transplant. The essential lesion appeared to be increased permeability of blood vessels and the syndrome was characterised by a fever with fluid retention, a low central venous pressure and low serum albumin usually leading to dyspnoea, cyanosis, massive pulmonary oedema and death despite assisted ventilation. Associated features were convulsions, probably due to foci of localised cerebral oedema. In addition there was also seen a renal lesion characterised by intravascular haemolysis and oliguric renal failure although this latter complication resolved if patients were dialysed. Some features, particularly fluid retention, low serum albumin and renal impairment occurred in most of these first 8 patients. Because pulmonary oedema with leaky vascular problems had not been seen in the original series of 50 patients given mismatched transplants and methotrexate in Seattle (2) we explored the possibility that methotrexate may have been inhibiting a cellular immune reaction occurring immediately after transplant (an in vivo MLR). Laboratory data showed that cyclosporin levels in our patients were not sufficient high during the first two weeks after transplant to inhibit an MLR in vitro. In an attempt to prevent this syndrome the next 15 patients treated in the original series of 35 patients were given methotrexate in addition to Cyclosporin A during the first two weeks after transplant. Nevertheless, 5 of these patients died of this complication, and 6 of the 15 patients required re-grafting because of graft failure presumably attributable to the methotrexate. The use of methotrexate was therefore abandoned and thereafter patients in the study received only Cyclosporin A and an attempt was made using the radioimmune assay to keep the peak serum Cyclosporin A levels at around 1,000ng/ml. These patients also received infusions of concentrated albumin daily and some received prophylactic Acyclovir to prevent possible herpes infections. Pulmonary oedema was a major factor in the death of 4 of the remaining 12 patients and in the whole series of 35 patients 12 patients died of the problem.

UP-DATE ON THE ORIGINAL MISMATCHED PATIENTS

Between June 1979 and July 1982 35 patients were transplanted and 11 remain alive between 2½ to 4½ years after transplant with the latest death in the series occurring 629 days post transplantation. As originally reported the incidence of acute skin graft versus host disease was approximately 80%. However, most of these rashes disappeared on treatment and GvHD affecting the gut and the liver was uncommon. Only one patient died of a direct consequence of GvHD although in another 5 it was a contributing cause. Chronic graft versus host disease developed in another 3 patients and in two cases this responded to treatment with steroid plus Azathioprine or resumption of Cyclosporin A. One patient remains alive with very mild chronic graft versus host disease which is continuing to improve. Four patients in the series relapsed with their original disease and all died.

ANALYSIS OF GENETIC FACTORS INFLUENCING THE FIRST MISMATCHED STUDY

Of the 34 patients who shared one haplotype with no other antigenic matching, 5 of 16 survive and amongst those with shared antigens at any locus of the non-identical haplotype, 6 of 18 survive.

Thirteen of the whole series of 35 patients received marrow from their father and 7 are alive (54%) whreas only 4 of 16 sibling recipients are alive and none of the 6 patients who received marrow from their mother or child survived. However, for logistic reasons the fathers were generally taken in preference to the mothers as possible donors and the recipients of the fathers were inevitably younger than for siblings. In consequence examination of the effect of age on survival shows that 8 of 15 (53%) patients under the age of 19 years survive whereas only 38% of 8 patients between 20 years and 29 years survive, and none of 12 patients over the age of 30 years survive.

RECENT STUDIES

As a consequence of the seemingly strong influence of age on outcome of our programme from July 1982 was confined to recipients of mistmatched bone marrow transplant under the age of 20 years. Twelve patients received mismatched transplants and only CyA prophylaxis and only one survives. The causes of death in general were multi-organ failure although pulmonary oedema was a major factor in the terminal events for 5 patients. All patients had died within 110 days of transplant.

REMOVAL OF T-LYMPHOCYTES FROM DONOR MARROW

Purging marrow of T-lymphocytes has been mooted as a possible method of preventing graft versus host disease for some time, but it has only been the recent availability of good specific monoclonal antibodies that have made such maneouvres practially feasible. Early studies have been encouraging in matched transplants showing that good engraftment occurs with minimum GvHD without additional immunosuppression and long term survivors seem likely (6). However, time to adequate engraftment ($0.5 \times 10^9/l$ granulocytes) is longer than seen with Cyclosporin and controlled trials will be required to determine the advantages and disadvantages (including cost) of the various regimens now available.

At the University of Wisconsin, Madison, a pilot study of the use of monoclonal antibody for the purging of marrow prior to mismatched bone marrow transplantation ws undertaken, and the results presented at the ISEH meeting in London in July 1983 (6). This group used in vitro treatment of donor bone marrow with an anti-E rosette receptor antibody (CT2) and complement (C) prior to bone marrow transplantation. CT2 is a mouse monoclonal antibody directed against a 50,000 dalton E-rosette antigen. Baby rabbit serum was used as the C1 source. This in vitro treatment in general was found to remove greater than 99% of the E-rosette positive marrow cells and greater than 98% of the T3 positive cells; nevertheless, within 14 days after bone marrow transplantation donor T-lymphocytes could be found in the recipient peripheral blood in matched transplants and GvHD, albeit mild, also occurred. This group reported the results of a total of 10 mismatched family donor transplants in which no immunosuppression was given after transplant. In general they found that engraftment occurred although for some patients there was considerable delay of many weeks before reconstitution was sufficient to allow the patients to leave hospital. In our initial study of 35 mismatched patients, those patients who received Cyclosporin A alone were found to have prompt engraftment (comparable with matched transplants). The possibility therefore exists that if a mismatched (purged) marrow is given without further immunosuppression to the recipient, then remaining host T-cell immunity is sufficient to suppress graft take. This delay in engraftment is not so marked in matched transplants, presumably because of a quantitative effect due to the degree of matching. In summary, the use of CYA alone has been found to be associated with prompt engraftment, but serious problems occurred in the vascular endothelium. This latter problem did not occur in the patients receiving T-cell depleted marrow (without CYA) but slow engratment often occurred. Although the vascular endothelial lesion may be related to CYA (see below), because it only rarely occurs in matched transplants the involvement of an immune component to the pathogenesis also needs to be considered. It therefore seemed reasonable that we should study a group of patients in which we combined both approaches.

MONOCLONAL ANTIBODY PLUS CYCLOSPORIN A FOR MISMATCHED BONE MARROW TRANSPLANTS

In our recent programme four patients have received mismatched bone marrow transplants from family members after the marrow has been treated to remove immunocompetent cells. Three patients had marrow treated with a monoclonal anti-human T-cell antibody designated UCHT 1. One patient received marrow treated with a rat IgM monoclonal antibody (CamPath I) (7) which stains both T and B lymphocytes. In all four patients the mononuclear fraction of the marrow was treated with antibody at 4°C, incubated for 20 minutes and then washed once in the cold and infused into the patient. GM-CFC assessment showed no loss of bone marrow colony growth by the procedure. All four patients received CYA from the day prior to transplant. The 3 patients who received marrow treated with UCHT 1 had engraftment (two promptly 12-16 days) but two died of haemorrhage and one of renal failure. The patient who received marrow treated with CamPathI had failure of engraftment in spite of excellent GM-CFC activity and two further untreated transplants from the same donor. None of these patients developed the pulmonary oedema problem

MISMATCHED BONE MARROW TRANSPLANTS FOR FIRST REMISSION AML

An observation made by us and others is that matched bone marrow transplantation produces very long term results (8) and the same factors appear to be important for mismatched transplants. We have now conducted 51 mismatched bone marrow transplants, and 16 of these were for patients with AML in first remission at the time of the graft. Eleven of these patients were under the age of 30 years and 7 (64%) remain alive from 1½ to 4½ years. The five 1st remission AML patients who received transplants over the age of 30 years all succumbed. If we extrapolate lessons we have learnt from our matched programmes it seems reasonable to suppose that true assessment of mismatched bone marrow transplantation can only really be adequately determined if we initially confine our programme to young AML patients in their first remission. The fact that 64% of these patients in our initial study are alive and well on a plateau of survival between 1½ and 4½ years compares very favourably with other alternative methods of treatment such as chemotherapy (9) or matched transplants (3). However, further improvement will depend upon defining the nature of the pulmonary oedema/leaky vascular problem.

THE LEAKY VASCULAR PROBLEM

In our patients receiving mismatched transplants, because they are such a heterogenous group, it has proved impossible to define any factors associated with the leaky vascular problem. However, we have a large homogenous group of patients receiving matched transplants for first remission AML in which the same problem occurred (albeit much less commonly) and so we have attempted to see which factors may be important for the pathogenesis of this lesion in this group of patients. Seventy two patients with first remission AML received matched transplants from sibling donors over a period of 5 years until May 1983. 18% of these patients died of a lesion that could be attributed to the vascular endothelium.

We examined the whole group of 72 patients to see if there was any correlation between the dose of Cyclosporin A given and survival. Only 9 patients remained exactly on protocol dose of Cyclosporin A but a further 14 patients had at least this dose of Cyclosporin A although at some time during the first two months after transplant the dose was increased for a short period of time either because of transient graft versus host disease or because of inadequate serum levels. Thus 23 patients had at least the protocol dose of Cyclosporin A. A further 29 patients had their dose of Cyclosporin A consistently reduced and this was nearly always because of impaired renal function. An additional 20 patients had Cyclosporin A doses increased because of the reasons stated previously and in addition subsequently had to have their dose of Cyclosporin A reduced below protocol doses and they are not included in the analysis below. 21 of the 23 (91%) patients who received at least protocol dose remain alive and well compared with only 16 of the 29 (55%) patients in which the dose of Cyclosporin A was reduced (p<0.01). Of the 20 patients who had the dose of Cyclosporin A raised and subsequently reduced only 40% survived. Cyclosporin A levels conducted on over 3,000 occasions in these patients showed no correlation with survival and so we looked for other factors that may be responsible for causing this inverse relationship between Cyclosporin A dose and vascular endothelial damage. We were particularly concerned that other drugs may be additive to the Cyclosporin in producing endothelial damage. We could find no correlation between the total cumulative dose of the antileukaemic drugs (anthracycline, cytosine arabinoside or 6-thioguanine) given prior to transplant and the tolerated dose of Cyclosporin A after transplant. There was also no difference in the number of days from diagnosis to transplant and the tolerance of Cyclosporin. The only real correlation we could find was between the amount of Gentamycin and/or Amikacin recieved during the two months after bone marrow transplant. In the 23 patients who received at least the protocol dose of Cyclosporin A only 6 patients had more than 10 days of Aminoglycoside treatment and no patient had more than 15 days (mean 4.35 days), whereas, for the 29 patients who had their dose of Cyclosporin A reduced 13 had more than 10 days of these antibiotics and 9 had more than 15 days. These differences were significant (p<0.05). We cannot say if there is a definite inter-relationship between nephrotoxic antibiotics and Cyclosporin A because the patients requiring the extra antibiotics were selected in that they were sicker. We have also found that patients who died of the pulmonary oedema leaky vascular problem in this matched series of remission AML patients also have evidence of abnormal liver function prior to developing oedema. Fifty nine patients with bilirubin levels of less than 100mmol/l (normal < 17mmol/l) during the first three months after transplant had a 73% chance of survival whereas patients with bilirubin levels of >100mmol/l (13 patients) had only a 24% chance of survival (p = <0.05). We know that Cyclosporin A (and GvHD) in some instances produces a rise in serum bilirubin level but the cause of death in patients with bilirubins of >100mmol/l was not liver failure but predominantly pulmonary oedema with or without infection and renal failure.

It seems likely that approximately 20% of the patients who receive matched transplants die of a generalised vascular lesion and this problem is certainly more dominant in the mismatched bone marrow transplants. Therefore priority must be given to examining the nature of the vascular endothelium after transplantation particularly with reference to the inter-relationship between Cyclosporin and the chimeric state and possible immune reaction directed against the endothelial cells. Since the advent of Cyclosporin A the classical triad of graft versus host disease is not a major problem but we may have unmasked an entirely new lesion, the pathogenesis of which remains obscure.

THE FUTURE ROLE OF BONE MARROW TRANSPLANTATION

The ability to extend the procedure of bone marrow transplantation to patients other than those with HLA matched donors is going to determine its long term role as a therapeutic modality. Although the preliminary results of mismatched transplants are encouraging, much progress is required if this procedure is to become generally more accepted. As yet there is no indication that the degree of MLC antigeneic difference for one haplotype mismatches influences results, but studies of larger numbers of patients may reveal important antigens. In general it seems useful to regard the three broad disease groups treated separately, because the optimal procedures and problems occurring for aplastic anaemia, leukaemia, and SCID seem different. Patients with SCID appear to engraft more easily and with less problems than the others and methodology successful for SCID may not be applicable to, for example, leukaemia. Likewise, methods that work easily in matched transplants (i.e. T-lymphocyte purging) encounter unexpected problems when applied to mismatched transplants. Obviously extensive basic scientific studies are required to understand better the immunobiology of the mismatched chimeric state and we feel that central to this understanding is the vascular endothelium. Throughout the world there are now sufficient patients off all treatment with longstanding stable mismatched chimeras to make the prospect of success in solving their problems a distinct possibility in the not too distant future.

REFERENCES

1. Report of the Working Group on Bone Marrow Transplantation, Chairman, Sir Douglas Black. London H.M. Stationery Office, 1982.
2. Clift RA, Hansen JA, Thomas ED, et al: Transplantation of marrow from an unrelated donor to a patient with acute leukaemia. N Eng J Med (303): 565-567.
2. Powles RL, Morganstern G, Clink HM, et al: The place of bone marrow transplantation in acute myelogenous leukaemia. Lancet (1): 1047-1050,

1980.

4. Powles RL, Morganstern GR, Kay HEM, et al: Mismatched family donors for bone marrow transplantation as treatment for acute leukaemia. Lancet (1): 612-615, 1983.

5. Lumley H, Powles RL, Morgenstern GR, et al: Pseudosyngeneic transplantation as a treament for recurrent leukaemia following allogeneic bone marrow transplantation. In: Touraine, Gluckman and Griscellie (eds) Bone Marrow Transplantation in Europe, Proceedings of the 5th European Symposium on Bone Marrow Transplantation, Courchevel, March 1981, Excerpta Medica, Amsterdam, Vol II, pp 24-28, 1981.

6. Finlay JL, Trigg ME, Billing R, et al: Bone marrow transplantation following in vitro treatment of donor marrow with anti-T lymphocyte (E-rosette receptor) antibody and complement. Ex Haem Supp (14): 3, 1983.

7. Hale G, Bright S, Chubley G, et al: Removal of T cells from bone marrow for transplantation: A monoclonal antilymphocyte antibody that fixes human complement. Blood (62): 873-882, 1983.

8. Thomas ED, Buckner CD, Banaji M, et al: One hundred patients with acute leukaemia treated by chemotherapy, total body irradiation and allogeneic bone marrow transplantation. Blood (49): 511, 1977.

9. Mayer RJ, Weinstein HJ, Coral FS, et al: The role of intensive postinduction chemotherapy in the management of patients with acute myelogenous leukaemia. Cancer Treatment Rep (66): 1455-1462, 1982.

PROSPECTS FOR IMMUNOTHERAPY

P. ALEXANDER

Conflicting evidence for immune reactions by the patient with cancer.
Immune reactions have been invoked to explain the very rare instances
of complete spontaneous regression of malignant tumours and the more
frequent spontaneous disappearance of some, but not all, metastatic
deposits which is most readily observable with melanomas. The cura-
bility by chemotherapy of aggressive and metastatic choriocarcinoma
and the occasional cure of Burkitt's lymphoma by a single treatment with
cytotoxic agents has also been ascribed to a contribution by immune
factors, as has the precipitation of cancer by stress, if indeed this
is a real phenomenon. Changes in the histological appearance of nodes
which drain a tumour, but which are not involved with tumour and the
presence within tumours of leukocytes, especially macrophages, are
consistent with an immunologically mediated host response in certain
cancers. The clinical and pathological data is not decisive and much
of the attention which has been devoted to tumour immunology stems from
studies of experimental tumours in animals in which tests involving
transplantation provide definitive proof of the existence of tumour
specific antigens for some but by no means all of the cancers studied.
Such transplantation tests can not be applied to man and the *in vitro*
tests for anti-tumour antibody and cytotoxic lymphocytes are for most
human cancers conflicting and, in general, cannot be interpreted
because of confounding factors. The one example of a truly tumour
specific antigen in human cancer is the B-cell lymphoma which produce
an immunoglobulin molecule which is unique to each tumour.

The increased incidence of malignant disease in immune depressed individuals is largely caused by an excess of some rare malignancies such as
non-Hodgkin's lymphomas and Kaposi sarcomas and relatively benign skin
cancers. The incidence of the common carcinomas which constitute 80%
of cancer is not increased by immune suppression. The available data

43

is consistent with the hypothesis that immune suppression in general promotes the occurence of cancers in the aetiology of which a virus is implicated. It is the virus and not the cancer which is under immune surveillance.

The most satisfactory evidence for an immune response to cancer would be effective immunotherapy. Within the last fifteen years there have been hundreds of claims that immunological manoevres based on augmenting or inducing an immunological host response alone or in conjunction with other therapies, are therapeutically useful but almost none of the claims made have withstood the test of prospective randomised controls and, there is as yet, no role for any of the immune procedures tested in the treatment of cancer except in an investigational setting. Well conducted randomized trials have failed to support earlier claims made for immunotherapy in the treatment of melanoma (except for the destruc- tion of superficial tumours by intra-lesional injection of agents which cause inflammation), lung cancer, colon cancer and gynaecological can- cers. In the acute leukaemias immunotherapy during remission may be better than no treatment at all, but do not equal the results of intensive chemotherapy and other measures such as total body irradiation and bone-marrow grafting. The exceptions are the B-cell lymphomas in which therapy which uses the idiotypic immunoglobulin as a highly specific target is both logical and promising.

New immunological approaches to cancer treatment

Recent developments in immunology provide a solid basis for new types of passive immunotherapy which do not rely on the presence of tumour specific antigens and their recognition by the host. It is now well worth testing whether a useful response may be induced by laboratory produced monoclonal antibodies -- and more in the future by clones of specific T-cells grown *in vitro* -- that are directed against antigens which are associated with the cancer cell but which do not evoke a host response because they are not novel to the host. Such antigens can provide a target for therapy if they are present in cancer cells in much larger amounts than in normal cells or if the antigen is only present in normal cells which are capable of replacement. For example, a differen- tiation antigen present both on lymphomas and on mature lymphocytes would constitute a good target since the loss of the mature lymphocytes which would accompany the destruction of the cancer would be tolerable as they would be replaced because their stem cells would not be killed.

Monoclonal antibodies could be used to interfere with tumour growth to kill cancer cells via antigens in the plasma membrane by either immuno-phagocytosis (particularly if the cancer cells are in the circulation) or **lysis** due to binding of complement or leukocytes. A serious limita-tion is the readiness with which Ag-Ab complexes internalise before these cytotoxic reactions can occur. One of the advantages of using antibodies that carry bound toxins (such as ricin) or cytotoxic agents is that internalisation should assist and not hinder the anti-tumour activity. Antibodies can be made that bind to extra cellular poly-saccharides or glycolipids and these may provide a good target for localising to the tumour chemotherapeutic agents bound to antibodies by a bond that is hydrolysed by enzymes in extra-cellular fluid.

There are also prospects for therapy which uses the selective cyto-toxicity of products of immunologically stimulated leukocytes such as **the lymphokine** leukotoxin and possibly also products deriving from phagocytes. These agents rely for their selectivity not on an immuno-logically specific reaction but on the physiology of certain cancer cells which render these more susceptible than many normal cells. We have evidence to indicate that a product released by T-cells and belonging to the class of lymphotoxins is responsible for the selective killing of some types of cancer cells at sites of inflammation induced by injecting BCG or *C. parvum*. The production of such factors by gene cloning technique is on the cards and raises the prospect of systemic applica-tion.

2. CURRENT CLINICAL PROGRESS WITH NEW AGENTS

PLATINUM ANALOGS

S.K. CARTER

Cisplatin (cis-platinum diamminedichloride) is one of the most important new cancer drugs of recent years. It has a broad spectrum of activity and has proven to be a compound easily combined with other cytotoxic agents. Analog development has been vigorously approached in the platinum area. Currently three analogs are under active evaluation by the Bristol-Myers Company (Table 1). The data are still preliminary but this paper will attempt an impressionistic view of the current interim status.

The clinical evaluation of platinum analogs is a complicated process. In the first place each analog must be compared with cisplatin. In the second place competing analogs must also be compared with each other. With at least three analogs under simultaneous evaluation, the process of choosing the best one requires an intricate clinical evaluation strategy with clearly defined decision-making criteria.

Three broad factors need to be analysed for each compound: 1) efficacy; 2) toxicity; and 3) cross-resistance. Efficacy breaks down into the effect against cisplatin sensitive and cisplatin resistant tumors. In cisplatin sensitive tumors this involves a requirement for superiority to cisplatin in at least one of the following parameters: 1) complete response rate; 2) overall response rate; 3) time to failure; 4) duration of response; 5) survival from initiation of chemotherapy; and 6) survival from first diagnosis of metastatic disease. Initially, the efficacy comparison may require combination chemotherapy testing. It is not impossible to conceive a scenario which would involve a discordancy of results between single agent tests and combination results.

In cisplatin resistant tumors the process is a bit simpler. In tumors such as large bowel cancer, non small cell lung cancer and malignant melanoma, any meaningful activity with an analog would be important and indicative of the need for further study.

49

Table 1. Cisplatin and cisplatin analogs: physico-chemical properties.

derivative	chemical name	formula molecular weight	solubility g/l	mmol/l
Cisplatin NSC 119875	cis-diamminedichloro-platin (II)	 Pt (II) (NH$_3$)$_2$Cl$_2$ molecular weight: 300,1	1 (0,9 % NaCl)	3
JM8 NSC 241240 CBDCA Carboplatin	diammine [1,1-cyclo-butan(dicarboxylato)] platin(II)	 Pt(II) (NH$_3$)$_2$(C$_4$H$_6$) (COO)$_2$ molecular weight: 371,2	18 (H$_2$O)	50
TNO 6 NSC 311056	1,1 diaminemethyl-cyclohexan(sulfato) platin(II)	 PtII (NH$_2$)$_2$(CH$_2$)$_2$ C$_6$H$_{10}$(SO$_4$) molecular weight: 433,4	20-40 (H$_2$O)	46-92
JM9 NSC 256927 CHIP	cis-dichloro-trans-dihydroxy-bis-iso-propylamin-platin (IV)	 Pt(IV)Cl$_2$(OH)$_2$ (C$_3$H$_7$NH$_2$)$_2$ molecular weight: 418,2	10-20 (0,9 % NaCl)	24-48

Toxicity end-points would focus on four broad areas: 1) renal toxicity; 2) nausea and vomiting; 3) marrow suppression; and 4) neurologic toxicity including ototoxicity and peripheral neuropathy. For each toxicity parameter there would be potentially either a qualitative or quantitative difference in comparison to cisplatin. The qualitative difference would involve a complete absence of the parameter. The quantitative difference would involve the toxicity being found with the analog but with an incidence and/or severity less than that observed with cisplatin.

A lack of cross-resistance involves a meaningful response rate for the analog in the face of clear cut resistance to cisplatin. This resistance can be defined in one of two ways: 1) progressive disease while on cisplatin treatment; and 2) progressive disease after a response to cisplatin while on cisplatin containing maintenance therapy.

To date, the three analogs which have received significant study have only partially answered the many questions which were proposed in the prior discussion. Many trials are currently on-going and so the data may well change by the time this paper is published.

Concerning the efficacy in platinum sensitive tumors, the most data are available in ovarian cancer. It appears from the phase I and early phase 2 data that both JM-8 and JM-9 have activity in ovarian cancer which appears equivalent to that observed with cisplatin. The most advanced drug is JM-8 which is now in phase 3 study at the Royal Marsden Hospital under the direction of Eve Wiltshaw. Dr. Wiltshaw is performing a randomized phase 3 study in women with advanced ovarian cancer and no prior therapy with cytotoxic chemotherapy. The randomization is to cisplatin versus JM-8. Over 100 patients have been entered and the preliminary analysis of over 60 evaluable patients demonstrates comparable, complete and overall response rates with the two drugs. The phase 3 studies with JM-9 are now just ready to begin. The data with TNO-6 is disappointing with evidence of a distinctly inferior response potential in this tumor.

When other platinum sensitive tumors are examined, JM-8 shows evidence of activity as well. This is particularly true in small cell lung cancer and testicular cancer at the Royal Marsden and bladder cancer in a trial being performed under the aegis of the Medical Research Council. The preliminary data on TNO-6 from the Bristol-Myers multi-center trial indicates that this analog has minimal activity against the range of cisplatin sensitive tumors and that the activity will be inferior to that observed with cisplatin. There is not enough data available for JM-9 to make any statement in this area.

When toxicity is examined for the three analogs, a pattern, significantly different in a quantitative sense from cisplatin, emerges. All three analogs are dose-limited by myelosuppression with thrombocytopenia being a bit more severe than leukopenia. When renal toxicity is examined then a true separation is observed. Both JM-8 and JM-9 appear to be devoid of any meaningful renal toxicity. Both drugs can be administered without hydration, and given in repeated courses, without any significant elevations of serum creatinine, or diminishment of creatinine clearance, being observed. The study with TNO-6 is quite different. With this drug, erratic but significant renal toxicity has been observed. Some cases have developed renal failure after one or two courses of drugs while other patients have demonstrated no evidence of renal damage. An attempt to ameliorate renal toxicity through the utilization of hydration has not been successful. It appears, from the preliminary data available to date, that the incidence of renal toxicity, after TNO-6, is the same with or without hydration. This would indicate a mechanism of renal toxicity which is different from that of cisplatin. An early hint of this was available from the phase I studies which demonstrated high levels of proteinuria which is not a common feature of cisplatin renal toxicity.

Nausea and vomiting is a severe problem with cisplatin and usual anti-emetic therapies are only partially successful at best in ameliorating the problem. It is not uncommon for patients to refuse continued cisplatin therapy because of the emetogenic potential of the drug. A very positive aspect of JM-8 in the studies to date is that the nausea and vomiting, which results from therapy, is both less severe and more responsive to anti-emetic treatment in comparison to cisplatin. Data emerging from the Royal Marsden group demonstrates that patients who have received both cisplatin and JM-8 clearly prefer the latter drug from the perspective of tolerance. Similar data, but with less detail, indicates lessened nausea and vomiting, which also exist for JM-9 and TNO-6. It still remains too early to meaningfully speak about ototoxicity and peripheral neuropathy but the early impression is favorable for both JM-8 and JM-9 in this regard.

In summary for toxicity, JM-8 appears to have two significant advantages over cisplatin: 1) a lack of meaningful renal toxicity; and 2) diminished, and more treatable, nausea and vomiting. This drug is dose limited by myelosuppression which is quantitatively more severe than that reported for cisplatin. A similar pattern also appears evident for JM-9 but not for TNO-6 which has significant renal toxicity and so appears to be the distinctly inferior analog.

The final factor for analysis is cross-resistance. The impression to date, from available information, is favorable to JM-8, neutral to JM-9 and unfavorable for TNO-6. Hilary Calvert in his extensive phase 1-2 study, at the Royal Marsden with JM-8, has observed a series of patients with ovarian cancer resistant to cisplatin who have subsequently responded to JM-8. On the opposite side of the spectrum an ovarian cancer study with TNO-6 specifically designed to treat cisplatin resistant cases has shown absolutely no activity and has been stopped. No data on this question are available, as yet, with JM-9.

CONCLUSION

KNTH

At this current moment, tremendous clinical activity exists with platinum
analogs. While a great deal of data exist, they are preliminary and extensive
new information should be available by the time this paper is published. What
can be said about the clinical study material now available for analysis is
highly favorable to JM-8 as the leading analog and encouraging as well about
JM-9. JM-8 appears to be at least equivalently active in cisplatin sensitive
tumors with two significant toxicologic advantages - no renal toxicity and
lessened emetogenic potential. JM-9 has the same toxicologic advantages but
the efficacy data are much less mature. TNO-6 appears to be inferior as
regards both efficacy and toxicity and has a dubious future.

MITOXANTRONE: A PROMISING NEW AGENT FOR THE TREATMENT OF HUMAN CANCER

COLIN P. TURNBULL[1] AND DAVID JACKSON[2]

Mitoxantrone (1,4-dihydroxy-5,8-bis((2-(2-hydroxyethyl)amino)ethyl-amino)-9, 10-anthracenedione hydrochloride NOVANTRONE*) was first synthesized by Murdock[1]. Based on its antitumor activity in mice and the observation that it did not cause progressive irreversible cardiotoxicity in animals, mitoxantrone was selected for clinical evaluation. An independent effort at the University of Kansas[2] also identified mitoxantrone and confirmed the observations of the Lederle investigators in transplantable murine tumors.

Because of structural similarities between doxorubicin and mitoxantrone, much of the early enthusiasm for the development of mitoxantrone lay in the hope that this agent would have the antitumor activity of the anthracyclines without their cardiotoxicity. There are several important differences between mitoxantrone and the anthracyclines, preclinically and clinically, such that mitoxantrone may be considered representative of a new class of anticancer agents. Mitoxantrone and doxorubicin have significantly different spectra of activity in animal tumor models[3]. Cytotoxicity studies with P-388 cells in vitro have shown that, unlike doxorubicin, mitoxantrone produced true first order cell kill kinetics, cell kill being independent of duration of exposure[3]. Mitoxantrone and doxorubicin exhibit different propensities for enzymatic reduction to semiquinone free radicals, with reactive oxygen formation and intracellular lipid peroxidation, mechanisms implicated in the pathogensis of myocardial lesions observed with doxorubicin and daunorubicin. In biological systems containing NADPH and reductive enzymes such as NADPH cytochrome P-450 reductase, mitoxantrone, in contrast to doxorubicin, has variously been shown to inhibit lipid peroxidation[4], decrease oxygen consumption and hydrogen peroxide formation[5], and does not significantly stimulate NADPH consumption or superoxide formation[6]. Studies on the electrochemical reduction of mitoxantrone and

---

*Trademark American Cyanamid Company

[1]American Cyanamid Company   [2]Lederle Laboratories
   One Cyanamid Plaza   Division of American Cyanamid Company
   Wayne, NJ 07470   Middletown Road, Pearl River, NY 10965

daunorubicin show a high reduction potential for the former relative to daunorubicin with insignificant free radical and superoxide formation. Kharasch and Novak reported that mitoxantrone inhibits doxorubicin induced lipid peroxidation and suggested studies involving the coadministration of the two agents be undertaken to determine if mitoxantrone could afford protection against the cardiotoxicity of doxorubicin[8]. The lack of complete cross resistance between the two agents, preclinically[9,13] and clinically[10-12,27,28] further supports the view that mitoxantrone represents a unique new class of antitumor agent.

A number of studies on the mechanism of action of mitoxantrone have been performed[3,13,14,15]. Mitoxantrone inhibits both DNA and RNA synthesis and binds to DNA by intercalation and by electrostatic interaction with the anionic exterior of DNA[14]. Mitoxantrone also induces chromatid breakage[16], sister chromatid exchanges and chromosomal aberrations in Chinese hamster ovary cells[17]. At the level of the cell, mitoxantrone causes a block in cell cycle progression in G2 with a two-fold increase in RNA content[18]. While cells in S-phase are most sensitive to the blocking activity of mitoxantrone, cell-killing activity is non-cell cycle specific.

CLINICAL STUDIES

Pharmacokinetics

The pharmacokinetics of mitoxantrone have been studied by a number of investigators[19,20,21,22,23]. While significant differences in certain parameters have been reported reflecting differences in methodology, a number of features have consistently been observed. Following intravenous administration, mitoxantrone rapidly disappears from the plasma and is extensively distributed to tissues with a large volume of distribution; this has been variously reported as 13.8 L/kg[20] (approximately 522 L/M^2) and 1875 L/M^2 [22]. In most patients, the plasma disappearance of mitoxantrone can be described by a three component exponential curve with a long terminal half-life of at least 38 hours. Studies utilizing both radio-labeled drug and HPLC methodology indicate that mitoxantrone undergoes a significant degree of metabolism[22]. Three metabolites of unknown structure were detected by HPLC in the urine of a patient treated with the drug[22]. Renal excretion of mitoxantrone does not appear to be a major route of elimination as determined from the low recovery of drug in the urine ($<$ 10% after five days). Indeed, renal impairment has not been found to affect the pharmacokinetics of the drug[23]. Conflicting results, however, have been obtained on the effect of hepatic impairment of mitoxantrone pharmacokinetic parameters. Savaraj et al[20] have reported that the terminal plasma t 1/2 was increased from a mean of 38 hours in "normal" patients to 70 hours in patients with hepatic dysfunction or third spaces, whereas Malspeis and Neidhart[23] found no significant difference in patients with varying degrees of hepatic dysfunction. Clinical experience to date indicates that dosage adjustment in cases of hepatic dysfunction may not be required. Analysis of tissue content of mitoxantrone at various periods after dosing indicated that the drug persists in the body for extensive periods; Alberts[22] has reported that 15% of an administered dose was retained 35 days after dosing in seven organs analyzed. Despite this,

repeat dosing for four courses each at three weekly intervals in one
patient did not appreciably alter the pharmacokinetic parameters of
the drug[20].

Phase 1

Results of Phase I studies of mitoxantrone have recently been reviewed
by Smith[24]. In summary, neutropenia was found to be dose limiting
in all schedules. On the basis of the apparent lack of schedule
dependency, a dose and schedule of 12-14 mg/M^2 every three weeks was
selected for Phase II evaluation in solid tumors in adults.

Phase II

Breast Cancer

Patients with advanced breast cancer were entered into Phase II
studies, results from certain of which have been reported in the
literature[24,10,11,25]. The following summary is based on the
American Cyanamid Data Base. In 88 evaluable patients previously
untreated by chemotherapy for advanced disease

given mitoxantrone 14 mg/M^2 q. 3-4 weeks, there were six complete
responses (CR) and 27 partial responses (PR) for a total response rate
of 38%. Responses occurred in all dominant sites of metastatic
disease (there were no patients with central nervous system or
lymphangytic lung disease in this study) and were unaffected by the
length of the disease-free interval, or performance status. The mean
times to response were six weeks for skin and regional nodes,
nine weeks for primary tumor, and 21 and 24 weeks for liver and bone,
respectively. The median duration of response in this study (from
start of treatment) was approximately 10 months. In patients
previously treated with chemotherapy for advanced disease response
rates (CR + PR) have variously been recorded between 10% and 27%.
Analyzing these response rates by dose level, the collective response
rate from the three studies at doses   11 mg/M^2 was 9%; at
12-13 mg/M^2 17%; and at a dose of 14 mg/M^2 was 31%.

In a randomized comparative study at Ohio State University with
doxorubicin, 5/20 patients responded to mitoxantrone 12 mg/M^2
compared with 6/20 to doxorubicin 60 mg/M^2. This difference was not
statistically significant. On crossover, 3/10 patients responded to
mitoxantrone (2/6 initially unresponsive to doxorubicin and 1/4 who
relapsed on treatment) and 1/10 responded to doxorubicin (0/8
unresponsive to mitoxantrone and 1/2 progressing on treatment)
indicating incomplete cross resistance between the two drugs.

With a regimen consisting of cyclophosphamide 500 mg/M^2
5-fluorouracil, 1,000 mg/M^2 and mitoxantrone 10 mg/M^2, all drugs
on day 1 of a 21 day treatment cycle, 2 CR and 19 PR (total PR + CR
72%) were recorded in 27 patients, the remaining six patients
achieving stable disease[26]. Patients were previously untreated by
cytotoxic chemotherapy for advanced breast cancer and had
predominantly visceral disease (20/27), with 26/27 having estrogen
receptor negative tumors.

Acute Leukemias

Using a dosage schedule of 10 mg/M^2 daily x 5 Prentice et al[27] reported three CRs and one PR in seven evaluable patients with acute myelocytic leukemia (AML) in first relapse and two PRs in five patients with refractory AML. One CR and one PR occurred in two patients with refractory acute lymphocytic leukemia (ALL). None of four patients with chronic myeloid leukemia (CML) in blast crisis achieved a response nor did one patient with ALL in first relapse. Pacciuci et al[28] reported six CRs in 12 patients with generally refractory ALL at doses ranging from 8-14 mg/M^2 daily x 5. In 12 patients with AML, one CR and one PR were observed. Arlin et al[29] have recently reported two CRs in seven patients with AML and one CR in three patients with chronic granulocytic leukemia in blastic crisis (CGL in BC) all treated with mitoxantrone 12 mg/M^2 daily x 5. At a lower dose of 10 mg/M^2 day x 5, one of five patients with ALL, one of 12 with AML and one of seven with CGL in BC achieved CR. These data indicate considerable activity of mitoxantrone in previously treated patients with acute leukemias and confirm early observations of activity in Phase II screening trials[30].

Lymphomas

At a dose schedule of 14 mg/M^2 q. three weeks, Gams et al[31] have reported five PRs and one stable disease in eight patients with various histological grades of non-Hodgkins lymphoma (NHL) whereas only three PRs were observed in 32 evaluable patients treated at a dose of 5 mg/M^2 weekly. Coltman et al[32] have treated at total of 58 patients (16 Hodgkins (HD) and 42 NHL) with mitoxantrone 12 mg/M^2 q. three weeks. Patients had been heavily pretreated with cytotoxic drugs. Two PRs and one CR occurred in 13 evaluable HD patients and seven PRs and one CR in 37 evaluable NHL patients.

Other Tumors

Responses have been observed in primary liver cell cancer, tumors of the head and neck and multiple myeloma[33] in Phase II studies. Sufficient data are available on colon carcinoma, melanoma and renal cell carcinoma to conclude that mitoxantrone is not active in these tumors.

Toxicity

Hematological

Dose limiting toxicity with mitoxantrone is leukopenia. White blood cell (WBC) nadirs have mostly occurred 10-14 days after dosing, with recovery usually by day 21. In 120 evaluable patients previously untreated by chemotherapy for advanced breast cancer treated with an initial dose of mitoxantrone 12-14 mg/M^2, the mean WBC nadir after the first course of therapy was 3.200/cm^3. In patients previously treated by cytotoxic chemotherapy, WBC nadirs were similar. While only a relatively small number of patients have received substantial cumulative doses of mitoxantrone, the available data do not suggest that cumulative neutropenia will be a clinical problem.

Thrombocytopenia has not been a problem with mitoxantrone. Platelet recovery follows a similar timescale to that of the WBC. In 677 evaluable courses, 1% showed a platelet nadir $< 50,000/cm^3$.

Non Hematological Toxicity

Acute non-hematological toxicity with mitoxantrone has consistently been reported to be low in incidence and generally mild. For a cytotoxic drug, mitoxantrone is exceptionally well tolerated. In 957 patients treated on the once every three week schedule, the incidence and severity of the most frequent side effects are listed in the Table.

	Mild	Moderate	Severe	Very Severe
Stomatitis	3.9%	1.7%	0.3%	
Nausea and vomiting	21%	12%	3%	4%
Alopecia	11%	3%	1%	0%

Thus, it is apparent that 94% of patients did not experience stomatitis; 60% of patients did not experience nausea and/or vomiting and 85% of patients did not experience alopecia. Additionally, of more than 3,000 patients treated with mitoxantrone worldwide, there have been no reports of tissue necrosis as a result of extravasation As noted recently by Holland[35], these pooled data from the American Cyanamid data base do not differ signficantly from those reported individually from small series of patients.

Cardiac Episodes

Considerable attention has been focused on the incidence and severity of cardiac episodes associated with mitoxantrone therapy in man. A number of reports of cardiac episodes including congestive heart failure (CHF), occurring in patients treated with mitoxantrone, have now appeared in the literature. Almost exclusively, these events have occurred in patients with either prior anthracycline therapy and/or other known predisposing factors, thus making a rational assessment of the cardiotoxic potential of mitoxantrone per se somewhat difficult. A comprehensive analysis of 88 such cardiac events occurring in some 3,360 patients was recently made by Crossley[36]. From this analysis, it is apparent that for the patients who had not received previous anthracycline therapy, there appears to be minimal risk for cardiotoxicity up to cumulative doses of 140 to 160 mg/M^2. This corresponds to about one year of therapy. In patients who had prior anthracycline therapy, there appears to be minimal risk up to cumulative doses of 120 mg/M^2.

While very few of the patients have had endomyocardial biopsies, there have been a few reports of anthracycline-like pathological changes, being Grades 1 to 2.5. Conclusions based on biopsy interpretations are not currently possible.

Where clinical CHF has occurred in association with mitoxantrone therapy, it has generally been responsive to standard therapy.

Conclusion

Mitoxantrone is a fascinating new anticancer agent with considerable promise for the treatment of human cancer. The drug has single agent activity in advanced breast cancer comparable to the most active currently available agents and also appears to be highly active in refractory leukemias and lymphomas. The low incidence of severe acute subjective side effects and the apparent reduced propensity for clinical cardiotoxicity of mitoxantrone relative to the anthracyclines hold the prospect of an improved quality of life for patients requiring cytotoxic chemotherapy.

References

1. Murdock, K. C., Wallace, R. E., Durr, F. E., Child, R. G., Citarella, R. V., Fabio, P. F., and Angier, R. B. Antitumor Agents I. 1,4-bis-(aminoalkyl amino)-9,10-anthracenediones. J. Med. Chem. 22, 1024-1030, 1979.

2. Zee-Cheng, R. K. Y., and Cheng, C. C. Antineoplastic Agents: Structure-Activity Relationship Study of bis(substituted aminoalkylamino)anthraquinones. J. Med. Chem. 21, 291-294, 1978.

3. Johson R. K., Broome, M. G., Howard, W. S., Evans, S. F., and Pritchard, D. F. Experimental Therapeutic and Biochemical Studies of Anthracenedione Derivatives, in "New Anticancer Drugs: Mitoxantrone and Bisantrene," edited by M. Rozencweig et al, Raven Press, New York, 1983.

4. Mimnaugh, E. G., Trush, M. A., Ginsburg, E., Gram, T. E. Differential Effects of Anthracycline Drugs on Rat Heart and Liver Microsomal Reduced Nicotinamide Adenine Dinucleotide Phosphate Dependent Lipid Peroxidation. Cancer Res., 42, 3574-3548, 1982.

5. Doroshow, J. H. Comparative Cardiac Oxygen Radical Production by Anthracycline Antiobiotics, Mitoxantrone, Bisantrene, m-AMSA, and Neocarcinostatin. Clinical Res., 31, 67A, 1983.

6. Kharasch, E. D. and Novak, R. F. Biochemical Pharmacoloy, 20, 2881-2884, 1981.

7. Sinha, B. K., Motten, A. G. and Hanck, K. W. The Electrochemical Reduction of 1,4-bis (2-(2-hydroxyethyl)amino)ethylamino) anthracenedione and daunomycin: Biochemical Significance in Superoxide Formation. Chem. Biol Interactions, 43, 371-377, 1983.

8. Kharasch, E. D. and Novak, R. F. Inhibition of Adriamycin-Stimulated Microsomal Lipid Peroxidation by Mitoxantrone and Ametantrone, two New Anthracenedione Antineoplastic Agents. Biochemical and Biophysical Research Communications, 108 (3), 1346-1352, 1982.

9. Fujimoto, S and Ogawa, M. Antitumor Activity of Mitoxantrone Against Murine Experimental Tumors: Comparative Analysis Against Various Antitumor Antibiotics. Cancer Chemother. Pharmacol, 8, 157-162, 1982.

10. Neidhart, J. A., Gochnour, D., Roach, R. W., and Young, D. C. Mitoxantrone Versus Doxorubicin in Advanced Breast Cancer: a Randomized Cross-Over Trial. Abstracts 13th ICC, 1983. Cancer Treatment Reviews, in Press.

11. Stuart-Harris, R. C. and Smith, I. E. Mitoxantrone: A Phase II Study in the Treatment of Patients with Advanced Breast Carcinoma and Other Solid Tumors. Cancer Chemotherapy and Pharmacology 8, 179-182, 1982.

12. Yap, H-Y, Blumenschein, G. R., Schell, F. C., Buzdar, A. U., Valdivieso, M., and Bodey G. P. Dihydroxyanthracenedione: a Promising New drug in the Treatment of Metastatic Breast Cancer. Ann. Int. Med., 95, 694-697.

13. Johnson, R. K., Zee-Cheng, R. K-Y., Lee, W. W., Acton, E. M., Henry, E. W., and Cheng, C. C. Experimental Antitumor Activity of Aminoanthraquinones. Cancer Treatment Reports 63, 425-439, 1979.

14. Foye, W. O., Vajragupta, O. P. A., and Sengupta, S. K. DNA-Binding Specificity and RNA Polymerase Inhibitory Activity of bis-(aminoalkyl)anthraquinones and bis(methylthio)vinylquinone iodides. J. Pharm. Sci., 71 (2), 253-257, 1982.

15. Kapuschinski, J., Darzynkiewicz, Z., Traganos, F., and Malamed, M. R. Interactions of a New Antitumor Agent, 1,4-dihydroxy-5, 8-bis ((2-(2-hydroxyethyl)amino)ethylamino)-9,10-anthracenedione with nucleic acids. Biochem. Pharmacol., 30, 231-240, 1981.

16. Hsu, T. C., Cherry, L. M., and Pathak, S. Induction of Chromatid Breakage by Clastogens in Cells in G_2 Phase. Mutation Research, 93, 185-193, 1982.

17. Nishio, A., DeFeo, F., Cheng, C. C., and Uyeki, E. M. Sister-Chromatid Exchange and Chromasomal Aberrations by DHAQ and Related Anthraquinone Derivatives in Chinese Hamster Ovary Cells. Mutation Research, 101, 77-86, 1982.

18. Traganos, F., Evenson, D. P., Staiano-Coico, L., Darzynkiewicz, Z., and Melamed, M. R. Action of Dihydroxyanthraquinone on Cell Cycle Progression and Survival of a Variety of Cultured Mammalian Cells. Cancer Res., 40, 671-681, 1980.

19. Reynolds, D. L., Ulrich, K. K. Patton, T. F., Repta, A. J., Sternson, L. A., Myron, M. C., and Taylor, S. A. Plasma Levels of 1,4-dihydroxy-5,8-bis ((2-((2-hydroxyethyl)amino)ethyl)amino)-9, 10-anthracenedione dihydrochloride (DHAD) in Humans. Int. J. Pharmaceutics, 9, 67-71, 1981.

20. Savaraj, N., Lu, K., Valdivieso, M., Burgess, M., Umsawasdi, T., Benjamin, R. S., and Loo, T. L. Clinical Kinetics of 1,4-dihydroxy-5,8-bis ((2-(2-hydroxyethyl)amino)ethyl)amino)-9 10-anthracenedione. Clin. Pharmacol Ther. 312-316, 1982.

21. Stewart, J. A., McCormack, J. J., and Krakoff, I. H., Clinical and Clinical Pharmacologic Studies of Mitoxantrone. Cancer Treat. Rep. 66, 1327-1331, 1982.

22. Alberts, D. S., Peng, Y. M., Leigh, S., Davis, T.P., and Woodward, D. L. Pharmacokinetics of Mitoxantrone in Patients. Abstracts 13th ICC. Cancer Treatment Reviews in Press.

23. Neidhart, J. A. and Malspeis, L. Pharmacokinetics of Mitoxantrone Following Administration of a Single Intravenous Dose. Data on file, Lederle Laboratories.

24. Smith, I. E., Mitoxantrone (NOVANTRONE): A Review of Experimental and Early Clinical Studies. Cancer Treatment Reviews, <u>10</u>, 103-115, 1983.

25. Mouridson, H. T., Van Oosterom, A. T., Rose, C., and Nooi, M. A. A Phase II Study of Mitoxantrone as First Line Cytotoxic Therapy in Advanced Breast Cancer. 13th ICC Abstracts. Cancer Treatment Reviews, in Press.

26. Yap, H. Y., Esparza, L., Blumenschein, G. R., Hortobagyi, G. N., and Bodey, G. P. Combination Chemotherapy with Cyclophosphamide, Mitoxantrone, 5-Fluorouracil in Patients with Metastatic Breast Cancer. 13th ICC Abstracts. Cancer Treatment Reviews, in Press.

27. Prentice, H. G., Robbins, G., Hulhoven, R., and Michaux, J. L., Therapeutic Activity, Toxicity, and Pharmacokinetics of Mitoxantrone. A Phase I/II Study in Patients with Acute Leukemia. 13th ICC Abstracts. Cancer Treatment Reviews, in Press.

28. Paciucci, P. A., Ohnuma, T., Cuttner, J., and Holland, J. F. Mitoxantrone in Refractory Acute Leukemia. 13th ICC Abstracts Cancer Treatment Reviews, in Press.

29. Arlin, Z., Silver, R., Cassileth, P., Armentrout, S., Gams, R., Ersler, A., Amare, M., Brown, G., Schoch, I., and Dukart, G. Phase I/II Trial of Mitoxantrone in Adult Acute Leukemia (AL) Abstracts. 2nd European Congress of Clinical Oncology, 1983.

30. Data on file, Lederle Laboratories.

31. Gams, R. A., Keller, J., Colomb, H. M., Steinberg, J., and Dukart, G. Mitoxantrone in Malignant Lymphoma. 13th ICC Abstracts. Cancer Treatment Reviews, in Press.

32. Coltman, C.A., Jr., McDaniel, T. M., Balcerzk, S. P., Morrison, F. S., and Von Hoff, D. D. Mitoxantrone Hydrochloride in Lymphoma. 13th ICC Abstracts. Cancer Treatment Reviews, in Press.

33. Data on file, Lederle Laboratories.

34. Data on file, Lederle Laboratories.

35. Holland, J. F., Chairman's Summary on the 13th ICC Symposium on Mitoxantrone. Cancer Treatment Reviews, in Press.

36. Crossley, R. J. Clinical Safety and Tolerance of Mitoxantrone 13th ICC Abstracts, Cancer Treatment Reviews, in Press.

CURRENT CLINICAL PROGRESS – PODOPHYLLOTOXINS

Brian F. Issell

Podophyllotoxin is a compound derived from the roots or rhyzomes of certain plants of the genus Podophyllum (Mandrake, American May apple). VP-16, or etoposide, and VM-26, or teniposide, are semisynthetic derivatives of podophyllotoxin. They differ from the parent compound podophyllotoxin and other classical spindle poisons such as colchicine, vincristine, and vinblastine by not interacting with tubulin or interfering with microtubule assembly (1).

VP-16, VM-26 COMPARISON

VP-16 and VM-26 differ chemically only by a methyl for thenylidine substitution on the glucopyranoside moiety. After more than 10 years of clinical development, it seems that there is no meaningful significant difference between the clinical activity or toxicity profiles of these drugs. VP-16 has historically been tested in mainly adult tumors while the use of VM-26 has been emphasized in pediatric malignancies.

CLINICAL ACTIVITIES

Table 1 lists the tumor types where activity has been demonstrated for VP-16 and VM-26. The tumors are further divided according to whether the drug appears to have contributed a meaningful benefit to patients in more than one reported study or where contribution to patient benefit is still not clearly established.

TABLE 1: VP-16 – VM-26 ACTIVITIES

VP-16	VM-26
Contribution Established	
Small Cell Lung Cancer	Pediatric ALL
Testicular	Non-Hodgkin's Lymphoma
Non-Hodgkin's Lymphoma	
Contribution Less Established	
Kaposi's Sarcoma	Neuroblastoma
Acute Leukemia	Brain Tumors
Hodgkin's Disease	
Breast Cancer	

65

Small Cell Lung Cancer

VP-16 is amongst the most active single agents for this disease (2). Although earlier reports of high response rates in refractory patients were encouraging (3-4), more recent studies in patients who have failed prior intensive chemotherapy suggest only a 10-20% response rate (5-6). However, the addition of cisplatin to VP-16 in the salvage setting has resulted in response rates approaching 50% at several centers (6-8). Since cisplatin as a single agent appears to have similar activity to etoposide in comparable patients, it seems that the therapeutic synergy between VP-16 and cisplatin observed in murine tumor system may also be relevant in human cancer. VP-16-213 is now included in the majority of large cooperative group front-line chemotherapy regimens for small cell lung cancer (9). Its combination with cyclophosphamide and Adriamycin has given results which are amongst the best reported for this disease; although, it is not always possible to evaluate the contribution of VP-16 in these studies (10). VM-26 has not been adequately studied in small cell lung cancer, but evidence of activity comparable to VP-16 was reported from one Phase 2 study (11).

Testicular Cancer

Single agent VP-16 appears to be active in testicular cancer patients who are refractory to front-line combination chemotherapy. In one study, 46% of 24 assessable patients responded including 3 patients (12.5%) who remained disease free for over 2 years and may represent cures (12). Testicular cancer is a further tumor where there may be a therapeutic synergy between cisplatin and VP-16. Combining the two drugs in this setting has resulted in long-term complete remissions in 47% of 30 patients with germ cell malignancy in one study (13). VM-26 has not been adequately tested in testicular cancer.

Malignant Lymphomas

Impressive single agent activity was observed for VP-16 in diffuse histio-cytic lymphoma where 42% of 19 evaluable patients who had failed front-line combination chemotherapy responded to VP-16 (14). In addition, VP-16 containing combination regimens have given beneficial results in the salvage therapy of Hodgkin's disease and non-Hodgkin's lymphomas (15-16) and in the front-line therapy of non-Hodgkin's lymphomas (17).

Similarly, VM-26 as a single agent appeared active in patients with refractory lymphoma (18). VM-26 has also been studied in front-line combination chemotherapy for non-Hodgkin's lymphoma patients and appears a useful drug in this setting (19).

Acute Leukemia

VM-26 appears to be an important drug in the management of pediatric acute lymphoblastic leukemia. An apparent synergy between cytarabine (araC) and VM-26 appears useful. This combination resulted in 9 of 14 patients achieving complete remissions after they had failed remission induction with standard drugs. In addition, six of these patients had also been treated with prior cytarabine (20). The role of VP-16 in leukemia has been explored more in adult myelogenous disease, and it has been suggested that this compound may have a special place where monocytoid cells have failed to clear with front-line combination chemotherapy (21).

Other Tumors

As a single agent VM-26 has shown activity in refractory pediatric neuroblastoma and appears to be usefully combined with cisplatin in this setting (22). VM-26 also appears to be active in brain tumors (23-24). Although it was added to BCNU in one comparative study (25), its contribution to the definite management of this disease is difficult to assess.

VP-16-213 may be a useful drug in breast cancer management. Durable partial responses have been seen as a single agent (26); and when combined with doxorubicin in the salvage setting (27-28). Of recent interest has been the reported activity of etoposide single agent therapy in early stage disseminated Kaposi's sarcoma. Of 22 evaluable patients studied in one trial, 45% attained a complete response and 41% a partial response (29).

TABLE 2: VP-16; VM-26 CLINICAL TOXICITIES

MYELOSUPPRESSION
- Leukopenia dose limiting & predictable.
- Thrombocytopenia less frequent.

ACUTE (UNCOMMON)
- Fever, chills, bronchospasm.
- Hypertension, cardiorespiratory compromise.
- Hypotension (with rapid infusion).

GASTROINTESTINAL
- Nausea & vomiting.
- Infrequent diarrhea & mucositis.

ALOPECIA
- Common & reversible.

PERIPHERAL NEUROPATHY
- Mild & infrequent.

CHRONIC PULMONARY
- 1 case for teniposide.

CLINICAL TOXICITIES

The clinical toxicities for both compounds are similar and are listed in Table 2. Both compounds are well tolerated and easily managed with predictable leukopenia being the dose–limiting effect. Other rare but severe acute reactions include allergic–like episodes and cardiopulmonary collapse. Although one case of pulmonary hyaline membrane disease has been reported as related to VM–26 dosing (30), no other chronic cumulative toxicities have been recognized with either drug.

REFERENCES:

1. Locke, J.D. and Horwitz, S.B.: Effect of VP–16–213 on Microtubule Assembly in vitro and Nucleoside Transport in HeLa Cells. Biochemistry 15: 5435, 1976a.
2. Comis, R.L.: Small Cell Carcinoma of the Lung. Cancer Treat. Rev. 9: 237-258, 1982.
3. Cohen, M.H., Broder, L.E., Fossieck, B.E., Ihde, D.C., Minna, J.D.: Phase II Clinical Trial of Weekly Administration of VP–16–213 in Small Cell Bronchogenic Carcinoma. Cancer Treat. Rep. 61: 489-490, 1977.
4. Tucker, R.K., Ferguson, A., VanWyk, C., Sealy, R., Hewitsen, R., and Levin, W.: Chemotherapy of Small Cell Carcinoma of the Lung with VP–16–213. Cancer 41: 1710-1714, 1978.
5. Tempero, M., Kessinger, A., and Lemon, H.M.: VP–16–213 Therapy in Patients with Small Cell Carcinoma of the Lung After Failure on Combination Chemotherapy. Cancer Clin. Trials 4: 155-157, 1981.
6. Evans, W.K., Osoba, D., Feld, R., and Shephard, F.A.: VP–16 Alone and in Combination with Cisplatin (P) for Relapse in Small cell Lung Cancer (SCLC). Proc. The III World Conference on Lung Cancer, p. 218, 1982.
7. Tinsley, R., Comis, R., DiFino, S., Ginsberg, S., Gullo, J., Hickes, R., Poiesz, B., Rudolph, A., Issell, B., and Lee, F.: Potential Clinical Synergy Observed in the Treatment of Small Cell Lung Cancer (SCLC) with Cisplatin (P) and VP–16–213 (V). Proc. ASCO 2: 198, 1983.
8. Lopez, J.A., Mann, J., Grapski, R., and Krikorian, J.G.: Salvage Chemotherapy of Refractory Small Cell Lung Cancer (SCLC) with VP–16 and Cis-Platinum (DDP). Proc. ASCO 1: 151, 1982.
9. U.S. Dept. Health & Human Service. Compilation of Experimental Cancer Therapy Protocol Summaries, 7th edition, 1983.
10. Aisner, J., Whitacre, M., VanEcho, D.A., Wesley, M, and Wiernik, P.H.: Doxorubicin, Cyclophosphamide and VP–16–213 (ACE) in the Treatment of Small cell Lung Cancer. Cancer Chemother. Pharmacol. 7: 187-193, 1982.
11. Woods, R.L., Fox, R.M., Trattersall, M.H.N.: Treatment of Small Cell Bronchogenic Carcinoma with VM–26. Cancer Treat. Rep. 63: 2011, 1979.
12. Fitzharris, B.M., Kaye, S.B., Saverymuttu, S., Newlands, E.S., Barrett, A., Peckham, M.J., and McElwain, T.J.: VP–16–213 as a Single Agent in Advanced Testicular Tumors. Eur. J. Cancer 16: 1193, 1980.
13. Williams, S.D., Einhorn, L.H., Greco, F.A., Oldham, R., and Fletcher, R.: VP–16–213 Salvage Therapy for Refractory Germinal Neoplasms. Cancer 46: 2154-2158, 1980.
14. Bender, R.A., Anderson, T., Fisher, R.T., and Young, R.C.: The Activity of the Epipodophyllotoxin VP–16 in the Treatment of Combination Chemotherapy Resistant Non–Hodgkin's Lymphoma. Am. J. Hematol. 5: 203, 1978.
15. Cabanillas, F., Hagemeister, F.B., Bodey, G.P., and Freireich, E.J.: IMVP–16: An Effective Regimen for Patients with Lymphoma who have Relapsed after Initial Combination Chemotherapy. Blood 60: 693-697, 1982.

16. Santoro, A., Bonfante, V., and Bonadonna, G.: Third-Line Chemotherapy with CCNU, Etoposide and Prednimustine (CEP) in Hodgkin's Disease (HD) Resistant to MOPP and ABVD. Proc. ASCO 1: 165, 1982.

17. Fisher, R.I., DeVita, V.T., Huybbard, S.M., Longo, D.L., Wesley, R., Chabner, B.A., and Young, R.C.: Diffuse Aggressive Lymphomas: Increased Survival After Alternating Flexible Sequences of ProMACE and MOPP Chemotherapy. Annals of Int. Med. 98: 304-309, 1983.

18. Chiuten, D.F., Bennett, J.M., Creech, R.H., Glick, J., Falkson, G., Brodovsky, H.S., Begg, C.G., Muggia, F.M., and Carbone, P.O.: VM-26, A New Anticancer Drug with Effectiveness in Malignant Lymphoma: An Eastern Cooperative Oncology Group Study (EST 1474). Cancer Treat. Rep 63: 7, 1979.

19. The Australian and New Zealand Lymphoma Cooperative Chemotherapy Study Group: Comparison of the Use of Teniposide and Vincristine in Combination Chemotherapy for Non-Hodgkin's Lymphoma. Cancer Treat. Rep. 66:49-55, 1982.

20. Rivera, G., Dahl, G.V., Bowman, W.P., Avery, T.L., Wood, A., Aur, R.J.: VM-26 and Cytosine Arabinoside Combination Chemotherapy for Initial Induction Failures in Childhood Lymphocytic Leukemia. Cancer 46: 1727, 1980.

21. Bernasconi, C., Lazzarino, M., and Morra, E.: The Use of an Epipodophyllotoxin Derivative (VP-16-213) in the Treatment of Acute Monocytic and Myelomonocytic Leukemias. In: Stacher, A., Hocker, P. (Hrsg) Erkrankungen der Myelopoese-Leukemien, Myeloproliferatives Syndrom, Polyzythamie. Urban and Schwarzenerg, Muchen, Berlin, S 224.

22. Hayes, F.A., Green, A.A., Casper, J., Cornet, J., and Evans, W.E.: Clinical Evaluation of Sequentially Scheduled Cisplatin and VM-26 in Neuroblastoma: Response and Toxicity. Cancer 48: 1715-1718, 1981.

23. Spremulli, E., Schulz, J.J., Speckhart, V.J. and Wampler, G.L.: Phase II Study of VM-26 in Adult Malignancies. Cancer Treat. Rep. 64: 147, 1980.

24. Gerosa, M.S., DiStefano, E., and Olivi, A.: VM-26 Monochemotherapy Trial in the Treatment of Recurrent Supratentorial Gliomas: Preliminary Report. Surg. Neurol. 15: 128, 1981.

25. Sweet, D.L., Hendler, F.J., Hanlon, K., Hekmatpanah, J., Griem,M.L., Duda, E.E., Mulligan, B., and Wollman, R.L.: Treatment of Grade III and IV Astrocytomas with BCNU Alone and in Combination with VM-26 Following Surgery and Radiation Therapy. Cancer Treat. Rep. 63: 1707-1711, 1979.

26. Schell, F.C., Yap, H.Y., Hortobagyi, G.N., Issell, B., and Esparza, L.: Phase II Study of VP-16-213 (Etoposide) in Refractory Metastatic Breast Carcinoma. Cancer Chemother. Pharmacol. 7: 223-225, 1982.

27. Vaughn, C.B., Greb, E.M., Lockhard, C., Groshko, G., Enochs, K., Duffin, H., and Demitrish, M.: VP-16 and Adriamycin in Patients with Advanced Breast Cancer. Am. J. Clin. Oncol. (CCT) 5: 505-507, 1982.

28. Konits, P.H., VanEcho, D.A., Aisner, J., Morris, D., and Wiernik, P.H.: Doxorubicin Plus VP-16-213 for the Treatment of Refractory Breast Carcinoma. Am. J. Clin. Oncol. (CCT) 5: 515-519, 1982.

29. Laubenstein, L.J., Krigel, R.L., Hymes, K.B., and Muggia, F.M.: Treatment of Epidemic Kaposi's Sarcoma with VP-16-213 (Etoposide) and a Combination of Doxorubicin, Bleomycin, and Vinblastine (ABV). Proc. ASCO 2: 228, 1983.

30. Commers, J.R., Foley, J.F.: Pulmonary Hyaline Membrane Disease Occurring in the Course of VM-26 Therapy. Cancer Treat. Rep. 63: 1093, 1979.

PHARMACOLOGY OF NITROSOUREA ANTICANCER AGENTS

ANN L. WANG AND PHILIP S. SCHEIN.

In 1959, 1-methyl-1-nitroso-3-nitroguanidine (MNNG) was reported to have a measurable and reproducible antitumor activity against the murine ascitic leukemia, L1210 (1). This observation resulted in extensive study of the N-nitroso compounds of antitumor activity. It was demonstrated that the nitroso group was required for activity and that substitution of a chloroethyl on the terminal methyl group enhanced antitumor activity. This led to the development of 1-(2-chloroethyl)-nitrosourea (2).

Concurrently, the group at the Southern Research Institute began studying compounds with a structural similarity to MNNG which could release diazomethane. 1-Methyl-1-nitrosourea (MNU) was the first nitrosourea studied from this series. MNU showed an increased activity towards i.p. implanted L1210 as compared to MNNG and had activity towards intracranially implanted L1210 due to its lipid solubility (3). This work led to the synthesis of over 200 congeners of MNU and subsequently the development and clinical use of the chloroethyl nitrosourea derivatives, which included 1,3-bis(2-chloroethyl)-1-nitrosourea (BCNU) (4), 1-(2-chloroethyl)-3-cyclohexyl-1-nitrosourea (CCNU), and methyl-CCNU. These chloroethyl derivatives are recognized as an important class of chemotherapeutic agents with established clinical antitumor activity for a broad range of human malignancies including, acute lymphocytic leukemia, lymphomas, myeloma, melanoma, gliomas and gastrointestinal neoplasms (5). However, these same agents produce a delayed and cumulative bone marrow toxicity which limits their clinical application. Attachment of a sugar carrier to a methyl- or chloroethylnitrosourea cytotoxic group, as with streptozotocin (6) and chlorozotocin, resulted in a marked reduction in bone marrow toxicity.

Nitrosoureas spontaneously decompose under physiological conditions (8,9) with chemical half lives ranging from 5 min for CNU to 2 hrs for CCNU (10). Following decomposition, two electrophilic species are formed, both of which are capable of alkylation; these are diazohydroxide and a carbonium ion (11).

71

The other major product of decomposition is an organic isocyanate (11), the structure of which is determined by the N-3 substituent of the parent nitrosourea. These isocyanates undergo carbamoylation reactions with intra-cellular nucleophiles, primarily amino acids (12).

Alkylation has been widely accepted as the principal mechanism of anti-tumor activity, but studies have failed, with a wide range of nitrosoureas, to show a linear relationship between in vitro alkylating activity and the chloroethyl antitumor activity for the murine L1210 leukemia (13,14). Studies with water-soluble analogues have suggested a parabolic relationship with an optimal relative alkylating activity of 60% that of chlorozotocin (13,14).

Kohn has proposed that the single alkylation function of the chloroethyl nitrosoureas can cross-link DNA as determined by inhibition of alkali-induced strand separation (15). This cross-linking is the result of a chloroethylation of a nucleophilic site on the first strand, followed by a displacement of Cl^- by a nucleophilic site either on the same or on an opposing DNA strand, forming an ethyl bridge. There also can be linkage between DNA and nuclear proteins, as demonstrated by binding to specific proteins. This process of DNA-DNA and DNA-protein cross-linking may contribute to the overall mechanism of toxicity, along with a combination of macromolecular alkylation and carbamoylation.

It remains to be determined whether both alkylation and carbamoylation are required for antitumor activity. Many biological consequences of nitrosourea carbamoylation have been documented. These include: (1) prolong-ation of the S phase synthesis of L1210 cells (16); (2) inhibition of repair of X-irradiated DNA by 2-chloroethyl isocyanate (17); (3) inhibition of DNA polymerase II (18) and glutathione reductase (19) by the isocyanates produced by BCNU and CCNU has been demonstrated; (4) binding of the cyclohexylisocyanate generated by CCNU with the histone fractions of HeLa cells (20); (5) inhibition of processing of nucleolar and nucleoplasmic RNA (21). In clinical studies it has been shown that patients undergo a marked loss of erythrocyte glutathione reductase after BCNU therapy (22). Glutathione reductase inactivation has been shown to be the result of 2-chloroethyl-isocyanate which is released by BCNU decomposition (19). Recent studies with Walker 256 rat mammary carcinoma cells, which are resistant to alkylating agents but not cross resistant to nitrosoureas (23), indicate that there is a specific effect on the glutathione reductase (24). This gives further credence to the idea that the contribution of carbamoylation to cytotoxicity is not negligible.

It has been possible to identify qualitative regions of nitrosourea binding within the chromatin substructure. Chromatin is composed of nucleosomes, which are double tetrameric cores of histones H2a, H2b, H3 and H4 (25) in association with $\sim$140 base pairs of DNA. The nucleosomes are separated by linker regions consisting of up to 60 base pairs of DNA with histone H1.

Limit digests of specific regions of chromatin by micrococcal nuclease and DNase I have provided further data on the relative accessibility of chromatin substructures for alkylation: micrococcal nuclease results in preferential digestion of internucleosomal DNA with the production of nucleosomal subunits; in contrast, treatment of chromatin with DNase I produces a somewhat random digestion of nucleosomal core DNA and concomitantly in a preferential cleavage of transcriptional regions of chromatin (26).

Studies with ^{14}C-chloroethyl chlorozotocin and ^{14}C-chloroethyl-CCNU (20) have shown that the alkylation appears to take place on DNA associated with the nucleosomal core particles. Methyl-^{14}C-MNU, in contrast to the chloroethyl nitrosoureas, reacts with the linker regions of DNA between the nucleosomes. It is possible that the dissimilar chromatin binding regions of the methyl and chloroethyl nitrosoureas contribute to the differing cytotoxicity and carcinogenic potentials of these two classes of nitrosoureas.

It has been demonstrated that there is a preferential alkylation of extended (probably transcriptional) chromatin subfractions in HeLa cells by chloroethyl nitrosoureas (27). The quantitative alkylation of functional chromatin regions may prove important to the cytotoxic properties of these drugs, although there is need for convincing evidence that differences between tissues such as tumor cells and bone marrow exist. Indications from human bone marrow studies (28) provide preliminary information that transcriptional chromatin does indeed provide a primary target for nitrosourea alkylation.

The employment of traditional biochemical and pharmacological concepts, together with the development of original molecular approaches, has created a more comprehensive understanding of the mechanism of action of nitrosoureas. For example, it is clear that all nuclear macromolecules are susceptible to alkylation and/or carbamoylation by nitrosoureas. The relative importance of these respective processes is equivocal. The structural organization of nuclear chromatin, either at the nucleosomal or functional level, is a critical determinant when considering specific macromolecules as potential targets for nitrosourea interaction. Perhaps a more complete understanding of the nuclear architecture of specific cell types will lead to a more precise understanding of nitrosourea selectivity, especially with respect to the nonmyelotoxic properties of chlorozotocin. Such knowledge could also assist in the rational development of novel nitrosourea analogues.

REFERENCES

1. Greene MO and Greenberg J: The activity of nitrosoguanidines against ascites tumors in mice. Cancer Res (20):1166-1173, 1960.
2. Hyde KA, Acton E, Skinner WA, Goodman L, Greenberg J, Baker BR: Potential anticancer agents. LXII. The relationship of chemical structure to antileukemic adults with analogs of 1-methyl-3-nitroguanidine (NSC-9369). J Med Pharm Chem (5):1-14, 1962.
3. Skipper HE, Schabel FM, Trader MW, Thomson JR: Experimental evaluation of potential anticancer agents. VI. Anatomical distribution of leukemic cells and failure of chemotherapy. Cancer Res (21):1154-1164, 1961.
4. Johnston TP, McCaleb GS, Montgomery JA: The synthesis of antineoplastic agents, XXXII. N-nitrosoureas. Int J Med Chem 6:669-681, 1963.
5. Wasserman TH, Slavic M, Carter SK: Clinical comparison of the nitrosoureas. Cancer (36): 1258-1268,1975.
6. Rakieten N, Rakieten M, Nadkarni M: Studies on the diabetogenic action of streptozotocin (NSC-37917). Cancer Chemother Rep (29):91-98, 1963.
7. Johnston TP, McCaleb GG, Montgomery JA: The synthesis of chlorozotocin, the 2-chloroethyl analogue of the anticancer antibiotic streptozotocin. J Med Chem (18): 104-106, 1975.
8. Colvin M, Brundhett RB, Cowens W, Jardin I, Ludlum D: A chemical basis for the antitumor activity of chloroethylnitrosoureas. Biochem Pharmacol (25): 695-699, 1976.
9. Montgomery JA, James R, McCaleb GS, Kirk MC, Johnston TP: Decomposition of N-(2-chloroethyl)-N-nitrosourea in aqueous media. J Med Chem (18):568-571, 1975.
10. Schein PS: Nitrosourea antitumor agents. In: Advances in Cancer Chemotherapy (Umezawa H, ed) Baltimore, University Park Press, 1978 pp 95-106.
11. Montgomery JA, James R, McCaleb GS, Johnston TP: The modes of decomposition of 1,3-bis(2-chloroethyl)-1-nitrosourea and related compounds. J Med Chem (10):668-674, 1967.
12. Wheeler GP, Bowdon BJ, Struck RT: Carbamoylation of amino acids, peptides and proteins by nitrosoureas. Cancer Res (35):2974-2994, 1975.
13. Panasci LC, Green D, Nagourney R, Fox P, Schein PS: A structure-activity analysis of chemical and biological parameters of chlorethylnitrosoureas in mice. Cancer Res (37):2615-2618, 1977.
14. Heal JM, Fox P, Schein PS: A structure-activity study of seven new water soluble nitrosoureas. Biochem Pharmacol (28):1301-1306, 1979.
15. Kohn KW: Interstrand cross-linking of DNA by 1,3-bis(2-chloroethyl)-1-nitrosourea and other 1-(2-haloethyl)-1-nitrosourea. Cancer Res 37:1450-1454 1977.
16. Bray DA, DeVita VT, Adamson RH, Oliverio VT: Effects of 1-(2-chloroethyl)-3 cyclohexyl-1-nitrosourea (CCNU NSC-79037) and its degradation products on progression of L1210 cells through the cell cycle. Cancer Chemother Rep (55):215-220, 1971.
17. Kann HE, Kohn KW, Lyles JM: Inhibition of DNA repair by the 1,3-bis(2-chloroethyl)-1-nitrosourea breakdown product, 2-chloroethylisocyanate. Cancer Res (34):398-402, 1974.

18. Baril BE, Baril EF, Laszlo J, Wheeler GP: Inhibition of rat liver DNA polymerase by nitrosoureas and isocyanates. Cancer Res (35):1-5, 1975.
19. Babson JR and Reed DJ: Inactivation of glutathione reductase by 2-chloroethyl nitrosourea-derived isocyanates. Biochem Biophys Res comm (83):754-762, 1978.
20. Tew KD, Sudhakar S, Schein PS, Smulson ME: Binding of chlorozotocin and 1-(2-chloroethyl)-3-cyclohexyl-1-nitrosourea to chromatin and nucleosomal fractions of HeLa cells. Cancer Res (38):3371-3378, 1978.
21. Kann HE, Kohn KW, Widerlite L, Gullion A: Effects of 1,3-bis(2-chloroethyl) -1-nitrosourea and related compounds on nuclear RNA metabolism. Cancer Res (37):1450-1454, 1977.
22. Frischer H and Ahmad T: Severe generalized glutathione reductase deficiency after antitumor chemotherapy with BCNU (1,3-bis(chloroethyl)-1-nitrosourea).
23. Tew KD and Wang AL: Selective cytotoxicity of haloethylnitrosoureas in a carcinoma cell line resistant to bifunctional nitrogen mustards. Mol Pharm (21):729-738, 1982.
24. Wang AL and Tew KD: Carbamoylation of glutathione reductase as a toxic property of nitrosoureas in an alkylating agent resistant cell lines. Submitted.
25. Thomas JO and Kornberg RD: An octamer of histones in chromatin and free in solution. Proc Nat Acad Sci USA (72):2626-2630, 1975.
26. Garel A and Axel R: Selective digestion of transcriptionally active ovalbumin gene for oviduct nuclei. Proc Nat Acad Sci USA 73:3966-3970, 1976.
27. Tew KD, Schein PS, Lindner DJ, Wang AL, Smulson ME: Hydrocortisone modification of chromatin structure alters nitrosourea binding within the nucleus. Cancer Res (40):3697-3703, 1980.
28. Byrne P, Tew K, Jemionek J, MacVittie T, Erickson L, Schein, PS: Cellular and molecular mechanisms of bone marrow sparing effects of the glucose chloroethylnitrosourea chlorozotocin. Blood: In press.

CURRENT CLINICAL PROGRESS WITH NEW AGENTS: ALKYLATING AGENTS

S.ECKHARDT

INTRODUCTION

The first report on the biological effect of alkylating
agents was published as early as in 1887 /1/. Almost fifty
years elapsed until it became known that sulphur mustard had
antitumor effect against experimental solid tumors /2/, and
the first clinical observations on the potential usefulness
of alkylating agents were recorded in 1946 /3/. Since the
first successful application of nitrogen mustard in haemopoietic malignancies thousands of molecules with alkylating
capacity were synthetized and most of them have shown remarkable antitumour properties. Nevertheless, it became very
soon obvious that their selectivity is poor and their therapeutic activity, therefore, was limited. Consequently the
view is now being expressed that the future progress would
seem to lie in the discovery of compounds that are toxic
towards a limited range of neoplasms /4/. Such substances do
exist among the methanesulfonates /busulphan/, hexitol derivatives /dibromomannitol/ or nitrosoureas /streptozotocin/
and were recently synthetized in other classes of alkylating
agents as well /quinones, acridines/. This review deals with
those alkylating agents which are currently undergoing clinical
trials. From the survey nitrosoureas are omitted being
previously discussed.   However, some of the recently
produced compounds with unidentified mechanism of action
are incorporated into the review.

Cyclophosphamide analogues

Cyclophosphamide /CPM/, one of the most well tolerated
cytostatic agents acted as parent compound for the synthesis

77

of further analogues such as ifosfamide, trofosfamide,
sulfosfamide, ASTA B 516 and ASTA B 707. Among them only
ifosfamide /Holoxan/ deserved special attention. This drug
[/3-/2-chloroethyl/2-/2-chloroethylamino/-tetrahydro-H-
-1,2,3-oxaphosphorine-2 oxide/] was found to be inactive
in vitro and for antitumour activity requires metabolism by
liver microsomal enzymes. The metabolic procedure is, however, prolonged and so is its action in comparison to CPM.
Animal data showed favourable antitumour properties identical
to that of the parent compound. The uroepithelial toxicity of
ifosfamide could be dramatically reduced by sodium-2-mercap-
toethanesulphate /MESNA/ /5/. Thus, its clinical use was
promising. According to broad phase II studies it is active
in breast, ovarian and small cell lung cancer. Recent phase
III studies demonstrated its effectiveness in combination
with VP-16213 in therapy resistant lung, ovarian and testicular cancer as well /6/.

Nitrogen mustard analogues

Among these analogues steroid-N-nitroso-omega-haloalkyl-
-carbamates have to be discussed due to their clinical significance. In a series of chemicals containing a glucocorticoid
esterified with nitrogen mustards prednimustine became of
wide clinical interest. The rationale in designing this
compound was to combine two individually active antitumour
agents, in this case prednisone and chlorambucil /7/. A broad
phase II trial organized by the EORTC revealed antitumour activity in malignant lymphomas, and marginal tumor responses
were also seen in melanoma and bronchial cancer. In another
trial 35 % response rate was observed in hormone resistant
advanced prostatic cancer /8/.

Dialkyltriazenes

Among dialkyltriazenes DTIC /5-/3,3-dimethyl-triazino/-
-imidazol-4-carboxamide is still the only widely used antitumour agent. Its di-2-chloroethyl analogue: BTIC has been
subjected to phase I trials without convincing results. The
clinical application of dialkyltriazenes seems to be

justified only in melanoma, soft tissue sarcoma and neuroblastoma. In Hodgkin's disease DTIC might be used as a component of several second choice regimens /9/. Pyrazolo-
imidazole /IMPY/ is not yet classified as an alkylating
agent. It probably inhibits ribonucleotide reductase. In
animal experiments there is no cross resistance between DTIC
and IMPY. The drug penetrates into the glioblastoma tissue.
Phase I trials are in progress /10/.

Halogenated hexitols

As early as in 1961 Hungarian authors were able to demonstrate the antitumour activity of halogenated hexitols
/11/. In a series of compounds 1,6-dibromo-1,6-dideoxy-D-
-mannitol /DBM/ was the first clinically applied, This drug
exhibited a highly selective antitumour effect in myeloproli-
ferative disorders and became a standard second choice drug
for the therapy of CML in many countries /12, 13/. Dibromodulcitol /DBD, Mitolactol, Elobromol/ the stereoisomeric
analogue of DBM inhibited the growth of numerous ascitic and
solid tumours /14/. Based on these findings a broad phase II
study was performed in Hungary and in the USA. Among 1414
patients CR+PR were observed in head and neck /33.05 %/,
breast /28.05 %/, bladder /23.7 %/, melanoma /23.2 %/ and
lung cancer /20.08 %/ /15/. Similar results were compiled by
US authors in 1981 /16/. Since the drug exerted antitumour
effect by oral route and its toxicity was well tolerated, it
became presently a target of various polychemotherapy
studies. So far, its beneficial effect in combination with
Adriamycin seems to be proven in advanced breast cancer /17/.
Among the analogues of dibromodulcitol the dianhydro-deriva-
tive has undergone phase I-II investigations. This compound,
dianhydrogalactitol /DAG/ is one of the metabolites of the
parent compound possessing two epoxy groups with alkylating
capacity. According to various authors the anhydride formation might be one explanation for the cytostatic effect of
halogenated hexitols /18/. DAG, however, did not possess
higher antitumour activity than that of DBM. In a broad

phase II investigation on 933 patients suffering from various malignancies only 6 % response rate /CR+PR/ could be observed. Nevertheless, the capacity of DAG to penetrate through the blood/brain barrier has been repeatedly confirmed and therefore the drug is currently a target for study in relapsing brain malignancies /15, 16/. More recently some new halogenated hexitol analogues have been synthetized in Hungary. Among them 1,2,5,6-dianhydro,3,4-di-O-acetylgalactitol /DADAG/ was the first candidate for clinical trial showing striking antitumour properties against a series of experimental melanomas and possessing a well tolerated toxicity. In phase I and early phase II studies activity was found in patients with melanoma and brain tumours. 1,2,5,6-dianhydro-3,4 di-O-succinylgalactitol /DisuDAG/ an even more active compound in experimental solid tumour models awaits clinical study /15/.

Miscellaneous compounds

Although triethyleneiminoquinones were synthetized in the early sixties and found to be alkylating DNA of tumour cells. Their toxicity was so high that they never reached broad clinical trials. More recently anthraquinones with antitumour activity were developed which, however, cannot be classified as alkylating agents due to their similarity in action to adriamycin. Nevertheless Dihydroxyanthracendione /DHAD/ and Ametantrone /1,4-bis 2/2 hydroxyethylamino/-ethyl/amino 9,10 anthracendione diacetate have to be mentioned here. While the former proved to be effective in phase I-II studies against leukemias and lymphomas, the latter was active against experimental colon cancer. So far no evidence of such activity exists in human GI tract malignancies /19/. Among aziridinylbenzoquinones the 1,4 cyclohexadiene-1,4 dicarbamic acid 2,5-bis-1-azaridinyl/-3,6-dioxodiethylester /AZQ/ underwent phase I study and produced some PR-s in relapsing gliomas /20/. A derivative of TEM /triethylenmelamine/ the pentamethylmelamine /PMM/ was also subjected to phase I studies. The most likely area for clinical investigation is ovarian cancer. Nevertheless, the compounds has considerable GI and CNS toxicity /21/.

CONCLUSIONS

After the great explosion in the research of alkylating agents in the fifties and sixties only few useful new compounds with alkylating capacity were developed. Most of them are analogues with modified activity or reduced toxicity. In this respect we might cite the great scientist Kretschmer: "Science is a question of character, strict discipline and renunciation, a question of honesty, unflagging persistance integrity and an unquenchable ambition to succeed." This statement is particularly valid for cancer chemotherapy.

REFERENCES

1. Meyer V: Medizinisch-chemische Notizen. II. Physiologische Wirkung der gechlorten Schwefelaethyle. Brichte der Deutsch. Chem. Ges. /20/: 1729-1731, 1887.
2. Adair F.E., Bagg H.J.: Experimental and clinical studies on the treatment of cancer by dichloroethylsulfide. Ann. Surg. /93/: 190-199, 1931.
3. Gilman A., Philips F.S.: The biological actions and therapeutic applications of the β-chloroethylamines and sulfides. Science /103/: 409-415, 1946.
4. Ross W.C.J.: Rational design of alkylating agents. In: Sartorelli A.L., Johns D.G. /ed/ Antineoplastic and Immunosuppressive Agents I. Springer Verlag, Berlin, Heidelberg, New York. 1975, pp. 33-51.
5. Brock N.: Konzeption und Wirkungsmechanismus von Uromitexan /Mesna/. In: Burkert H., Nagel G.A.: Neue Erfahrungen mit Oxazaphosphorinen unter besonderer Berücksichtigung des Uroprotektors Uromitexan. Karger Verlag. Basel, München, Paris, London, New York, Sidney. 1980. pp. 1-11.
6. Welleus W., Mussgung G., Habets L., Schäfer E., Westerhausen M.: Die Kombination Ifosfamid/VP-16213 bei der Therapie des kleinzelligen Bronchialkarzinoms und anderer Malignome. In: Burkert H., Nagel G.A.: Neue Erfahrungen mit Oxazaphosphorinen unter besonderer Berücksichtigung des Uroprotektors Uromitexan. Karger Verlag. Basel, München, Paris, London, New York, Sidney. 1980. pp. 84-90.
7. Könyves I., Fex H., Högberg B., Jensen C., Stamwik A.: Steroid-N-nitroso-omega-haloalkyl carbamates. In: Davis W., Harrap K.R.: Characterization and Treatment of Human Tumours. Proc. VII.Internat.Symp. on the Biological Characterization of Human Tumors, Budapest. Excerpta Med. Amsterdam 1977. pp. 303-307.
8. Könyves I., Wåhlby S.: Review on clinical experiences

with prednimustine. In: Davis W., Harrap K.R.: Characterization and Treatment of human tumours. Proc. VII. Internat.Symp. on the Biological Characterization of Human Tumours, Budapest. Excerpta Med. Amsterdam 1977. pp. 303--307.

9. Hickman J.A.: Investigation of the mechanism of action of antitumor dimethyltriazenes. Biochimie /60/: 997-1006, 1978.

10. Stanbus A.E., Ken T.A., Balcerzak S.P., Randall G., Neidhart J.A.: Pharmacokinetics of pyrazolo-imidazole /IMPY/ in humans. Proc.Amer.Ass.Cancer Res. /20/: 204, 1979.

11. Institóris L., Horváth I.P., Csányi E.: Activité cytostatique de certains dérivés halogénés de polyalcools. In: Proc. of the II. Symp. Internat. Chimiotherapy, Naples 1961. Karger, New York 1963. pp. 250-253.

12. Eckhardt S., Sellei C., Horváth I.P., Institóris L.: Effect of 1,6-dibromo-1,6-dideoxy-D-mannitol on chronic granulocytic leukemia. Cancer Chemother. Rep. /33/: 57-61, 1973.

13. Dibromomannitol Cooperative Study Group Report. Survival of CML patients treated by Dibromomannitol. Europ. J. Cancer /9/: 583-589, 1973.

14. Kellner B., Németh L., Horváth I.P., Institóris L.: 1,6--dibromo-1,6-dideoxydulcitol: A new antitumoural agent. Nature /213/: 402-406, 1967.

15. Eckhardt S.: Current status of anticancer drug development in the CMEA countries. In: Hilgard P., Hellmann K.: Anticancer Drug Development. Prous J.R. publishers, Barcelona, 1983. pp. 181-194.

16. Chiuten D.F., Rozencweig M., von Hoff D.D., Muggia F.M.: Clinical trials with the hexitol derivatives in the US. Cancer /47/: 442-451, 1981.

17. Eckhardt S.: Dibromodulcitol. Medicina Publisher, Budapest 1982.

18. Elson L.A., Jarman M., Ross W.C.J.: Toxicity, haematological effects and antitumour activity of epoxides derived from disubstituted hexitols. Mode of action of mannitol myleran and dibromomannitol. Europ. J. Canc. /4/: 167-171, 1968.

19. Kuhn J.G., von Hoff D.D., Myers J.W.: New anticancer drugs. In: Pinedo H.M.: Cancer Chemotherapy 1981. Excerpta Medica, Amsterdam-Oxford. 1981. pp. 131-165.

20. Kahn A.H., Driscoll J.S.: Potential CNS antitumour agents. VI. Aziridinylbenzoquinones. J.med.Chem. /19/: 313-319, 1976.

21. von Hoff D.D., Kuhn J., Harris G.J.: New anticancer drugs. In: Pinedo H.M.: Cancer Chemotherapy 1980. Excerpta Medica, Amsterdam-Oxford. 1980. pp. 126-127.

INTERFERON

J L TOY

Although there is a large body of information concerning the biological behaviour of the interferons, the transposition of that knowledge into the clinical trials arena is not a simple affair. The kernel of the problem for the physician wishing to design the most rational clinical study is that the fundamental mechanism of anticancer action of the interferons is not known, and so obviously it becomes the case that choosing a strategy with a high degree of probability of success is very difficult. The constrained consequently have chosen to tread the empirical road. The majority of early Phase I studies were designed to determine maximum tolerated doses (MTD) of interferons when given in various schedules and routes. Perhaps two philosophies underpinned such a strategy, one being that it is important to know as much as is possible about basic pharmacological properties of a drug, and another being the implied suggestion that there exists a dose cytotoxic response relationship with the biological modifier as with the common cancer chemotherapeutic drugs. An early study which explored the latter concept was one based upon the experimental evidence that concentrations of interferon greater than 10^3 units per ml inhibit greater than 50% of cultured myeloblasts and that such concentrations of interferon could be achieved in blood by administering 50×10^6 units $/m^2$ over 24 hours by continuous IV infusion [1]. It proved to be however that no significant therapeutic benefit was observed in the subsequent Phase II study in AML [2].

The assignment of the MTD of interferon has been made by investigators after having considered toxicities both of an objective and subjective nature; the latter often being patient-determined. One study [3] suggested $2.5-5.0 \times 10^6$ units $/m^2$ IM daily was acceptable whilst another [1] using the same interferon suggested 100×10^6 units $/m^2$ by continuous IV infusion for 7 days to be the MTD. However, by and large, different authors are making similar conclusions about schedule-dependent doses of different interferons they consider to be acceptable; as might be expected short pulses of treatment allow for higher doses, circa 30×10^6 units/m^2 daily, than do daily prolonged treatments when only approximately 5×10^6 units/m^2 are tolerated.

The Phase II interferon cancer studies have been extensive and wide-ranging in their designs and tumour selections although not exhaustive simply because of the very large number of alternatives that are possible when embarking from an uncertain stance. A large number of tumour types have seemingly shown an objective response to various interferons. Yet it is not possible, I feel, to have an absolute confidence in these data partly because of the inherent variability that will naturally accrue in a large series of studies with different protocol designs and also because of variable investigators' interpretations of results obtained and their placing of the responses on the map of meaningful clinical benefit. It is better, I believe, to consider a list of tumours reported to have shown a complete response to interferon treatment (Table 1). Although even here I should not wish to imply there to be a definite absence of possible caveats, I would proffer this list is still a rather impressive one.

TABLE 1

DISEASES IN WHICH CRS HAVE BEEN OBTAINED WITH INTERFERONS

Metastatic renal carcinoma	HLBI, Gamma:	USA, Japan
Nasopharyngeal carcinoma	Fibro:	Germany
Head and Neck carcinoma	Leucocyte:	Yugoslavia
Bladder, transitional cell	Leucocyte:	USA
Pleural mesothelioma	Leucocyte:	Germany
Malignant melanoma	Rec α:	USA
Multiple myeloma	Rec α, HLBI:	USA, Japan
Non-Hodgkin's lymphoma	Leucocyte, Fibro, HLBI:	USA, Germany, Japan
ALL	Leucocyte:	France
Kaposi's sarcoma	Rec α, HLBI:	USA

Pundits of interferon clinical research have suggested that the most responsive tumour types to this class of biological modifiers are renal cancer, NHL, myeloma and Kaposi's sarcoma. More recently one drug company has proclaimed that it hopes to be able to register an IFN-alpha clone for use in the treatment of malignant melanoma.

Metastatic renal cell carcinoma has been studied at several centres and the published studies are shown in Table 2. Much interest has been aroused by the responses obtained in this disease because of its lack of an identified successful treatment regime. The cumulative response rates to interferons are a CR of 2.3% and a PR of 12.5%. Additionally, it is possible that there may be a dose-response relationship identified by certain of the studies and if one should choose to consider only those studies which obtained responses then an overall response rate of 16.7% is calculated. It is of note that responses would seem to occur in only soft tissues such as lung. Trials in this disease are continuing with combination treatment modalities being presently investigated with optimism.

TABLE 2

STUDIES OF INTERFERON IN RENAL CANCER

CENTRE	TYPE	DOSE (IM unless stated otherwise)	EVALUABLE	CR	PR
MD Anderson	Leuc	3Mu daily	38	2	10
Illinois	Leuc	1Mu tiw	15	0	0
		10Mu tiw	15	1	1
UCLA	Leuc	2Mu 5d/week	43	1	6
Scandinavia	Leuc	20Mu intralesional	2	0	0
		4-16Mu daily	5	0	0
MSKCC	Rec A	50Mu/m^2 tiw	33	0	5
MD Anderson	Rec A	2Mu/m^2 daily	15	0	0
		20Mu/m^2 daily	15	0	4
Westminster	HLBI	2.5Mu/m^2 daily	21	0	1
ECOG	HLBI	3-20Mu/m^2 dx10 21d cycles	33	1	6
Ohio	HBLI	5Mu/m^2 tiw	33	0	5
Duke-BRMP	HLBI	3Mu tiw	20	0	1
Japan NCI	HLBI	3Mu daily	54	3	4

Non-Hodgkin's lymphoma was one of the first malignancies to show response to interferon. Nodular or favourable histology lymphomas are most responsive (Table 3). The objective response rate for these histologies is an impressive 43.9% whilst for DHL and unfavourable histologies it is only 8.7%. There is one follow-up report on which an assessment of the durability of the remissions can be made. The Stanford Group [4] reported unmaintained remissions of between 6 and 12 months, and also described two patients in whom a second response was obtained with interferon after relapse off treatment.

TABLE 3

STUDIES OF INTERFERON IN NON-HODGKIN'S LYMPHOMA

CENTRE	TYPE	DOSE (IM unless stated otherwise)	EVALUABLE	CR	PR
Stanford	Leuc	5Mu bd daily	7 Nodular	1	2
			3 DHL	0	0
MD Anderson	Leuc	3Mu daily	6 Nodular	1	2
			1 DHL	0	0
USA multi	HLBI	5Mu/m^2 tiw	10 Nodular	0	2
			5 DHL	0	0
Japan NCI	HLBI	3Mu daily	15	1	2
USA multi	Rec α2	10-25Mu/m^2 tiw	7 favourable	0	2
USA multi	Rec α2	50Mu/m^2 IV daily x5 every 2-3/52	11 unfavourable	0	2
USA NCI	Rec A	50MU/m^2 tiw	11 favourable	0	8
			3 unfavourable	0	0

Multiple myeloma, like NHL a B cell neoplasm, is also an interferon-responsive tumour. As tabulated in Table 4 the objective response rate is not high but it should be noted that most of the patients in these studies will have received interferon when their disease was already resistant to available therapies and when, as occurs with this illness, their general health would have been exceedingly poor. There are data, however, which report previously untreated myeloma patients entered into a randomised trial designed to compare interferon with standard melphalan plus prednisone therapy. The trial was conducted by the Myeloma Group of Central Sweden [5], who have shown that while there is a statistically significant advantage conferred by conventional treatment over interferon (40% vs 12% response rate p<0.05), and markedly so for IgG class myeloma (48% vs 4% response rate p<0.001), that there is an appreciable response rate to interferon. IgA shows a 25% response rate and Bence-Jones a 21% response rate even when interferon is being used in a manner, unlikely by chance alone, to be optimal.

TABLE 4

STUDIES OF INTERFERON IN MULTIPLE MYELOMA

CENTRE	TYPE	DOSE (IM unless stated otherwise)	EVALUABLE	CR	PR
M D Anderson	Leuc	3-9Mu daily	10	0	3
Sweden	Leuc	3Mu daily	75	0	9
Villejuif	Fibro	6Mu IV weekly	16	0	0
Leuven	Fibro	30Mu weekly	3	0	0
Galveston	Rec A	$3 \rightarrow 100Mu/m^2$ IV daily x14. Then $10Mu/m^2$ SC tiw	21	1	4
London	HLBI	4Mu daily	20	0	0
Japan NCI	HLBI	3Mu daily	44	1	8

Kaposi's sarcoma, associated with AIDS, is a disease which is difficult to treat with conventional cytotoxic drugs because exacerbation of immunodeficiency results, with severe opportunistic infection as an almost invariable consequence. Interferon, appears not to precipitate major episodes of infection and is showing high promise of being helpful for this disease (Table 5). Here, as with renal carcinoma, a dose response relationship possibly exists. It should not go unnoticed that the treatment time to achieve complete response has been as long as 9 months. In most other Phase II studies interferon has been administered for a 28 day treatment period only at the time of response assessment, and it is conceivable that such a period is too short.

TABLE 5

STUDIES OF INTERFERON IN AIDS-ASSOCIATED KAPOSI'S SARCOMA

CENTRE	TYPE	DOSE (IM unless otherwise stated)	EVALUABLE	CR	PR
UCLA	Rec α2	$1Mu/m^2$ SCx5d alt weeks x4	9	0	1
		$50Mu/m^2$ IVx5d alt weeks x4	26	2	14
MSKCC	Rec A	36 or 54Mu daily	34	5	8
NIH	HLBI	$7.5Mu/m^2$ daily	7	0	2
MD Anderson	HLBI	$20Mu/m^2$ daily	9	1	2±5

Many interferon trials in various malignant diseases report minimal and stable disease responses and several experienced in the evaluation of cytotoxics suggest such reports represent special pleading. Maybe they are correct. However, it is not without the bounds of possibility that what is being reported is a reflection of real effects to a biological modifier, insufficient alone to cure a patient, but possibly sufficient to supplement present anticancer treatments. Interferon must and will continue to be evaluated as a potential addition to the anticancer therapies.

References

Periodicals

1. Rohatiner AZS, Balkwill FR, Griffin DB, Malpas JS, Lister TA: A Phase I study of human lymphoblastoid interferon administered by continuous intravenous infusion. Cancer Chemother Pharmacol (9): 97-102, 1982.
2. Rohatiner AZS, Balkwill FR, Malpas JS, Lister TA: Experience with human lymphoblastoid interferon in acute myelogenous leukaemia (AML). Cancer Chemother Pharmacol (11): 56-58, 1983.
3. Priestman T: Initial evaluation of human lymphablastoid interferon in patients with advanced malignant disease. Lancet (ii): 113-118, 1980.
4. Louie AC, Gallagher JG, Sikora K, Levy R, Rosenberg SA, Merigan TC: Follow-up observations on the effect of human leucocyte interferon in non-Hodgkin's lymphomas. Blood (8): 712-718, 1981.

Books (edited by other than author of article)
5. Mellstedt H, et al, The Myeloma Group of Central Sweden, MGCS: Human leucocyte interferon (IFN-α) in the treatment of multiple myeloma (MM). In: De Maeyer E and Schellekens H (ed) Biology of the interferon system 1983. Elsevier Science Publishers B V, pp 519-525.

3. DRUG TREATMENT OF SPECIFIC CANCERS

CHEMOTHERAPY OF LUNG CANCER

H. H. HANSEN

Treatment of lung cancer continues to be one of the biggest challenges in oncology today - not only because the therapeutic advances remain modest but also because the incidence of lung cancer continues to rise rapidly. The increase is particularly observed among females, and it is expected that as many females will die from lung cancer as from breast cancer in the U.S. by the middle of 1980's (1).

Lung cancer can be separated into the four following major histologic types: epidermoid carcinoma, large cell anaplastic carcinoma, adenocarcinoma and small cell carcinoma. The percentage distribution among the various types is estimated to be 45, 15, 25 and 25% respectively.

Among these types, small cell carcinoma has emerged as the types of lung cancer, in which the main mode of therapy is combination chemotherapy. For the other cell types, surgery still remains the most important curative treatment modality. The treatment results, however, are discouraging and essentially unchanged within the last decade with only 7-8% of all patients with non-small cell lung cancer alive and disease-free five years after diagnosis.

CHEMOTHERAPY OF SMALL CELL CARCINOMA

The most frequently used and most active combination chemotherapy regimes include drugs such as VP-16-213, Cyclophosphamide or other alkylating agents, Vincristine, Doxorubicin, CCNU and Methotrexate (2).

Among the newer agents both Vindesine and Cis-platinum have shown some activity, also in patients having received prior chemotherapy (2).

The results obtained with combination chemotherapy have essentially been unchanged during the last 3-5 years with a complete or partial response observed within 1-2 months after initiation of treatment in 80-90% of all patients. Usually, the responses last for a median of 9-10 months

91

resulting in a median survival in most studies of 13-16 months in patients
classified initially as having limited disease compared to 10-12 months
for patients classified as having extensive disease. At least 5-8% of all
patients will achieve prolonged disease-free survival possibly representing cures (3).

Elimination of resistant cell lines after the initial response remains
still the main obstacle for improving therapy. At present, the major
therapeutic challenges and questions include the following:

1) Identification of new agents, which are non-cross-resistant to
   existing agents.

2) Is non-cross-resistant cyclic combination chemotherapy superior
   to non-cyclic combination chemotherapy with the same agents?

3) Which degree of toxicity is needed in the induction phase in order
   to achieve the highest complete response and duration of remission.

4) Is there a role for autologous bone-marrow transplantation combined
   with high-dose combination chemotherapy?

5) Does maintenance chemotherapy play a role?

6) Is there a role for surgery when combined with chemotherapy, and
      so, when is the optimal timing for surgery?

7) Identification of the role of prophylactic CNS-irradiation and
   radiotherapy to the primary tumor.

8) The treatment of patients relapsing on initial combination chemotherapy.

NON-SMALL CELL LUNG CANCER

Inspired by the successful application of combination chemotherapy
in small cell carcinoma obtained in the 1970's, it was not surprising
that some of this enthusiasm was transferred to the other cell types of
lung cancer.

In recent years many combination chemotherapy regimes have been
studied including from 2 to 7 different cytostatic agents. The therapeutic results of these combinations have resulted in conflicting data from
various investigators or cooperative groups using the same combinations.
Initial results for some of these combinations have been highly encouraging
with partial response rates varying from 30 to more than 40%.
However, follow-up studies by other investigators testing these combinations against single agents in randomized trials have shown a much lesser

activity with lower response rate, usually being less than 10%. Furthermore, toxicity from these combinations was frequently found to be considerable or excessive in view of the minimal response. In addition, there
has been a certain lack of reproducibility of results for some of the
combinations even in within the same cooperative groups (4).

More recently it has been observed, that the use of Cis-platinum with
either Vindesine (5) or VP-16 (6) consistant   results in a response rate
of more than 40% in previously untreated patients with epidermoid carcinoma
or adenocarcinoma. Whether these results also will result in an improved
survival rate and/or improved quality of life as compared to other supportive treatment alone or treatment with single agent chemotherapy and/or
radiotherapy independant of a number of predictive prognostic factors
such as performance status, extense of disease, prior weight loss and
prior treatment remains to be seen.

Until such a beneficial effect of combination chemotherapy is demonstrated it appears to be particularly useful to test new antitumor
agents in new combinations with active agents in previously untreated non-
small cell lung cancer in order to get the best assessment of antitumor
activity for these new agents or combinations. Hopefully, one of the
current available combinations or possibly a new combination of new and
active single agents will be identified that will be useful in prolonging
both the quality and duration of survival. Such a combination would then
be particularly useful as an adjuvant to localized treatment for stage
I and II lung cancer. Until such a treatment can be identified, chemotherapy for non-small cell lung cancer should remain at an investigative
level.

References

1. Stolley PD: Lung cancer in women - five years later,
    N Engl J Med (309): 428-429, 1983.

2. Hansen HH: Management of small cell anaplastic carcinoma 1980 - 1982.
    In: Ishikawa Y, Hayata Y, Suemasu K (eds) Lung Cancer 1982. Excerpta
    Medica - 1982, Amsterdam - Oxford - Princeton. International Congress
    Series 569.

3. Aisner J, Alberto P, Bitran J, Comis R, Daniels J, Hansen HH,
    Ikegami H, Smyth J: Role of chemotherapy in small cell lung cancer:
    A consensus report of the International Association for the Study of

Lung Cancer Workshop. Cancer Treat Rep (67): 37-43, 1983.

4. Aisner J, Hansen HH: Commentary: Current status of chemotherapy for non-small cell lung cancer. Cancer Treat Rep (65): 979-986, 1981.

5. Gralla RJ, Casper ES, Kelsen DP, Braun DW, Dukeman ME, Martini N, Young CW, Golbey RB: Cisplatin and vindesine combination chemotherapy for advanced carcinoma of the lung: A randomized trial investigating two dosage schedules. Ann Int Med (95) 414-420, 1981.

6. Klastersky J, Longeval E, Nicaise E, Weerts D: Etoposide and cis-platinum in non-small-cell bronchogenic carcinoma. Cancer Treat Rev (9): 133-138, 1982.

HORMONE-CHEMOTHERAPY IN TREATMENT OF ADVANCED BREAST CANCER

F. CAVALLI, A. GOLDHIRSCH, R. JOSS, K.W. BRUNNER

This paper will briefly review the current situation in the treatment of advanced breast cancer. Historically hormonotherapy was the first modality, which was used in the therapy of this disease. In an unselected population the results of endocrine treatment have remained stable in the last three decades: about 30% of the patients will achieve a partial remission, which will last between 10-20 months. In the last 10 years combination chemotherapy became the most widely applied treatment modality for advanced breast cancer. However nowadays it has been realised, that combination chemotherapy can only be palliative, whereas a few years ago it was hoped that with this treament at least some patients could be cured. With an optimal combination chemotherapy 50-70% of the patients will achieve a partial remission, which generally last 10-15 months. Because it is at present widely felt, that combination chemotherapy has reached a plateau in its effectiveness and because of the discovery of hormone receptors, hormonotherapy is presently experiencing an unexpected revival.

1. CURRENT RESULTS OF CHEMOTHERAPY

Table 1 summarises the result of some of the trials, which were prompted by the report of Cooper, who in 1969 observed a remission rate of 90% in 60 patients treated with a 5-drug combination (CMFVP) (1). These data can be shortly summarised as follows: none of the different modifications of the original 5-drug combination proved to be significantly superior (2). CMF is globally as active as the 5-drug combination (3-6). However, the addition of Prednisone to CMF improves most probably the global results through avoidance of excessive dose reductions (4,7). CMFVP is probably more active if given continuously than when an intermittent schedule is used (8). However, long term analyses of studies comparing the concurrent administration to the sequential use of the 5 cytotoxic drugs failed to demonstrate a significant superiority of the concurrent approach (9).

95

Table 1.   Combinations of cyclophosphamide (C), methotrexate (M), 5-fluorouracil (F), vincristine (V) and prednisone (P).

Combination	No. of Studies or Institution	No. of Pts.	Remission Rate (%)
CMFVP	9 studies	503	51
CMFV	3 studies	118	53
CMFP	ECOG	88	59
CMF	3 studies	366	50
CFP	3 studies	113	39
FVP	CALGB	82	36
CFV	Michigan Univ.	46	43
CMV	SAKK	46	32
CMP	SAKK	67	44

The next step in the evolution of the chemotherapeutic management of advanced breast cancer was the comparison of CMF(VP) and various adriamycin-containing regimens. Table 2 summarises the most important comparative studies (10-14). As it can be seen, no significant advantage for an adriamycin-containing regimen over CMF(VP) could be globally demonstrated. We shall address this question later on.

Table 2. Comparisons of CMF(VP) and CAF(VP) in breast cancer.

Reference	Treatments	No. Pts.	Response CR+PR	CR	Time to P(MOS)	Resp. DUR	Median Survival
Bull 1978	CMF	40	62	8	6	8	17
	CAF	38	82	18	10	10	27
Muss 1978	CMFVP	72	57	11	–	14	20
	CAFVP	76	58	13	–	16	33
Smalley 1980	CMFVP	107	42	8	4.3	5.5	14.0 good
	CAF	106	60	19	8.0	8.0	16.7 risk
							11.0 good
							13.0 risk
Carmo-Pereira 1981	CMFP	26	65	19	–	12	22
	CAF	25	56	16	–	12	18
ECOG 1982	CMFP	76	53	5	5.7	6.3	15.8
	CAF	79	53	17	7.8	11.0	18.6

Historically the next step can be seen in the development of so-called "non-cross-resistant". Since CMF(P) and AV were felt to be not cross-resistant, their sequential use was evaluated in two studies (15-16). So far an advantage for the sequential use of two different non-cross-resistant regimens could not be demonstrated.

2. COMBINED HORMONO-CHEMOTHERAPY

Breast cancer tissue is thought to be composed of at least two different cellular types, one which is responsive to hormone treatment and one which is sensitive to cytotoxic drugs. A combination of both treatments should therefore improve the results of treatment of advanced breast cancer. The first trials evaluating the efficacy of a combined endocrine and cytotoxic treatment yielded conflicting results (17-19). Lately Cocconi et al (20), who compared CMF + Tamoxifen to CMF alone, demonstrated that the higher response rate for the combined approach does not translate into a prolonged survival, provided that endocrine treatment is given upon relapse to the patients treated primarily only CMF. If so, the sequential approach elicits even a somewhat longer survival as compared to CMF + Tamoxifen (p = 0.25). Nevertheless there is a widespread tendency to treat many patients with a combination of both treatments simultaneously. The Swiss Group for Clinical Cancer Research (SAKK) performed therefore a trial comparing the concurrent to the sequential use of cytotoxic chemotherapy and hormone treatment in the management of 464 patients with advanced breast cancer. In the treatment arm with the sequential use of both modalities, cytotoxic drugs were given only if the antitumour activity of the hormone treatment was inadequate. Hormone treatment consisted of oophorectomy for premenopausal and Tamoxifen administration for postmenopausal patients. The results of this trial have already been reported in detail (21-22). Length of survival was better, though not significantly, in premenopausal patients (p = 0.29) treated concurrently and in postmenopausal women (p = 0.17) treated sequentially. The difference in survival was, however, highly significant (p = 0.003) for postmenopausal women in the low-risk category (indolent disease), who received chemotherapy only after primary or secondary failure of the endocrine treatment. In all other subsets the differences in survival were statistically not significant between the two treatment strategies, even if generally there was a tendency for a longer survival in patients with a more aggressive disease when they were treated with a combined approach. On the contrary patients with a rather indolent disease seemed generally to profit from a treatment plan, encompassing hormonotherapy alone at first and the delayed use of chemotherapy (22). These findings suggest that postmenopausal women with metastatic breast cancer should probably be treated primarily by carefully monitored hormone treatment, while worst prognostic subsets among premenopausal women should probably receive a combined chemo-hormonotherapy. In this trial we were also able to confirm among the patients receiving a delayed chemotherapy, that endocrine treatment is able to influence the response rate and the duration of remission of the following chemotherapy. Patients responding to hormonotherapy showed also a statistically longer survival as compared to patients showing only a no change or a progressive disease with the endocrine treatment ($p < 0.05$).

3. A RANDOMIZED TRIAL OF 3 DIFFERENT REGIMENS OF COMBINATION CHEMOTHERAPY

In the SAKK trial which we have just presented above (concurrent versus sequential chemo-hormonotherapy), at the time of the randomization, the patients were also randomly allocated to three different chemotherapy regimens, representing a low-dose (1mfp = I), a more conventional (LMP/FVP = II) and a somewhat intensive cytotoxic treatment (LMFP/ADM = III). The drug programs are illustrated in Table 3. Considering all 397 patients who

Table 3. Regimens of combination chemotherapy.

I "MINIMAL" (1mpf)	CLB	$5mg/m^2/d$	d 1-14	p.o.		q 4 wks
	MTX	$10mg/m^2/w$	d 1+8	p.o. (1 dose!)		= INTERMITTENT
	5-FU	$500mg/m^2/w$	d 1+8	p.o.		
	PDN	$30mg/m^2/d$	d 1-14	then		
II "MEDIUM" (LMP/FVP)	CLB	as in I				
	MTX	$15mg/m^2/w$	subdivided in 3 daily doses			q 4 wks
			d 1-3, d 8-10 p.o.			= CONTINUOUS
	PDN	$30mg/m^2/d$	d 1-14			
	5-FU	$500mg/m^2/w$	d 15+22	i.v.		
	VCR	$1,2mg/m^2/w$	d 15+22	i.v.		
	PDN	$30mg/m^2/d$	d 5-28	then		
III "MAXIMAL" (LMFP/ADM)	CLB	as in I				
	MTX	$40mg/m^2/w$	d 1+8	i.v.		q 8 wks
	5-FU	$600mg/m^2/w$	d 1+8	i.v.		= INTERMITTENT
	PDN	$30mg/m^2/d$	d 1-14	then		
	ADM	$60mg/m^2$	d 28			

received chemotherapy either concurrently with or sequentially to the endocrine treatment, we observed that statistically significant differences in the response rate elicited by the three chemotherapeutic regimens were only marginally translated into different survival curves (21). We decided therefore in a subsequent analysis of this study to limit our evaluation to the patients, who received chemotherapy concurrently with an endocrine treatment. This restriction permits to analyse a more homogenously treated patient population and also eliminates the influence of a possible hormone-induced remission upon the therapeutic result of a subsequent cytotoxic treatment (21,23,24). We have already reported this new analysis in more detail (25).

Among the 216 evaluable patients treated concurrently with hormono-chemotherapy, the patients receiving the low-dose regimen lmfp showed a response rate (CR + PR) of 32% (24/70). The response rates were 52% (36/70) and 54% (38/72) for the women treated with the two more intensive regimens of chemotherapy. The low-dose, peroral combination of cytotoxic drugs (lmfp) elicited a lower response rate ($p < 0.01$) and a shorter survival ($p = 0.03$) as compared to the results registered in all patients receiving the two more intensive chemotherapies, which showed very similar therapeutic results as regards response rate, time to progression and survival.

We further analysed various subsets of patients in order to evaluate the impact of the treatment upon different prognostic groups (Tables 4 and 5).

Some of the differences registered may in fact be due to statistical artefacts generated by the multiplicity of statistical analyses in small groups. Some of our findings can, however, be considered as rather obvious, e.g., the superiority of a more intensive chemotherapy in patients with a poor performance status and/or visceral lesions. Furthermore we found that in patients with only bony metastases neither the response rate nor the median survival (approximately 2 1/2 years) are influenced by the intensity of the chemotherapy given concurrently with an endocrine manipulation.

But some of our findings were quite unexpected. Particularly striking are the essentially similar survival courses in all premenopausal patients, notwithstanding the different intensities of the chemotherapy. On the contrary, we observed a statistically significant advantage for the more intensive chemotherapies in postmenopausal women and, even more surprisingly, in this group the difference was almost completely confined to the patients older than 60 years. This finding cannot be considered an artefact, since postmenopausal patients represent more than 3/4 of the evaluable cases and since all prognostic factors were extremely well-balanced among the three different regimens of chemotherapy.

Table 4. Influence of prognostic factors upon response rate in different regimens of chemotherapy.

| | Response Rate (% CR + PR) | | |
	Treatment I	Treatment II + III	p value
Premenopausal	40	58	0.054
Postmenopausal	30	50	<0.05
Low risk	24	47	n.s.
High risk	36	54	<0.05
No. of sites:			
1	30	49	n.s.
2	16	55	<0.01
⩾3	57	52	n.s.
Performance status:			
0-1	39	51	n.s.
2-4	17	56	<0.01
Age (years):			
⩽50	33	62	0.058
50-60	37	40	n.s.
⩾60	28	57	<0.01
Free interval (months):			
0-12	33	46	n.s.
12-60	31	57	<0.01
⩾60	36	50	n.s.
Site of metastases*:			
Osseous only	31	39	n.s.
Visceral + local	18	69	<0.05
Visceral only	20	73	<0.05
Lung (dominant)	26	55	<0.05

*Patients broken down according to 2 different systems (see Table 2)

Table 5. Influence of prognostic factors upon survival in patients treated with different regimens of chemotherapy*.

| | Median Survival (months) | | |
	Treatment I	Treatment II + III	p value
Premenopausal	26	25	n.s.
Postmenopausal	17	28.5	0.018
Low risk	26	31	0.043
High risk	19.5	27	n.s.
No. of sites:			
1	28.5	33	n.s.
2	13.5	25	0.02
⩾3	15	26	n.s.
Performance status:			
0–1	27.5	33.5	n.s.
2–4	13	22.5	0.002
AAge (years):			
⩽50	25	26	n.s.
50–60	18	19	n.s.
⩾60	19	33	0.03
Free interval (months):			
0–12	16.5	19	n.s.
12–60	25	33.5	0.05
⩾60	17.5	32.5	0.04
Site of metastases**:			
Osseous only	28	31	n.s.
Osseous + local	26.5	30.5	n.s.
Visceral + local	8	21.5	0.05
Osseous + visceral	12	22	n.s.
Liver (dominant)	7	20.5	0.004
Lung (dominant)	16	32.5	0.03

*besides degree of response
**patients broken down according to 2 different systems (see Table 2).

4. ARE THE CURRENT TRIALS IN ADVANCED BREAST CANCER CONFUSING THE ISSUE?

If one analyses the two most important studies among the 5 comparing an adriamycin-containing regimen to CMF(P) - the one of the Southwest Oncology Group - SWOG (26) an the one of the Eastern Cooperative Oncology Group - ECOG (27) - then some interesting features are appearing (Table 6). As regards to

Table 6. Results of SWOG and ECOG with CMFP(V) vs. CAF in different survival risk categories of breast cancer.

Category of Metastases	SWOG	ECOG
0 Bone only	Too few cases	Survival ↑ with CMFP
1 Loco-regional (± bone)	CAF better:	Survival ↑ with CMFP
2 Nodular lung	− rem. rate	
3 Soft tissue progr. to liver	− TTP	
4 Untreated primaries	− survival	No significant differences
5 Ipsilateral pleural ± bone		
6 Lymphangitic pulmonary	No signif. differences	
7 Liver ± other metas.		Survival ↑ with time to P↑ CAF

the site of metastases, in the SWOG study CAF produces an higher remission rate, a longer time to progression and survival in patients with loco-regional metastases ± bony metastases, nodular secondaries in the lung as well as soft tissue metastases. No difference was seen among patients presenting ipsilaterial pleural metastases, lymphangiatic lung involvement or liver metastases. In the ECOG-study the median survival is significantly longer if patients with bony metastases or loco-regional disease receive CMFP instead of CAF. To the converse, women with liver ± other sites live longer if they were treated with CAF.

The ECOG-study was then further analysed taking into consideration other prognostic factors such as estrogen receptors, age, number of sites, performance status. The more intensive therapy with CAF tends to elicit better results as compared to CMFP in patients showing a more aggressive disease (ER−, visceral metastases, poor performance status, 4 or more sites of disease). Concerning the age of the patients the findings of the ECOF are quite similar to those of the SAKK-study: CAF tends to be superior to CMFP in women below 50 or above 60 years, while in patients between 50 and 59 years CMFP seems to be superior.

In advanced breast cancer the only hard parameter is survival. Looking at survival, at least in the ECOG- and SWOG-studies, the more interesting chemotherapy does not produce a statistically longer survival. However in subsets those statistically significant differences are observed: in fact, in some subsets they are in favour of CAF, in some other of CMFP(V). Similar trends were observed in the already mentioned analysis of the SAKK study.

Therefore the current tendency to merge all patients with advanced breast cancer in the same trial is probbly hampering the solution of the therapeutic problems by nullifying the differences among different subsets.

REFERENCES

1. Cooper R: Combination chemotherapy in hormone resistant breast cancer. Proc Am Ass Cancer Res (10):15, 1969.
2. Brunner KW: Present status of combination chemotherapy in advanced breast cancer. In: Application of Cancer Chemotherap. Antibiotics Chemother. (24):173-188, Karger, Basel, 1978.
3. Canellos GP, Pocock SJ, Taylor SG, et al: Combination chemotherapy for metastatic breast carcinoma. Cancer (38):1882-1886, 1976.
4. Tormey D, Carbone P and Band P: Breast cancer survival in single and combination chemotherapy trials since 1968. Proc Am Ass Cancer Res (18):64, 1977.
5. Broder LE and Tormey DC: Combination chemotherapy of carcinoma of the breast. Cancer Treat Rev (1):183-203, 1974.
6. Band PR, Tormey DC and Bauer M for the ECOG: Induction chemotherapy and maintenance chemo-hormonotherapy in metastatic breast cancer. Proc Am Ass Cancer Res (18):228, 1977.
7. Brunner KW, Sonntag RW, Martz G, Senn HJ, Obrecht P and Alberto P: A controlled study in the use of combined drug therapy for metastatic breast cancer. Cancer (36): 1208-1219, 1975.
8. Smalley RV, Murphy S, Huguley CM, et al: Combination versus sequential five-drug chemotherapy in metastatic breast cancer. Cancer Res (36):3911-3916, 1976.
9. Chlebowski RT, Irwin LE, Pugh RP, Sadoff L, et al: Survival of patients with metastatic breast cancer treated with either combination or sequential chemotherapy. Cancer Res (39):4503-4506, 1979.
10. De Lena M, De Palo GM, Bonadonna G, Beretta G and Bajetta E: Terapia del carcinoma mammario metastatizzato con ciclofosfamide, methotrexate, vincristina e fluorouracile. Tumori (59):11-24, 1973.
11. Bull JM, Tormey DC, Li SH, et al: A randomized trial of Adriamycin versus Methotrexate in combination drug therapy. Cancer (41):1649-1657, 1978.
12. Muss HB, White DR, Richards F, et al: Adriamycin versus Methotrexate in five drug combination chemotherapy for advanced breast cancer. Cancer (42):2141-2148, 1978.
13. Smalley RY, Carpenter J, Bartolucci A, et al: Comparison of cyclophosphamide, methotrexate, 5-fluorouracil (CAF) and cyclophosphamide, methotrexate, 5-fluorouracil, vincristine, prednisone (CMFVP) in patients with metastatic breast cancer. Cancer (40):625-632,1977.
14. Carom-Pereira J, Cost FL, Henriques E: Chemotherapy of advanced breast cancer. A randomized trial of vincristine, adriamycin and cyclophosphamide (VAC) versus cyclophosphamide, methotrexate, 5-fluorouracil and prednisone (CMFP). Cancer (48):1517-1521, 1981.
15. Brambilla C, Valagussa P, Bonadonna G: Sequential combination chemotherapy in advanced breast cancer. Cancer Chemother Pharmacol (1):35-39, 1978.

16. Tormey DC, Gelman R, B and P and Carbone P for the ECOG: Comparison of single to alternating combination therapy in metastatic breast cancer. Am Ass Cancer Res 171 (Abstract), 1980.

17. Brunner KW, Sonntag RW, Alberto P, et al: Combined chemo- and hormonal therapy in advanced breast cancer. Cancer (39):2923-2933, 1977.

18. Carter SK: The interpretation of trials: combined hormonal therapy and chemotherapy in disseminated breast cancer. Breast Cancer Research and Treatment (1):43-52, 1981.

19. Tormey DC, Falkson G, Cowley J, Falkson HC, Voelkel J and Davis TE: Dibromodulcitol and adriamycin + tamoxifen in advanced breast cancer. Am J Clin Oncol (5):33-39, 1982.

20. Cocconi G, De Lisi V, Boni C, et al: Chemotherapy versus combination of chemotherapy and endocrine therapy in advanced breast cancer. Cancer (51):581-588, 1983.

21. Cavalli F, Beer M, Martz G, et al: Gleichzeitige oder sequentielle hormono-chemotherapie sowie vergleich verschiedener polychemotherapien in der behandlung des metastasierenden mammakarzinoms. Schweiz Med Wschr (112):774-783, 1982.

22. Cavalli F, Beer M, Martz G, Jungi WF, Alberto P, Obrecht JP, Mermillod B and Brunner KW: Concurrent or sequential use of cytotoxic chemotherapy and hormone treatment in advanced breast cancer: report of the Swiss Group for Clinical Cancer Research. Brit Med J (1):286,5-8, 1983.

23. Legha SS, Buzdar AU, Smith TL, Swenerton KD, Hortobagyi GN and Blumenschein GR: Response to hormonal therapy as a prognostic factor for metastatic breast cancer treated with combination chemotherapy. Cancer (46):438-445, 1980.

24. Manni A, Trujillo JE and Pearson OH: Sequential use of endocrine therapy and chemotherapy for metastatic breast cancer: effects on survival. Cancer Treat Rep (64):111-116, 1980.

25. Cavalli F, Pedrazzini A, Goldhirsch A, et al: Randomized trial of 3 different regimens of chemotherapy in patients receiving simultaneously hormone treatment for advanced breast cancer. Europ J Cancer and Clin Oncol (19,11):1615-1624, 1983.

26. Smalley RY and Bartolucci AA: Variations in responsiveness and survival of clinical subsets of patients with metastatic breast cancer to 2 chemotherapy combinations. In: Mouridsen HR and Palshoff T (eds) Breast Cancer - Experimental and Clinical. Pergamon Press, 1980. pp 141-146.

27. Cummings FJ, Gelman R, Horton J and Calman K: Comparison of CMFP with CAF in patients with metastatic breast cancer. In: Proceedings 13th Int Congress UICC, Seattle, 1982. Abstract C-186.

CHEMOTHERAPY OF OVARIAN CANCER

E. Wiltshaw

Ovarian cancer is one of the most interesting and challenging tumours for
the medical oncologist of the 1980s. Deaths from ovarian cancer amount to
approximately 4,000 per year and this figure has changed not at all over
the last 30 years.   Whilst there are many different histological types of
tumour, each with its own pattern of development, I shall only discuss two
groups. First, by far the most common malignancy, the epithelial tumour,
and second, the much rarer germ cell tumour.

FIGO stage	5 year survival
Stage I. Confined to one or both ovaries.	70%
Stage II. Confined to the pelvis.	40-60%
Stage III. Extending into the abdominal cavity.	5-10%
Stage IV. Blood borne metastatic spread.	0-1%

TABLE I

As with most cancers, prognosis in ovarian carcinoma is dependent on stage
at diagnosis, histological type and degree of differentiation. However,
by far the most important prognostic factor is stage (Table I). Unfortunately,
early ovarian cancer is very difficult to detect and surgery alone can only
hope to cure a few patients. Radiotherapy has been shown to be of value
in stage II disease and, less certainly, when there is minimal spread to
the abdominal cavity ('early' stage III).
    However, it is clear that effective chemotherapy is the only way to

radically change the overall survival of ovarian cancer.

My own department has been interested in the treatment of the epithelial tumours since 1958 when we first started using single alkylating agents, especially chlorambucil.

Early Studies in Stages III and IV disease.

In 1965 we published our first series of 62 cases. This series consisted of patients with stages III and IV disease plus recurrent tumour after radiotherapy. Crude clinical responses were seen in 61% of cases and the median length of remission was 7.5 months.[1] The results were similar to other later studies throughout the world using melphalan, cyclophosphamide and chlorambucil as single agents given by mouth. Although these results now seem wholly inadequate, it should be remembered that this was the first common epithelial cancer to show a consistent response rate to cytotoxic therapy. Unfortunately, however, the results were not good enough to prolong survival at any stage of the disease. Nevertheless, we had learned two important facts: namely, that complete clinical response was essential to long term survival, and failure to respond to an alkylating agent meant resistance to other single alkylating agents or, indeed, to combination chemotherapy.

Thus, in 1972, when cis-diammine dichloroplatinum (II) (cis-platin) first came to be tried at the Royal Marsden Hospital, we were excited to find that further remissions could be produced by this compound. Remissions were seen in 33% of cases when $30mg/m^2$ was given and in 52% when $100mg/m^2$ was subsequently used.[2]

Following this, in 1974, a trial was started comparing chlorambucil alone with chlorambucil plus cis-platin in previously untreated patients stages III, IV and with recurrent disease after radiotherapy.

Unfortunately, after 34 patients had been entered it became clear that the combination arm was very much better at achieving remissions than chlorambucil alone. Thus our group decided that the single agent should be dropped and be replaced by a combination of cis-platin plus chlorambucil plus Adriamycin. Results from this trial showed that remissions (52% and 54%) and survival were similar in both groups. Median survivals were 15 months and 17.5 months respectively.[3] Although the overall survival was again disappointing with only 10% alive at 5 years, the responses seen were of much better quality than in the past and second laparotomy with removal of residual tumour could be undertaken in about 50% of cases. Furthermore, the projected survival of complete remitters was now 70% at 5 years.

Our next trial was designed to answer the question: 'was cis-platin alone as good as combination chemotherapy?'. This question is important as the compound was now being introduced into use for ovarian cancer but almost always combined with other agents, thus adding to toxicity. The trial was closed in May 1981 but results so far show that cis-platin ($100mg/m^2$) alone is as good as chlorambucil ($0.15mg/Kg/day$ for 7 days) + cis-platin ($20mg/m^2$ day I) in stage IV disease and in patients after failure of radiotherapy, while in stage III disease cis-platin alone appears to be better than the combination in terms of survival.

The lessons learned from our trials and those of others, together with evidence from over 100 second look operations are as follows:

I. Complete remissions must be obtained in order to accomplish long-term survival.

2. Complete remission is easier to achieve if the bulk of the disease is small when chemotherapy begins.

3. Complete remission is evident in the majority of cases within six months of starting treatment.

4. The overall toxicity of high dose cis-platin is severe and long lasting.

5. Overall survival for stage III and IV disease treated at the Royal Marsden Hospital is now approaching 20%.

Present Studies. Stage III and IV disease.

It is rare for analogues of cytotoxic drugs to prove more valuable than the parent compound, but in 1980-81 the Institute of Cancer Research (Dr. Harrap) in collaboration with Johnson Mathey and Bristol Myers tested cis-diammine I,I cyclobutane dicarboxylate platinum (II) (JM8). They found this compound to be much less toxic in animals and still effective against some animal tumours. Then a phase I study was conducted by Dr. Calvert and later we collaborated in a phase II study in recurrent ovarian cancer following chemotherapy. Despite the fact that most patients had already received cis-platin, a response rate of 25% was seen in the first 30 patients.[4] As a result, a phase III study began and we now have approximately 100 patients in a randomised trial comparing cis-platin $100mg/m^2$ to JM8 $400mg/m^2$. Early results suggest similar response rates but much less toxicity for JM8.[5]

It is also possible that these drugs are not cross-resistant.

Thus in the whole population we hope to see an increased response rate with less toxic sequelae.

Treatment of Germ Cell Tumours

Germ cell tumours of the ovary are much rarer than their equivalents in the testis; they are also less easily diagnosed and therefore often more advanced when first treated. They occur in a younger age group in women than in men and have been managed, in the past, by gynaecologists rather than medical oncologists. For all these reasons the successful treatment of these tumours has lagged behind that of the male teratomas.

Thus, as recently as 1979, reports were still coming out which showed very poor survival although the use of drugs such as vincristine, actinomycin D and cyclophosphamide seemed to have cured a few patients.

TABLE II

I58 CASES OF EST FROM THE LITERATURE

(1976-79)

	No Cases	No. (%) surviving 2 yrs
Stage I	II2	22 (I8)
Stage II and III	46	9 (I7)
Surgery $\pm$ radiotherapy	III	9 (8)
Surgery + chemotherapy	47	22 (47)

One of the most rapidly lethal variants is the tumour containing yolk sac (endodermal sinus) elements. This tumour is associated with the production of alpha-foeto protein (AFP). A review of the literature from 1976-1979 shows that out of I58 cases only 3I survived more than 2 years despite the fact that II2 patients presented with FIGO stage I disease (Table II).

It is clear from these cases that aggressive surgery and radiotherapy are of no value. It is also striking that of the 3I patients surviving more than 2 years, 22 had additional chemotherapy. Our experience for this tumour had been similar until I977 when we began to use cis-platin, vinblastine and Bleomycin (PVB) for endodermal sinus tumour (EST). Since then we have treated 8 patients with the PVB regimen using the AFP level as a guide to successful therapy.

TABLE III

ROYAL MARSDEN HOSPITAL SERIES OF EST, 1977 - 1982.

Stage	No.	Survival in months
I	4	20+ 32+ 38+ 43+
III	3	41+ 45+ 50+
IV	I	5

7 of 8 patients are still alive and well despite the fact that minimal surgery was performed in all but one patient and radiotherapy was not used.

This treatment, whilst very toxic, is as successful as that seen in testicular teratoma and shows clearly that once there is an effective chemotherapy programme, other modalities can be discarded.

References

I. Wiltshaw E:
    a) Chlorambucil in the treatment of primary adenocarcinoma of the ovary.
    b) A retrospective comparison of Chlorambucil and radiotherapy in the treatment of ovarian adenocarcinoma.
    J.Obst.& Gynae. of Br.Commonwealth 72: 586-602, 1965.

2. Wiltshaw E, Subramanian S, Alexopoulos C, Barker G H:
    Cancer of the Ovary: A Summary of Experience with cis-dichlorodiammine platinum (II) at the Royal Marsden Hospital.
    Ca.Tr.Rep. 63: 1545-1548, 1979.

3. Barker G H & Wiltshaw E:
    Randomised Trial comparing low dose cisplatin and chlorambucil with low dose cisplatin, chlorambucil and Doxorubicin in advanced ovarian cancer.
    Lancet I: 747-750, 1981.

4. Evans B D, Raju K S, Calvert A H, Harland S J, Wiltshaw E.
    JM8 (Cis-Diammine 1,1-Cyclobutane Dicarboxylate Platinum II): A New Platinum Analogue Active in the Treatment of Advanced Ovarian Carcinoma.
    To be published Ca.Tr.Rep., 1983.

5. Wiltshaw E, Evans B D, Jones A C, Baker J W, Calvert A H.
    JM8, a Successor to Cisplatin in Advanced Ovarian Carcinoma.
    Lancet (letter) I: 587, 1983.

OBSTACLES TO IMPROVED END-RESULTS IN HEAD AND NECK CANCER

R.E. WITTES

The status of chemotherapy in the treatment of squamous cancers of the
upper aerodigestive tract has been the subject of several recent comprehensive
reviews (1,2,3). The drugs with measurable activity in these diseases have
been tested singly and in a multitude of combinations in patients with
relapsed or metastatic disease, and increasingly as the first form of therapy
in patients with advanced disease. In addition, many drugs have been administered simultaneously with radiotherapy in an effort to treat systemic disease
while sensitizing the locoregional lesion to radiation.

From this considerable clinical experience several generalizations are
possible. In disease which is <u>recurrent</u> after radiation and/or surgery,
single-agent chemotherapy produces significant objective responses in an
appreciable minority of patients. Since the duration of these responses is
almost always less than 6 months, the survivorship of the treated population
is not altered significantly. When drugs are used in combination, response
rates are probably somewhat higher than with single agents, though this is
clearly not always the case. Even with combinations of the most active
single agents, however, durations of response do not seem to be significantly
longer than with single drugs. In both single agent and combination trials,
the clinical complete response rate is very low.

When chemotherapy is used in <u>previously</u> <u>untreated</u> patients, the response
rate is in general higher than when the same regimens are used after failure
of other modalities. Many combinations containing cisplatin or methotrexate
are capable of inducing major degrees of tumor shrinkage in the vast majority
of patients so treated. Since most of these patients go on to surgery and/or
radiotherapy after one or two cycles of treatment, there are no reliable
data on the duration of these remissions, nor on the outcome of a policy of
continued chemotherapy treatment with local therapy withheld in the absence
of relapse. Since the vast majority of the trials in this patient population

111

have been uncontrolled pilot studies, each involving small numbers of patients, there is little information on the effect of initial chemotherapy on the natural history of the disease.

When chemotherapy is used simultaneously with radiation, one generally sees a non-selective radiosensitization within the treatment volume; the tendency to increased local control rates has in most trials been counter-balanced by substantially increased radiation toxicity, such that the "thera-peutic ratio" has not been greatly changed (1). Although some data suggest that tumors from certain anatomic sites may be more effectively treated by combined simultaneous therapy than by radiation alone, the enhanced toxicity of this approach together with the promise, still unrealized, of hypoxic sensitizers has dampened enthusiasm.

Why has progress been so modest despite a decade or more of widespread interest? The reasons are naturally complex and relate to considerations of the patient population, the disease itself, the available drugs, and the clinical trials methodology favored by many investigators.

The agents generally regarded as active for squamous head and neck cancer are methotrexate (M), cisplatin (P), and bleomycin (B). The activity of other agents frequently employed in combinations, such as vinblastine and hydroxyurea, is much less well documented, which of course does not mean that these agents are not active. Nevertheless, it must be said that the incor-poration of several classes of agents into combinations in past years - the bifunctional alkylating agents, nitrosoureas, vincristine - without adequate prior demonstration of single agent efficacy, resulted in combinations which were not more active than optimal single agent treatment but were a whole lot more toxic.

Now M, P, and B are not the easiest three drugs to administer together, chiefly because any nephrotoxicity induced by P can lead to accumulation of M and B, with disastrous consequences. Nevertheless, the construction of toler-able combinations of these drugs has been possible with careful attention to sequencing. Kaplan and Vogl (4), for example, have combined M, B, and P into a combination which is tolerable in the outpatient setting and whose activity seemed in a pilot study suggestively greater than what one might expect for single agent treatment. Indeed, if one assumes response proba-bilities of 30% for P, 30% for M, and 15% for B, then the response rate achieved by Kaplan and Vogl for CMB (65%) is very close to that expected (57%) if the three drugs are acting independently at their full single agent activity.   A randomized study in the Eastern Cooperative Oncology Group (5) subsequently confirmed that the response rate of MBP is superior to that of M alone, but the rate achieved in the group study was about 20 percentage points less than in the single institution pilot; also, the increased response rate did not translate into more durable remissions or into a survival advantage for patients treated with the combination.   It seems plain, therefore, that the quality of remissions, that is, the amount of tumor cell kill in responding patients, was roughly the same with the combination as with M alone.   This result, which seems to be generally true in head and neck cancer, since combinations do not increase the complete response rate, is obviously disappointing and probably sets a limit on what we can expect to achieve with existing drugs given according to empirical schedules.

We might be in a better position, of course, if we had a larger repertory of active agents which caused neither myelosuppression nor mucositis; such drugs would be ideal for combination with existing active agents.   Over the past few years Phase II testing has included the study of ftorafur, pyrazofurin, vindesine, maytansine, m-AMSA, methyl-GAG, dianhydrogalactitol, ICR 159, dibromodulcitol, VP-16, and AZQ; of these, methyl-GAG (6,7) has exhibited some activity (25% of 47 patients) and is without dose-limiting marrow or mucosal effects in most patients.

The tendency to short remissions in head and neck cancer is very frustrating clinically but is of great interest biologically.   The basis for this rapid emergence of drug resistance is unknown.   Perhaps the common prior use of radiation promotes the rapid generation of drug-resistant variants in vivo.   Whatever the cause, the phenomenon suggests that cultured cells derived from these tumors might be a useful in vitro model for studies of acquired drug resistance in human cancer.   Such a model is particularly attractive because much is known in other mammalian cell systems about mechanism of resistance to methotrexate, one of the few clinically useful agents in squamous head and neck cancer.

Since at a clinical level the identification of new active agents is the most urgent imperative, our procedures must minimize the chance of missing an active drug.   Inasmuch as conventional chemotherapy makes little impact on the course of the patient who has already failed local treatment, it makes good sense to concentrate the Phase II effort in patients who have received no prior chemotherapy.   Trials with new drugs which are identified as active in this population can then be extended to the previously treated group; in this way, previously treated patients will be spared the potential toxicity of inactive agents. Patients who appear to be failing the new agent after 1 or 2 cycles can be promptly switched to standard treatment.

The intensive investigation of chemotherapy as a preoperative or preradiation adjuvant is especially noteworthy. These studies, and particularly the use of chemotherapy as initial treatment, have been motivated by several observations. Control of locoregional disease, rather than distant metastases, is obviously the chief clinical challenge in the advanced head and neck cancers. The dramatic and rapid shrinkage of advanced primary tumors and cervical metastases with chemotherapy has led to the expectation that initial chemotherapy may improve end results essentially by upstaging the patient prior to local therapy. In addition, of course, since chemotherapy works systemically, it may also have a salutary effect on the evolution of distant metastases.

The question of which strategy is most worthy $(S \rightarrow R \rightarrow C, C \rightarrow S \rightarrow R, S \rightarrow C \rightarrow R)$ is probably unresolvable on theoretical grounds alone. It is certainly gratifying to watch large tumors dissolve. In addition, information on tumor responsiveness to chemotherapy may provide some guidance on whether such treatment might be useful subsequently. It may be sounder practice, however, to attempt maximal surgical cytoreduction prior to drug treatment; the chance of selecting out drug resistant cells probably decreases as the body burden of tumor decreases. Certain current hypotheses on optimal strategies for adjuvant therapy (8) suggest that treatment given after local therapy should begin immediately after surgery; this is certainly consistent with lessons from many laboratory models. Application to primary human head and neck cancer, however, may present a significant practical problem. The surgical procedures in head and neck cancer are often complex, require immediate or delayed reconstruction, and are not infrequently complicated by infection, wound or flap non-healing, and nutritional compromise. Moreover, even if chemotherapy can be started shortly after surgery, the need for repeated hospitalization and the recurrent side effects from treatment will surely affect patient compliance adversely. Experience in the National Cancer Institute's Head and Neck Contracts Program strongly suggests that patients will not comply with a regimen having these characteristics, at least not if it is administered after the $S \rightarrow R$ sequence. The improved technology of portable continuous infusion pumps may provide a very effective solution here, as may alteration of the sequence of postoperative modalities.

The question of the most appropriate endpoints for these studies is a very difficult one. Patients with head and neck cancer are an older population with a high prevalence of alcohol and tobacco abuse, a high prevalence and incidence of non-malignant co-morbid disease, and an impressive tendency to develop metachronous epithelial cancers. Many therapeutic trials in the past have documented an appreciable rate of death from causes other than the index primary tumor. Such results have led to the suggestion that survival may not be the appropriate endpoint for adjuvant trials at all.

Such criticisms have a certain validity. It may be difficult to measure improvements in survival from current baselines when there is so much "noise" from other causes of death. And it is probably also true that if chemotherapy only seems to improve local control rates over standard treatment, we might well count this achievement as a worthy therapeutic endpoint. Nevertheless, to the extent that these patients die of uncontrolled local or systemic disease, we may reasonably expect effective chemotherapy to improve survival. If it does not (i.e., if the improvement in survival is too small to be measured with statistical significance), then we are putting our efforts and our resources in the wrong place.

1. Million R, Cassizzi N, Wittes RE: pp. 301-386, In: Principles and Practice of Oncology, DeVita V, Hellman S, and Rosenberg S (Eds.), Philadelphia, J.B. Lippencott Company, 1982.

2. Wittes RE: Recent Results in Cancer Research 76:276, 1981.

3. Eisenberger M, Posada J, Soper W, Wittes R, In: Investigative Techniques in the Staging and Treatment of Head and Neck Cancer, Wittes R (Ed.), John Wiley, in press.

4. Vogl S, Kaplan B: Cancer 44:26, 1979.

5. Kaplan BH, Vogl SE, Cinberg J, Berenzweig M, O'Donnell M: Proc. Am. Soc. Clin. Oncol. 1:C-775, 199, 1982.

6. Thongprasert S, Bosl GJ, Geller NL, Wittes RE: Submitted for publication.

7. Perry DJ, Crain S, Weltz M, Wilson J, Davis RK, Woolley P, Forastiere A, Taylor HG, Weiss R: Cancer Treat. Rep. 67:91, 1983.

8. Goldie JH, Goldman AJ: Cancer Treat. Rep. 63:1727, 1979.

TREATMENT OF DISSEMINATED MALIGNANT LYMPHOMA

LISTER, T.A. and DHALIWAL, H.S.

It has been clear since the second half of the last
decade that a proportion of patients with disseminated
malignant lymphoma are curable (1,2,3). Since then strenuous
efforts have been made to increase that proportion. Selected
examples of the approaches taken to this end, and the results
achieved will be presented in this paper.

A. HODGKIN'S DISEASE

The major problems encountered in the treatment of
advanced Hodgkin's Disease are failure to achieve complete
remission and early recurrence.

In order to determine whether the latter is a function
of the former, and simply represents the inability of the tests
employed to detect minimal residual disease, a prospective
study of surgical re-staging following chemotherapy was undertaken at St. Bartholomew's Hospital, London (4). Staging
laparotomy with splenectomy was undertaken on 32 patients in
whom there was no clinical or radiological evidence of Hodgkin's
Disease after combination chemotherapy. Evidence that Hodgkin's
Disease had been present at any time was found in 12/32. In
four of the twelve (4/32 overall) it was active, as opposed to
'ablated', and in all cases the site of involvement was the
spleen.

These results suggest strongly, that early relapse is a
consequence of failure to eliminate minimal residual disease,
which is clinically undetectable and reinforces the argument
in favour of more effective early therapy.

This problem has been addressed by attempts to develop

117

combination chemotherapy which is non-cross resistant to
MOPP and then introduce alternating combination chemotherapy
into the initial treatment of patients with adverse prognostic
features. The most widely used combination is that of
adriamycin, bleomycin, vinblastine and dacarbazine (ABVD) (5).
This has been shown to induce complete remission in previously
untreated patients with a similar frequency to MOPP, with the
duration of first remission being the same for both treatments.
A comparative trial is now in progress in which MOPP alone is
being compared with MOPP alternating with ABVD (6). Although
the overall complete remission rate was the same for both
treatment groups, there was a significant advantage for those
patients receiving the alternating combinations in terms of
the duration of first remission, the probability of being
disease free at 5 years being 70% for MOPP plus ABVD compared
with 37% for MOPP alone. Further studies are now in progress
to confirm these results.

A spectrum of other combinations, reviewed by Canellos
et al (7), has been tested in patients failing MOPP with
variable results, and some have been introduced into alternating combinations with MOPP.

Large studies will be required to demonstrate whether the
use of 'non-cross resistant' combinations or the addition of
radiation therapy will improve the results of therapy for
advanced disease. The theoretical advantage of increasing
the intensity of the early therapy in those patients with
adverse prognostic features may be outweighed by the practical
consideration that advanced age correlates closely with a
poor prognosis and older patients tolerate very intensive
therapy badly.

B. NON-HODGKIN'S LYMPHOMA
(i) High grade - In general, the recent trend has been
to investigate increasingly intensive chemotherapy for patients
with disseminated high grade lymphoma. It must be emphasised
at the outset that the median age of the patients entered
into the studies at cancer centres tends to be lower than

that of the whole population of patients with the disease in
question and that the treatments being evaluated may not be
appropriate for a significant proportion of patients. Nonetheless the demonstration that an improvement can be achieved
for any of the patients is important.

Two very intensive multiple drug regimens have recently
been shown to yield results which in the first instance appear
better than those achieved elsewhere. Both are extremely
toxic and can only be prescribed within the context of a
major cancer centre. Skarin et al from the Dana Farber
Cancer Centre, Boston (8) treated 101 adults with cyclical
treatment comprising bleomycin, adriamycin, cyclophosphamide
and dexamethasone every three weeks with high dose methotrexate
($3g/m^2$) on day 14, followed by leucovorin rescue. Complete
remission was achieved in 72%, and 65% of those completing
therapy and being in CR at that time are predicted as being
without recurrence at five years. Fisher et al from the
National Cancer Institute, Betheseda (9), tested an alternative
programme comprising many cycles of prednisolone, methotrexate,
adriamycin, cyclophosphamide and VP16/213 and MOPP (ProMACE-
MOPP). Eighty one patients commenced therapy. Complete
remission was achieved in 55 with only 10 patients having
relapsed and a median follow up of 2½ years. Even though
the patient population in both studies was young and only
included 60% patients with stage IV disease, the results
are exciting.

The very grave outlook for those patients either failing
to enter complete remission following initial therapy or
relapsing, has prompted the investigation of lethal chemotherapy
and radiotherapy followed by bone marrow transplantation (10).
The numbers of patients treated to date remains very small.
However, the fact that there are any long term survivors is
encouraging and justifies further studies, since the prognosis
of this group is appalling.

(ii) Low grade - There is as yet no evidence that it is
possible to cure patients with advanced 'low grade' Non
Hodgkin's Lymphoma, although it is undoubtedly possible to

give many of them an excellent quality of life for many years with minimal intervention. It was clearly demonstrated in the 1970's that combination chemotherapy with cyclophosphamide, vincristine and prednisolone was no more effective at producing prolonged remission than either single agent chemotherapy or TBI (11,12,13,14). In addition, a small study testing high dose cyclophosphamide and prednisolone showed that even if complete remissions were achieved rapidly with this treatment, recurrences occurred quite quickly afterwards (14).

Attention has therefore been turned towards alternative approaches. Portlock and Rosenberg (16) from Stanford, have emphasised the importance of identifying those patients (still the minority) who may benefit from an expectant policy and be closely observed without treatment. Secondly, the use of interferon has been investigated. Chronic low dose interferon administration compatible with an ambulatory 'normal' home life has been shown to induce remission in between a quarter and a half of the patients treated (17,18), and its possible role in combination with alkylating agents is under consideration The third approach is at present applied to a very small number of patients. Miller and Levy (19) have reported the achievement of a complete remission in a patient with follicular lymphoma to treatment with anti-idiotypic serum. This remission has now continued unmaintained for nearly two years. If more early results are encouraging, the feasibility of extending this approach to large numbers of patients will have to be investigated.

ACKNOWLEDGEMENTS

We thank Jane Ashby for typing the manuscript.

REFERENCES

1. DeVita V. Jr., Serpick A, Carbone P: Combination chemotherapy in the treatment of advanced Hodgkin's disease. Ann. Int. Med. 73:881-895, 1979.

2. Sutcliffe S, Wrigley P, Peto J, et al: MVPP chemtherapy regimen for advanced Hodgkin's disease. Br Med J 1:679-683, 1978

3. DeVita VT, Chabner B, Hubbard SP et al: Advanced diffuse histiocytic lymphoma, a potentially curable disease. Lancet I:248-250, 1975.

4. Sutcliffe S, Wrigley P, Timothy A, et al: Post-treatment laparotomy as a guide to management in patients with Hodgkin's disease. Cancer Treat Rep 66 4:759-765, 1982.

5. Santoro A, Bonadonna G: Prolonged disease-free survival in MOPP-resistant Hodgkin's disease after treatment with adriamycin, bleomycin, vinblastine and decarbazine (ABVD). Cancer Chemother Pharmacol 2:101-105, 1979.

6. Santoro A, Bonadonna G, Bonfante V, et al: Alternating drug combinations in the treatment of advanced Hodgkin's disease. N Engl J Med 306:770-775, 1982.

7. Canellos G, Come S, Skarin A: Chemotherapy in the treatment of Hodgkin's disease. Semin Haemat 20:1-23, 1983.

8. Skarin A, Canellos G, Rosenthal D, et al: Improved Prognosis of diffuse histiocytic and undifferentiated lymphoma by use of high dose methotrexate alternating with standard agents (M-BACOD). J Clin Oncol 1:91-98, 1983.

9. Fisher R, DeVita V, Hubbard S, et al: Diffuse aggressive lymphomas: Increased survival after alternating flexible sequences of ProMACE and MOPP chemotherapy. Ann Int Med 98:304-309, 1983.

10. Appelbaum F, Thomas D: Review of the use of marrow transplantation in the treatment of Non-Hodgkin's lymphoma. J. Clin Oncol 1:440-447, 1983.

11. Portlock C, Rosenberg S, Glatstein E et al: Treatment of advanced Non-Hodgkin's lymphomas with favorable histologies: Preliminary results of a prospective trial. Blood 47:747-756, 1976.

12. Lister TA, Cullen MH, Beard MEJ et al:Comparison of combined and single agent chemotherapy in Non Hodgkin's lymphoma of favourable histological type. Br Med J 1:533-537, 1978.

13. Ezdinli EZ, Costello WG, Silverstein MN, et al: Moderate versus intensive chemotherapy of prognostically favorable Non-Hodgkin's lymphoma. Cancer 46:29-33, 1980.

14. Kennedy BJ, Bloomfield CD, Kiang DT et al: Combination versus successive single agent chemotherapy in lympho-cytic lymphoma. Cancer 41:23-28, 1978.

15. Bell R, Gallagher CJ, Ford J, Malpas JS, Lister TA: Phase II study of a high dose regimen of cyclophosphamide and prednisolone in advanced Non-Hodgkin's lymphoma of favorable histologic type. Cancer Treat Rep 66:377-380, 1982.

16. Portlock CS, Rosenberg SA: No initial therapy for stage III and IV Non-Hodgkin's lymphomas of favorable histologic type. Ann Int Med 90:10-13, 1979.

17. Gutterman JU, Blumenschein GR, Alexanian R, et al: Leukocyte interferon-induced tumor regression in human metastatic breast cancer, multiple myeloma and maligant lymphoma. Ann Int Med 93:399-406, 1980.

18. Louie AC, Gallagher JG, Sikora K, Levy R, Rosenberg SA, Merigan RC: Follow up observations on the effect of human leukocyte interferon in Non-Hodgkin's lymphoma. Blood 58:712, 1981.
19. Miller RA, Maloney DG, Warnke R, Levy R: Treatment of B-cell lymphoma with monoclonal anti-idiotype antibody. N Engl J Med 306:517-522, 1982.

MALIGNANT DISEASE IN CHILDHOOD

M.G. MOTT

1. INTRODUCTION

Cancer in childhood is fortunately rare, with an approximate annual incidence of 100 cases per million children in the developed world. It is, nevertheless, the commonest disease to kill children in our society and as effective treatment has become available for an increasing proportion of paediatric malignancies so it has become increasingly important to ensure that all effected children receive appropriate therapy. The spectrum of malignant disease is very different in children and adults. Whereas 85% of the tumours in an adult population are carcinomas, this is true of less than 5% of childhood malignancies. Almost half of the malignancies in childhood are leukaemias and lymphomas, and the rest consist primarily of a variety of primitive embryonal tumours that are rarely seen in adults. Failure to appreciate these differences was a major cause for the poor prognosis of paediatric tumours until recently. The primary reason for the improved prognosis in the last two decades has been the development of treatment protocols appropriate for these specific diseases. The overall incidence of childhood cancer has remained stable, but the death rate has fallen successively. The survival rate has more than doubled in the last 20 years (Table 1).

Table 1. Death rate from cancer and survival percentage in children.

Annual Death Rate per 100,000 (G.B.) Age 0-14 years		
Year	Rate	Survivors
1961	7.28	27.2%
1965	7.05	29.5%
1970	6.49	35.1%
1975	5.31	46.9%
1979	4.64	53.6%
Increase in survivors 1961-1979 = 50.7%		

OPCS, 1982

The increasing proportion of children cured of their disease has resulted in re-evaluation of our priorities for care. Escalation of treatment in order to cure a higher percentage of patients now has to be matched by concern to minimise the long-term sequelae of treatment for the survivors. The potential conflict between these two priorities demands a careful and rigorous scrutiny of the pros and cons of all treatment programmes if the best available option is to be offered to each patient. This is best illustrated by reviewing current treatment options for some of the more common childhood malignancies.

2. CURRENT TREATMENT OPTIONS

2.1. Acute Lymphoblastic Leukaemias

This is the most common group of malignancies seen in childhood and accounts for some 80% of all childhood leukaemia. The prognosis has improved steadily and the majority of affected children can now expect to be long-term survivors. A basic treatment programme has evolved which is used throughout most of the developed world. Treatment of large cohorts of children in the same manner has made it possible to identify prognostic factors which can be used to delineate groups of patients who are statistically likely to do more or less well with this treatment (1). Two factors which have consistently been found to be important are the age of the child at diagnosis and the presenting white count. There are in addition a number of other indices which have been found to be of variable importance (Fig. 1).

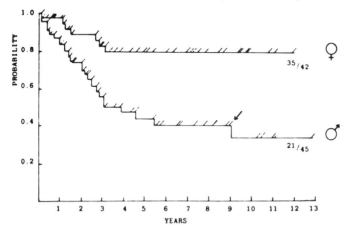

FIGURE 1. Comparison of complete remission duration of boys and girls with presenting WBC <20x 10^9/L and treated at Bristol Childrens Hospital 1969-1982.

The present trend is towards simplification of treatment for those patients who are likely to do well in order to reduce the morbidity. At the same time the intensity of treatment is being increased for those patients who are unlikely to do well with the standard treatment regimen. It should prove possible to provide a high cure rate for good risk patients with a regimen comprising: Induction treatment with prednisone, vincristing and asparaginase; CNA prophylaxis with intrathecal triple medication (methotrexate, hydrocortisone and cytosine arabinoside); and maintenance chemotherapy with daily oral mercaptopurine and weekly oral methotrexate for a two year period. On the other hand, patients who are at high risk of treatment failure when given standard treatment have been shown to have a better prognosis when treated with intensive schedules such as those pioneered by the West German BFM group (2). These treatment protocols result in substantial morbidity unless given by experienced paediatric oncologists with adequate backup facilities and should therefore only be given in specialist centres.

2.2. Hodgkin's Disease

The treatment of children with Hodgkin's disease has already been substantially refined. For the past decade many specialist centres have achieved 90% survival using a combination of low dose radiotherapy and chemotherapy with MOPP or a MOPP- variant (3). However, patients cured of their Hodgkin's disease by this means have a considerable risk of developing a second malignant neoplasm, usually acute myeloid leukaemia, which has a poor prognosis. Since many patients who fail primary treatment with either radiation or chemotherapy alone can be salvaged by re-treatment with the alternative modality, it should not be necessary to subject all patients to both modalities.

It is anticipated that this treatment approach will maintain the high cure rates achieved over the last decade while reducing the frequency of late complications.

2.3. Non-Hodgkin's Lymphoma

The non-Hodgkin's lymphomas of childhood are very different from those seen in adults and had in the past a poor prognosis with approximately 20% survival at 5 years. The introduction of intensive combination chemotherapy instead of radiation as primary treatment for these diseases has resulted in a dramatic improvement in prognosis; two-thirds of the 45 patients treated by us in 1977-83 are surviving and potentially cured of their disease (Fig. 2).

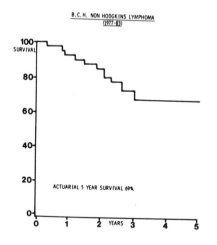

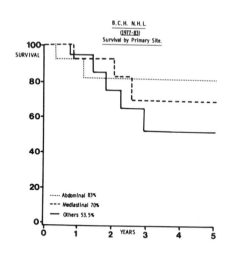

FIGURE 2. Actuarial survival of 45 children with NHL

FIGURE 3. Actuarial survival of 45 children with NHL by site

It is now possible to define groups of patients who have a low or high risk of treatment failure with these established treatment techniques, and future treatment can therefore be refined for different groups (Fig. 3). Treatment for patients with localised disease can probably be less intensive than before and can be completed within 6 months. Patients with unresectable B-cell malignancies presenting in the abdomen will require more intensive treatment, but this also can probably be completed within 6 months since later relapses in this disease are rare. Patients with mediastinal T-cell malignancies however might benefit from another approach (Fig. 4). They appear to have done even better in other centres when offered sustained intensive chemotherapy throughout the first few months of treatment followed by a simple leukaemia-type maintenance schedule, usually continued for a period of 2 years (2). This seems especially true for those with T-cell leukaemia, i.e. those with involvement of bone marrow, peripheral blood and/or CNS.

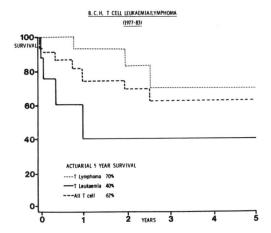

FIGURE 4. Actuarial survival of 23
children with T Cell leukaemia/lymphoma

2.4. Nephroblastoma

The kidney is one of the common sites for childhood tumours. We treated
32 patients in the years 1977-82 and Actuarial Survival for the whole
population is 90% at 5 years (Fig. 5, Table 2). Wilms' tumour is one of the

Table 2. Renal tumours 1977-82:
Survival by stage

<u>Wilms</u>

Stage 1	4/4	Stage 3	8/10
Stage 2	6/6	Stage 4	6/7
Stage 5	1/1	All stages	25/28

CMN   3/3

Adenocarcinoma   1/1

All Tumours 29/32

CMN = congenital mesoblastic nephroma

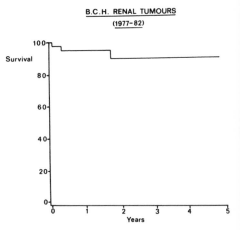

FIGURE 5. Actuarial survival
of 32 chidren with renal tumours

more common embryonal tumours and the evolution of successful treatment has
proved a prototype for the development of similar successful regimens for many
other tumours. Surgery alone cured only a small proportion of children with

Wilm's tumour and the addition of radiotherapy only raised the cure rate to approximately 50%, with substantial long-term morbidity in many of the survivors. The discovery and use of two highly effective chemotherapy agents, Actinomycin D and Vincristine, dramatically improved the cure rate, and the combination of both chemotherapy agents with surgery, with or without radiation, has made treatment failure for renal tumours a rare event in recent years (4). Cure rates in excess of 95% for patients with localised Wilms' tumour have permitted a progressive reduction in the amount of treatment given to these patients in successive trials. An example is the treatment plan for stage I Wilms' tumour (tumour confined to the kidney and completely resected by the surgeon) in the National Wilms' Tumour Study trials in the USA (Table 3). Recognition of histological features which indicate a relatively poor prognosis has likewise enabled the treatment to be refined for the majority who do not have those features (4).

Table 3. NWTS: Treatment plan - stage 1 nephroblastoma.

1969 NWTS I	Radiation 4000 rad Actinomycin D for 15 months 92% survival
1974 NWTS II	No radiation Actinomycin D + Vincristine for 6 months 95% survival
1979 NWTS III (favourable histology)	No radiation Actinomycin D + Vincristine for 10 weeks

2.5. Rhabdomyosarcoma

The treatment for this embryonal muscle tumour of childhood has likewise improved steadily and the combination of surgery, radiation and chemotherapy has made it possible to cure the majority of affected children. We have treated 28 patients in the years 1977-83 and Actuarial Survival at 5 years is 60% (Fig. 6). As was the case for nephroblastoma, the recognition of prognostic features led to the refinement of treatment in successive trials (5). Children who have an excellent chance of cure have been subjected to less intensive treatment (Table 4) while efforts at finding more effective treatment have been concentrated on those most at risk.

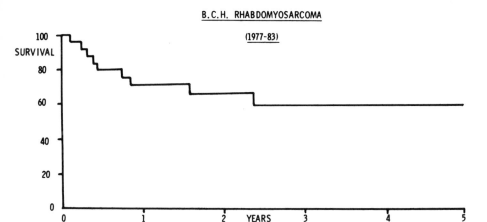

FIGURE 6. Actuarial survival of 28 children with rhabdomyosarcoma.

Table 4. I.R.S: Treatment plan - stage I rhabdomyosarcoma

1972 I.R.S. I	Radiation 5000-6000 rad VAC chemotherapy for 2 years 92% survival
1978 I.R.S. II	No radiation VA chemotherapy for 1 year 92% survival

VAC = Vincristine, Actinomycin D, Cyclophosphamide

2.6. Malignant Bone Tumours

Malignant tumours of bone have in the past carried a poor prognosis, especially in childhood, but the advent of effective chemotherapy has again substantially altered the prognosis. We have treated 27 patients in the years 1979-83 and Actuarial Survival at 3 years is 66.6%. Chemotherapy has also enabled clinicians to experiment with alternative modes of treatment. Osteosarcoma is an outstanding example of a tumour which in the past carried an appalling prognosis, patients with lesions of the distal skeleton having only a 20% chance of cure after primary treament with amputation (6). The great majority of patients developed progressive disease, usually with pulmonary metastases in the first instance. As effective chemotherapy became available it proved possible to prevent the development of pulmonary metastases in a substantial proportion of patients and to reduce considerably the number of metastases that developed in many of the remainder. Patients who develop a limited number of pulmonary metastases can often be salvaged by metastatectomy, multiple if required (7).

In addition to its effect on micro-metastases, chemotherapy can also result in substantial shrinkage of the primary tumour. This has made possible the application of more conservative surgery with resection of involved bone and the fitting of an endoprosthesis where necessary, rather than amputation (8). In children who have not completed bone growth it is necessary to make the prosthesis with the potential to increase in length as the child grows.

We adopted this experimental approach in 1979 in collaboration with Mr. R. Sneath in Birmingham and have treated 13 consecutive children with osteosarcoma with primary chemotherapy. The results to date are at least as good as those for patients who are offered primary amputation with or without subsequent chemotherapy (9). Although we still regard this procedure as experimental, we see no reason at present to doubt that many children can safely by offered limb saving procedures without increasing the risk to their life from metastatic disease.

Treatment with primary chemotherapy has the further advantage that the effect can be assessed histologiclly when the primary tumour is resected. Those patients whose tumour shows a marked chemotherapy effect continue to receive the same chemotherapy as maintenance, whereas those patients who have little histological change in their tumour are given alternative forms of chemotherapy (10).

2.7. Medulloblastoma

Brain tumours are the most common group of solid tumours of childhood and medulloblastoma has in the past proved a singularly difficult problem. Refinement of neurosurgical and radiotherapy techniques has resulted in a substantial improvement in the prognosis in recent years and approximately half of the children with medulloblastoma are now long-term survivors, though many pay a considerable price in terms of sequelae (Fig. 7). The development of successful chemotherapy for brain tumours has lagged behind the development of chemotherapy for other paediatric tumours but the results of a recent multi-centre trial organised on an internatinoal basis by SIOP (International

Society of Paediatric Oncology) suggest that here too we may be beginn
make headway (11).

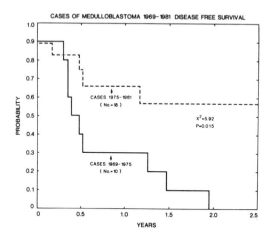

CASES OF MEDULLOBLASTOMA 1969–1981 DISEASE FREE SURVIVAL

FIGURE 7. Actuarial disease free survival of 28 children with medulloblastoma.

3. DISCUSSION

The treatment of childhood cancer has been progressively more successful
in recent years and an increasing proportion of children are long-term
survivors, cured of their primary malignancy. There is, however, an extra
dimension which has to receive high priority when considering what treatment
is appropriate for children, and that is the long-term effects of treatment on
growth and development, particularly the effects of radiation (12). It is,
however, apparent that it is not just physical growth which has to be
considered, but also growth in the intellectual and psycho-social spheres.
Many long-term survivors of childhood cancer in the past have paid a heavy
price for the eradication of their malignancy. Increasing malformations have
developed due to inadequate growth of bone and soft tissues; endocrine
deficiencies due to permanent damage to glands such as pituitary, thyroid, and
gonads; poor school performance either from intellectual impairment due to
cranial radiation or from loss of protracted periods of schooling. The need
to maintain a normal family environment despite the stresses and strains
imposed on everybody by the diagnosis and treatment is increasingly recognised
to be of vital importance if a child is to develop to his or her full
potential and to make the most of the life which is saved from cancer. All

st, therfore, be treated in a paediatric environment

s and expertise are available to deal with the many

of their illness, apart from the purely "oncologic"

radiation and chemotherapy. It is tempting to suggest that

patients requiring less intensive treatment no longer need the

ces of a specialist centre, but recent data about A.L.L. showed a

difference in 4 year survival of 58% vs. 40% (p<0.01) for patients treated in
conjunction with a specialist centre or not (13), and the importance of
receiving protocol treatment for Wilms' tumour has also been demonstrated
(14).

4. ACKNOWLEDGEMENTS

I am grateful to Jane Wadsworth and to Teresa Foxton for their help with
the statistical analyses. I also gratefully acknowledge the support of the
CLIC (Cancer and Leukaemia in Childhood) Trust and LRF (Leukaemia Research
Fund). The data presented are the results of the efforts of a large
multidisciplinary team, and I would like to thank the many people who
collaborate in our endeavours.

REFERENCES

1. Miller DR et al: Prognosic factors and therapy in acute lymphoblastic
    leukaemia of childhood: CCG-141. Cancer (51): 1041-1049, 1983.
2. Riehm H et al: The BFM studies 1970/76 and 1976/79 in childhood acute
    lymphoblastic leukaemia (ALL). In: Neth R (ed) Modern Advances in
    Leukemia IV. Springer-Verlag, Berlin, 1981, pp 87-93.
3. Donaldson SS: Hodgkin's disease. Treatment with low dose radiation and
    chemotherapy. Front Radiat Ther Onc (16): 122-133 (Karger, Basel), 1982.
4. D'Angio GJ et al: Wilms' tumour: An update. Cancer (45): 1791-1798, 1980.
5. Maurer H, Foulkes M, Gehan E: Intergroup rhabdomyosarcoma study (IRS)-II:
    Preliminary report. Proc. SIOP XV (Abstract): 103, 1983.
6. Price CHG, Jeffree GM: Metastatic spread of osteosarcoma. Br J Cancer
    (28): 515-524, 1973.
7. Rosen G et al: Chemotherapy and thoractomy for metastatic osteogenic
    sarcoma. A model for adjuvant chemotherapy and the rationale for the
    timing of thoracic surgery. Cancer (41): 841-849, 1978.
8. Marcove RC, Rosen G: En bloc resections for osteogenic sarcoma. Cancer
    (45): 3040-3044, 1980.
9. Burgers JMV, Voute PA, van Glabbeke M: OERTC-SIOP osteosarcoma trial. Proc
    SIOP XV (Abstract): 28-29, 1983.
10. Rosen G et al: Preoperative chemotherapy for osteogenic sarcoma. Selection
    of postoperative adjuvant chemotherapy based on the response of the
    primary tumour to preoperative chemotherapy. Cancer (49): 1221-1230, 1982.
11. Bloom HJG: Medulloblastoma in children: Increasing survival rates and
    further prospects. Int J Radiat Oncol Biol Phys (8): 2023-2027, 1982.
12. Rubin P, van Houtte P, Constine L: Radiation sensitivity and organ

tolerances in pediatric oncology: A new hypothesis. Front Radiat Ther Oncol (16): 62-82 (Karger, Basel), 1982.
13. Meadows AJ et al: Survival in childhood A.L.L. Cancer Investigation (1): 49-55, 1983.
14. Lennox EL et al: Nephroblastoma: The effect on survival of the first MRC trial. Brit Med J (2): 567-569, 1979.

CHEMOTHERAPY OF DISSEMINATED TESTICULAR CANCER

LAWRENCE H. EINHORN, M.D.

Testicular cancer is a relatively rare disease, accounting for only one percent of all male malignancy. Despite the relative paucity of new cases, testis cancer is an extremely important disease.

Platinum Plus Vinblastine Plus Bleomycin

In August, 1974, we began studies utilizing Platinum plus Vinblastine plus Bleomycin (PVB) in disseminated testicular cancer.

Thirty-three of 47 evaluable patients (70%) achieved complete remission. Five patients were rendered disease free following surgical removal of residual localized disease after significant reduction of tumor volume with chemotherapy.

These patients now have all been followed for seven years and they are all off chemotherapy for over five years.

From June, 1976, to June, 1978, we started a random prospective trial comparing our standard PVB with the same regimen using a 25% dosage reduction (0.3 mg/kg) for Vinblastine during remission induction.

Seventy-eight patients were entered on this study, and all patients have been followed for a minimum of four and a half years. The 25% reduction in the Vinblastine dosage resulted in the expected decrease in hematological toxicity.

The overall C.R. rate (68%) and surgical resection rate for localized residual disease (14%) were remarkably similar to our original PVB study. The therapeutic results are identical for the separate induction regimens. The relapse rate remained low, with all relapses occurring within one year of initiation of Platinum combination chemotherapy.

Fifty-three of 78 patients (68%) in this random prospective study remain continuously free of disease. In addition, five other patients are currently disease free with salvage chemotherapy with Platinum plus VP-16 plus combination chemotherapy (3). Thusly, 58 patients (74%) are currently alive and disease free, with minimum followup five years.

The role of maintenance therapy in disseminated testicular cancer had never been clearly established. It is quite possible that in a disease where remission induction therapy is so effective and C.R. can be defined so accurately (radioimmunoassay), HCG, AFP, lung tomograms, and computed abdominal tomography), maintenance therapy may be unnecessary. To test this hypothesis, we began a third generation study June, 1978, randomizing patients achieving C.R. to standard maintenance Vinblastine (0.3 mg/kg monthly for 21 months) vs. no maintenance therapy after the 12 weeks of remission induction therapy.

If a patient achieved a complete remission with chemotherapy alone, or if he had complete surgical resection of disease that histopathologically was teratoma, the patient was then eligible for the randomization for maintenance Vinblastine vs. no further therapy. Note is made of the fact that, if a patient had surgical resection of residual disease which was still viable carcinoma, even though the patient was then disease free following surgery, the patient was not placed on the maintenance program, as such patients receive two "adjuvant" courses of Platinum, Vinblastine, and Bleomycin.

One hundred and seventy-one evaluable patients were the subject of this study, and the minimum followup on this patient population is two and a half years. There was no obvious difference in the ability of either regimen to produce a complete remission or a disease free status with the addition of surgical resection of persistent disease, and maintenance therapy was found to be unnecessary.

Salvage Therapy

Although 80% of patients with disseminated testicular cancer will achieve a disease free status with Platinum plus Vinblastine plus Bleomycin (either with chemotherapy alone or surgical resection of residual disease), there still remains a patient population eligible for salvage therapy. These, of course, are those patients who fail to ever achieve a disease free status or those patients who relapse after complete eradication of disease with primary therapy.

Prior to the introduction of VP-16 in 1978, salvage chemotherapy consisted of a variety of treatment programs including Platinum plus Adriamycin, Platinum plus Adriamycin plus Vincristine plus Bleomycin, or if the patient was refractory to Platinum, Actinomycin-D-based chemotherapy, Adriamycin plus Cyclophosphamide, or numerous other treatment programs. Prior to 1978, we never achieved a one year continuous disease free survival with any treatment program. Furthermore, in 31 drug trials in 22 patients, we failed to ever achieve a partial remission or complete remission in any patient with non-platinum therapy (for example, Adriamycin plus Cyclophosphamide, etc.).

In a patient who has unresectable partial remission following Platinum plus Vinblastine plus Bleomycin, it has been our policy to maintain them on Vinblastine maintenance therapy until they show evidence of progressive disease. At the time they progress, they are refractory only to Vinblastine, and such patients are treated with salvage chemotherapy with Platinum plus VP-16 plus Bleomycin at that time. We prefer that approach in contrast to the immediate introduction of Platinum plus VP-16 plus Bleomycin after Platinum plus Vinblastine plus Bleomycin because there are occasional patients who are serologically negative and have an unresectable partial remission who, in reality, are already cured of their disease, because what we are visualizing radiographically is just necrotic fibrous tissue.

The two drug combination of Platinum plus VP-16 has been found to be highly synergistic in preclinical studies (4).

VP-16 has had more extensive single agent trials than Vinblastine, and with more impressive results, realizing the drug was utilized in an extremely refractory patient population. This response rate is quite remarkable when one considers that, in our extensive experience, we have never seen an objective response with any form of chemotherapy once a patient progressed on Platinum combination chemotherapy (i.e., actually progressed within four weeks of the last Platinum dosage).

The initial results with Platinum plus VP-16 plus Bleomycin plus Adriamycin salvage therapy have already been published (3). The updated results are shown below.

Response (N=45)

	Number (%)
C.R.	11 (24%)
P.R.	30 (67%)
NED with Surgery	13 (29%)
Teratoma	7
Carcinoma	6 (received 2 post-op courses of salvage therapy)

Current Status (N=45)

Continuously NED	17 (38%)
Presently NED	18 (40%)
Followup 24-51 months:	Median 37 months

We have deleted Adriamycin from the salvage therapy as we felt it added to the hematologic and mucosal toxicity without adding to the therapeutic efficacy.

Our present salvage program utilizes Platinum 20 mg/M^2 x 5 days plus VP-16 100 mg/M^2 x 5 days q 3 weeks x 4 plus Bleomycin 30 units on Day 1 every 3 weeks x 4 (total 120 units). This therapy is applicable for any patient who is not refractory to any of the three study drugs (i.e., no progression within four weeks of the last Platinum or Bleomycin therapy). This salvage program can produce formidable myelosuppression because it is employed in a heavily pretreated patient population. However, the 40% apparent cure rate in a patient population that previously had a zero cure rate is significant testimony to the activity of this regimen. At the present time, we are conducting our fourth generation study randomizing patients with testicular cancer to receive Platinum plus Vinblastine plus Bleomycin vs. Platinum plus VP-16 plus Bleomycin as first line therapy. Although VP-16 has more thrombocytopenia, it has no neuromuscular toxicity (compared to Vinblastine).

Summary

Testicular cancer has become a landmark tumor, as it is a model for a curable neoplasm. The serial development of accurate tumor markers, demonstration of apparent synergism of Vinblastine, plus Bleomycin, discovery of activity of Platinum, combination of PVB, application of surgical resection of post-chemotherapy residual disease, and the use of VP-16 salvage therapy have all been important. It is hoped that similar strategies may yield success in other solid tumors.

References

1. Mackay EN and Sellers AH: A statistical review of malignant testicular tumors based on the experience of the Ontario Cancer Foundation Clinics, 1938-1961. Can Med Assoc J 94:889-899, 1966.
2. Einhorn LH, Williams SD, Mandelbaum I, and Donohue J: Surgical resection in disseminated testicular cancer following chemotherapeutic cytoreduction. Cancer 48: 904-908, 1981.
3. Williams SD, Einhorn LH, Greco FA, Oldham R, and Fletcher R: VP-16-213 salvage therapy for refractory germinal neoplasms. Cancer 46:2154-2158, 1980.
4. Schabel FM Jr, Trader NW, Laster WR Jr: Cis-dichloro-diammineplatinum (II): Combination chemotherapy and cross-resistance studies with tumors of mice. Cancer Treat Rep 63:1549-1473, 1979.

RATIONAL APPROACH TO THE MANAGEMENT OF FEBRILE GRANULOCYTOPENIC PATIENTS.

H. LAGAST and J. KLASTERSKY.

It has been shown since 1966 (1) that infection is related to the absolute level of granulocytes. When the granulocyte count is below 100/μ 1, the patient is at the greatest risk of severe infections and gram-negative bacteremias are common (2).

Reducing the duration of neutropenia and the related risk of infection are the aim of various methods of prophylaxis. These methods can be classified into 4 groups : enhancement of host defense mechanisms, lowering of the acquisition of new potential pathogens, suppressing colonizing organisms and avoiding invasive procedures and damage to body barriers.

Prophylactic granulocyte transfusions and the J5 antiserum are 2 examples of the first type of prophylactic methods. Overall, there is no significant decrease of the infection rate among the patients receiving prophylactic granulocyte transfusions (3). When HLA matched donors are used for transfusion, they developed anemia (4); alloimmunization results from the transfusion of granulocytes from random donors.

Most of the gram-negative bacilli share an antigen core which is similar from species to species (5). By vaccinating normal volunteers with this antigen, it is possible to collect hyperimmnune plasma and to infuse it to patients with suspected or proven gram-negative septicemia. A large multicentric trial showed a significant reduction of mortality in patients with hypotension or profound shock (6). However, the reduction of mortality in patients with cancer and/or neutropenia did not reach statistical significance and needs therefore further investigation.

The combined use of a laminar air flow room and oral nonabsorbable antibiotics leads to a substantial reduction in the number of severe infections in cancer patients.(3). However, patient's survival does not increase as the result of these prophylactic measures. Only recently a

141

controlled study showed a decreased incidence of severe graft-versus-host disease leading to an increase of survival in bone marrow transplanted patients (7). It should be stressed that gastro-intestinal decontamination exerts only its maximum benefit when the patient is profoundly granulocyptopenic (less than 100 granulocytes/μl) and that the patient's compliance is a prerequisite for effectiveness.

When fever (temperature above 38°C) arises in a granulocytopenic patient without an obvious source such as blood products transfusion or chemotherapy including bleomycin, there is a need for a careful examination of the patient and a rapid collection of bacteriological specimens. Empiric antimicrobial therapy should promptly be initiated; gram-negative bacilli (E. coli, K. pneumoniae and P. aeruginosa) being the commonest pathogens in microbiologically documented infections, they should be covered by broad-spectrum combinations of antibiotics (8). These combinations should be synergistic and provide a highly bactericidal effect on the possible pathogens. Several studies showed a marked increase of clinical effectiveness of synergistic antibiotic regimens in gram-negative bacillary infections in granulocytopenic patients (9 - 12).

A serum bactericidal activity $\geqslant$ 1:16 is to be achieved in order to obtain a good chance of clinical success in profoundly granulocytopenic patients (13). On the fourth day of treatment with this type of therapy, 70 % of the patients will have an overall improvment. In some of these, granulocytopenia subsides and they should be treated as non granulocytopenic patients. When granulocytopenia persists, a prolonged therapy (until granulocytes > 500/μl) has no advantage over the same therapy administered for a total of 9 days only. The remaining patients (30 % of the treated patients), whether they have a documented infection or no focus of infection, do not respond to the empiric therapy.

When the infection is documented and empiric therapy is failing, antimicrobial therapy needs to be adjusted to the sensitivity of the pathogen and, if needed, the antibiotic dosage should be increased in order to achieve a serum bactericidal level $\geqslant$ 1:16. These patients should be investigated for localized infections and treated in consequence. Therapeutic granulocyte transfusions are to be considered and initiated, if available; several studies show a beneficial effect of granulocyte transfusions in patients with documented infection and no bone marrow recovery. (14).

If no microbiological source has been found for the febrile episode, occult fungal infection should be suspected and empiric amphotericin B initiated. Early empiric therapy with amphotericin B leads to a reduction of deaths due to fungal infection in this clinical situation (15). The combined use of granulocyte transfusion and amphotericin B was the cause of pulmonary infiltrates in one study (16). Nevertheless, this approach is now less frequently used.

To summarize the management of febrile granulocytopenic patients, the following scheme is recommended.

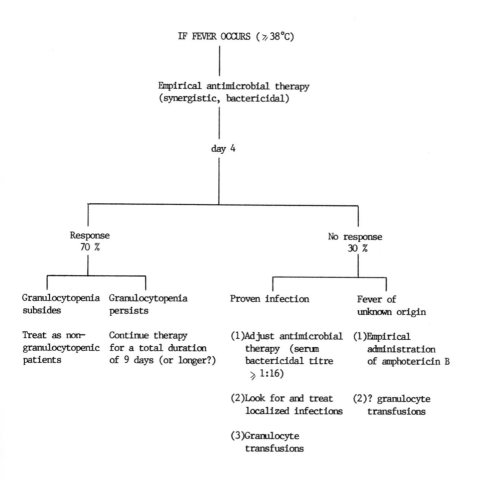

IF FEVER OCCURS (⩾ 38°C)

Empirical antimicrobial therapy
(synergistic, bactericidal)

day 4

	Response 70 %		No response 30 %
Granulocytopenia subsides	Granulocytopenia persists	Proven infection	Fever of unknown origin
Treat as non-granulocytopenic patients	Continue therapy for a total duration of 9 days (or longer?)	(1)Adjust antimicrobial therapy (serum bactericidal titre ⩾ 1:16) (2)Look for and treat localized infections (3)Granulocyte transfusions	(1)Empirical administration of amphotericin B (2)? granulocyte transfusions

References

1. Bodey GP, Buckley M, Sathe YS, Freireich EJ : Quantitative relationship between circulating leukocytes and infection in patients with acute leukemia. Am. Intern. Med. (64) : 328-340, 1966.
2. Schimpf SC, Hahn DM, Brouillet MD. Infection prevention in acute leukemia comparison of basic invection prevention techniques, with standard room reverse isolation or with reverse isolation plus added air filtration. Leuk Res (2) : 231-240, 1978.
3. Schimpf SC. Infection prevention during granulocytopenia. In Current Clinical topics in infectious diseases. Ed. JS Remington and MN Swartz, 1980, Mc Graw-Hill, New-York, pp 85-106.
4. Clift RA, Sanders JE, Thomas ED, Williams B, Buckner CD : Granulocyte transfusions for the prevention of infection in patients receiving bone- marrow transplants. New Engl. J. Med. (298) : 1052-1057, 1978.
5. Braude AI, Ziegler EJ, Douglas H, Mc CUtcham JA : Antibody to cell wall glycolipid of gram-negative bacteria : induction of immunity to bacteremia and endotoxemia. J. Infect. Dis. (136) : 167-173, 1977.
6. Ziegler EJ, Mc Cutchan JA, Fierer J, Glauser MP, Sadoff JC, Douglas H, Braude AI : Treatment of gram-negative bacteremia and shock with human antiserum to a mutant Escherichia coli. New Engl. J. Med (307) : 1225-1230, 1982.
7. Storb R, Prentice RL, Buckner CD, Clift RA, Appelbaum F, Deeg J, Doney K, Hansen JA, Mason M, Sanders JE, Singer J, Sullivan KM, Witherspoon, Thomas ED : Graft-versus-host disease and survival in patients with aplastic anemia treated by marrow grafts from HLA-identical siblings. N. Engl. J. Med. (308) : 302-307, 1983.
8. EORTC International Antimicrobial Therapy Project Group : Three antibiotic regimens in the treatment of infection in febrile granulocytopenic patients with cancer. Europ. J. Cancer & Clin. Oncol. (in press).
9. Klastersky J, Cappel R, Daneau D. Clinical significance of in vitro synergism between antibiotics in gram-negative infections. Antimicrob. Ag. Chemother. (2) : 470-475, 1972.
10. Klastersky J, Meunier-Carpentier F, Prevost JM. Significance of antimicrobial synergism for the outcome of gram-negative sepsis. Am. J. Med. Sci. (273) : 157-167, 1977.
11. Lau WK, Young LS, Black RE, Winston DJ, Linner SR, Weinstein RJ, Hewitt WL. Comparative efficacy and toxicity of amikacin/carbenicillin versus gentamicin/carbenicillin in leucopenic patients. A randomized prospective trial. Am. J. Med. (62) : 959-966 or 212-219, 1977.
12. Anderson ET, Young LS, Hewitt WL. Antimicrobial synergism in the therapy of gram-negative rod bacteremia. Chemotherapy (24) : 45-54, 1978.
13. Klastersky J. Clinical significance of the serum bactericidal activity. 13th International Congress of Chemotherapy, Vienna, 1983.
14. Klastersky J. Granulocyte transfusions as a therapy and a prophylaxis of infections in neutropenic patients. Europ. J. Cancer (15) : 15-22,1979.
15. Pizzo PA, Robichaud KJ, Gill FA, Witebsky FG. Empiric antibiotic an antifungal therapy for cancer patients with prolonged fever and granulocytopenia. Amer. J. Med. (72) : 101-111, 1982.
16. Wright DG, Robichaud KJ, Pizzo PA, Deisserath AD. Lethal pulmonary reactions associated with the combined use of amphotericin B and leukocyte transfusions. New. Engl. J. Med. 304 : 1185-1189, 1981.

CHAPTER II

CONTROL OF PAIN AND VOMITING IN CANCER PATIENTS

EFFECTIVE USE OF NARCOTIC ANALGESICS

R.G. TWYCROSS

Pain occurs in about 2/3 of patients with far-advanced cancer. It
is not always caused by the neoplasm itself; an important fact when
considering the place of narcotic analgesics in cancer pain management.
Further, some cancer induced pains are more responsive to narcotics than
others. For example, in metastatic bone pain a local high concentration
of prostaglandins "sensitizes" the nerve endings and, pharmacologically,
the best result is usually obtained by the combined use of a prostaglandin
synthetase inhibitor (aspirin, etc.) and a centrally acting narcotic.
The site of the neurological lesion, and the type of pain, also determine
how effective narcotics will be (Table 1). These factors are responsible
for the evolving science of "co-analgesics".

Table 1. Neurological classification of pain: implications for therapy

Type of pain	Treatment
1. Nociceptive	analgesics
2. Nerve compression	analgesics
	corticosteroids
	nerve blocks
3. Nerve destruction	psychotropic drugs
(dysaesthetic)	(especially antidepressants)
peripheral nerve-)	narcotics
occasionally useful;)	corticosteroids
cord lesion-)	nerve blocks
of no benefit)	cordotomy

There is need also to appreciate fully the "somatopsychic" nature
of pain. Pain is a dual phenomenon. One part is the perception of a

147

sensation and the other the patient's emotional reaction to it.
Attention must be given to factors that modulate pain sensitivity such
as anxiety, depression, fatigue, boredom, loneliness and hostility.
Failure to do so may result in potentially relievable pain remaining
intractable.

PRINCIPLES OF ANALGESIC USE

Analgesics, both nonnarcotic and narcotic, remain the backbone of
cancer pain management. Yet their use is not synonymous with analgesia.
Analgesics can never be more than part of a comprenhensive multi-modality
approach to pain control.

Keep it simple

The three basic analgesics are aspirin, codeine and morphine. The
rest should all be considered alternatives of fashion or convenience.
Appreciating this helps to prevent the doctor "kangarooing" from analgesic
to analgesic in a desperate search for some drug that will suit his
patient better.   If a nonnarcotic-weak narcotic preparation such as
aspirin-codeine or paracetamol-dextropropoxyphene fails to relieve, it
is usually best to move directly to a small dose of oral morphine sulphate.

It is necessary to be familiar with one or two alternatives for
use in patients who cannot tolerate the standard preparation. Aspirin
has two alternatives. Paracetamol (acetaminophen), which has no anti-
inflammatory effect, is one; nonsteroidal anti-inflammatory drugs, as a
group, is the other. Which alternative is appropriate depends on whether
there is need for a peripheral anti-inflammatory effect. The individual
doctor's basic analgesic ladder, with alternatives, should comprise no
more than 9 or 10 drugs in total. It is better to know and understand
a few drugs well than to have a passing **acquaintance** with the whole range.
The following should be noted:

    i. With mild or moderate pain, use a nonnarcotic initially.

    ii. It may be appropriate to continue to prescribe aspirin despite
        the use of a narcotic, especially in patients with bone pain.

    iii. It is logical to combine analgesics that act via different
        mechanisms. For example, aspirin and paracetamol; paracetamol
        and codeine; aspirin and morphine. Though it is not always wise
        to do so from the point of view of patient compliance, nor is
        it always therapeutically necessary.

iv. It is pharmacological nonsense to prescribe two weak narcotics simultaneously; likewise two strong narcotics.

v. It is sometimes justifiable for a patient on a strong narcotic to have another narcotic (weak or strong) as a second "as required" analgesic for occasional, troublesome pain. Generally, though, patients should be advised to take an extra dose of their regular medication if pain breaks through the "analgesic cover".

vi. If one weak narcotic preparation does not control the pain, do not waste time by prescribing an alternative; move to something definitely stronger.

vii. Morphine or an alternative strong narcotic should be used when nonnarcotics and weak narcotics fail to control the pain.

viii. "Morphine exists to be given, not merely to be withheld". The severity of the pain determines the choice of analgesic, not the doctor's estimate of life expectancy, which is often wrong. A patient should not be made to wait in pain until the last days of life.

ix. The top of the analgesic ladder is not reached simply by prescribing morphine. Morphine may be given in a wide range of doses from as little as 2.5 mg to more than 1g.

x. Do not use short acting preparations like pentazocine (weak), pethidine (intermediate) and dextromoramide (strong narcotic).

xi. Do not prescribe a narcotic agonist-antagonist (e.g. pentazocine), buprenorphine) with a narcotic agonist (i.e. codeine, morphine).

Use oral medication

The route of administration is a significant consideration because it has substantial impact on the patient's way of life. The patient taking oral medication is free to move around, travel in a car and, most important, be at home. Oral narcotics are effective provided the patient is not vomiting repeatedly.

Doses should be determined on an individual basis

The effective analgesic dose varies considerably from patient to patient. The right dose of an analgesic is that which gives adequate relief for at least 3 and preferably 4 or more hours. "Maximum" or "recommended" doses, derived mainly from post-operative parenteral single dose studies, are not applicable in cancer. The dose of morphine and other strong narcotic agonists can be increased almost indefinitely. On the other hand, the nonnarcotics, weak narcotic agonists and narcotic agonist-antagonist all reach a plateau of maximum effect after 2 or 3 upward dose adjustments. Thus, if the upper effective dose has been reached with one of these agents, the dose should not be increased further but a stronger drug should be prescribed.

Persistent pain requires prophylactic (preventative) therapy

To allow pain to re-emerge before administering the next dose not only causes unnecessary suffering but encourages tolerance. "Four-hourly as required" (PRN medication) has no place in the treatment of persistent pain. Whatever the cause continuous pain requires regular preventative therapy. The aim is to titrate the dose of the analgesic against the pain, gradually increasing the dose until the patient is pain-free. The next dose is given before the effect of the previous one has worn off and, therefore, before the patient may think it necessary. In this way it is possible to erase the memory and fear of pain.

For codeine and morphine a four hourly regimen is optimal. If a strong analgesic other than morphine is used, the physician must be familiar with its pharmacology. For example, pethidine is effective for an average of two to three hours. Yet, it is commonly boarded to be given every four or six hours. This is clearly insufficient, and forces the patient to be in pain for perhaps three out of every six hours. Levorphanol and phenazocine are often satisfactory when given every six hours; and methadone every 6-8 hours.

Not all pain is responsive to analgesics

Narcotics do not usually relieve pain caused by degenerative nerve damage (dysaesthetic and stabbing pains: Table 1), but the occasional patient does respond.

Adjuvant medication is generally necessary

Laxatives are almost always necessary for patients receiving a narcotic. Unless the doctor is fairly experienced, an antiemetic is best prescribed routinely with morphine or other strong narcotic, at least for the first 5-7 days. As already noted, there are many situations where a better result is obtained by adding a second drug rather than increasing the dose of morphine indefinitely.

Do not use mixtures routinely

At some centres, morphine is always prescribed with a second drug, either cocaine (a stimulant) or a phenothiazine (a tranquillizer). Sometimes both are added. In these circumstances, increasing the dose

of morphine can be hazardous if, by increasing the volume of the
mixture taken, the dose of the adjunctive medication is automatically
increased also, regardless of need.   Depending on the adjunctive drug,
this can lead to agitation and restlessness or to somnolence. It is
far better to give adjunctive medication separately. The dose of each
pharmacologically active substance can then be adjusted individually
against patient need.

Psychotropic drugs should not be used routinely

If the patient is very anxious, an anxiolytic should be prescribed.
If a patient remains depressed after 1-2 weeks of much improved pain
relief, an antidepressant may be necessary.

Insomnia must be treated vigorously

Discomfort is worse at night when the patient is alone with his
pain and his fears. The cumulative effect of many sleepless, pain-filled
nights is a substantial lowering of the patient's pain threshold with a
concomitant increase in pain intensity. Sometimes, it is necessary to
use morphine at night in patients well-controlled during the day by a
weak narcotic; or to use a much larger dose of morphine at bedtime to
relieve pains that are particularly troublesome when lying down for a
prolonged period.

It is sometimes necessary to balance degree of relief against unwanted
side effects

Examples include aspirin and gastric irritation, and morphine and
gastric stasis. Generally, there are ways round these problems but
occasionally a compromise is necessary.

Monitor progress

All cancer patients prescribed analgesics, whether nonnarcotic or
narcotic, need close supervision to achieve optimum comfort with minimal
side effects. Initial treatment review is sometimes necessary within
hours, normally within 1-2 days, and always after the first week.
Subsequent follow up will vary according to psychological and therapeutic
needs.   New pains develop and old pains may re-emerge. A fresh complaint
of pain demands re-assessment; not just a message to increase pain
medication, though this may be an important first-aid measure.

FURTHER READING

Twycross, RG and Lack, SA. Symptom control in far-advanced cancer:
pain relief. Pitman Books, London, 1983, 334 pp.

A DOUBLE BLIND CROSS-OVER STUDY OF TWO ORAL FORMULATIONS OF MORPHINE

J. WELSH, J.F.B. STUART, T. HAVESHAW, P. BILLIAERT AND K.C. CALMAN

1. ABSTRACT

Fifteen patients suffering pain as a result of various malignancies completed this study. Both MST Continus 30mg tablets and morphine sulphate solution (B.P.), were found to be acceptable and on a milligram equivalency shown to be comparable in their analgesic activity.

Both presentations improved sleep patterns significantly when compared with the duration of sleep recorded prior to the trial. The incidence and severity of side effects for each formulation followed almost identical patterns.

2. INTRODUCTION

There is widespread fear among cancer sufferers and relatives that during the natural history of the disease pain will become a significant, if not uncontrollable, problem. The incidence and severity of pain tends to be related to the extent, nature and stage of the malignancy. Several studies have shown that the incidence of pain in patients with advanced cancers is approximately 70% (1-4). It is a disquieting fact that many experiencing pain do not have this fully or adequately alleviated (3). It is possible with existing analgesics and pain treatment options to assure patients that if pain develops it can be removed or at least reduced in intensity.

Extracts from the opium poppy (Papaver somniferum) were used therapeutically by the Sumerians 4,000 years B.C. (5). The chief, active component of the extract, morphine, has been used over the centuries by the ancient Egyptians, Greeks and Romans but it was not until the Seventeenth Century that morphine was introduced to Britain (6).

Morphine has a half-life of 2.2 hours (7) and thus in patients with a persistent cause for their pain the drug must be administered frequently and regularly to prevent the occurrence of break through pain. Formulations containing morphine which have a longer duration of action have been produced

153

in the past few years. The principle of determining the pharmacokinetics, efficacy and toxicity of any new drug must equally apply to a novel formulation of an existing drug.

Hence this study was designed to determine the efficacy of M.S.T. Continus 30mg tablets in the control of severe pain secondary to cancer and also to assess the incidence and intensity of this preparation's side effects, in comparison with those of standard morphine sulphate solution B.P.

3. PATIENTS, METHODS AND MATERIALS

Eligibility for entry to the study involved the presence of pain of a severity judged to require opiates for control, in patients known to have a histologically documented malignant disease. Twenty-two patients commenced the trial having given their verbal informed consent.

There were nine males and thirteen females, median age fifty-five years. Of these seven were unable to complete the study (two males, five females; median age fifty-seven years). Urea and electrolytes, transaminase and bilirubin levels of all participants were within normal range.

Initially patients were stabilised on M.S.T. Continus 30mg tablets. As this was an outpatient study this procedure took one to two weeks to achieve satisfactory pain control. The patients were then randomised to receive either M.S.T. Continus 30mg tablets and placebo elixir or morphine sulphate solution B.P. in a milligram (mg) equivalent dose plus placebo tablets. After one week of treatment crossover was made to the other regime. Tablets were prescribed twice daily, twelve hours apart, and elixir every four hours. Apart from non-steroidal anti-inflammatory agents all other analgesics were discontinued upon entry. Assessment of pain relief was made by means of a Visual Analogue Scale (V.A.S.) completed by the patient at the following times: stabilisation period, day 0, 3 and 5; first week of study, day 2, 4 and 7; second week, day 9, 11 and 14. In addition duration of sleep was noted prior to stabilisation and throughout the study. Side-effects were scored, again by the patient, on a zero to three scale, three representing the most severe and zero no toxicity. Scoring was performed on a daily basis in a specially designed booklet which also had provision for recording drug compliance. All patients were reviewed weekly throughout the study period.

4. RESULTS

After completion of the trial the mean V.A.S. score after seven days of each arm was expressed as a percentage as shown in Table 1.

Table 1.   Mean V.A.S. score % after seven days therapy

	Stabilisation	Tablet	Elixir
Sleep	19.07	25.00	33.93
	SD $\pm$14.36	$\pm$27.45	$\pm$31.86
Night pain	21.64	25.57	28.79
	$\pm$15.26	$\pm$29.82	$\pm$28.99
Day pain	18.93	33.29	33.79
	$\pm$13.77	$\pm$26.35	$\pm$28.82

[n = 15.   No significant difference exists between scores for stabilisation, tablet or elixir.   (Students t-test)]

Three patients required fourteen days for stabilisation and thus score on day 14 was used in the calculation.

The effect of the two formulations on hours slept per night is shown in Table 2.

Table 2.

	Hours of sleep per night
Start of stabilisation	5.21 ± 1.78
After elixir for seven days	6.72 ± 1.54
After tablets for seven days	6.92 ± 2.06

Significance (Student's t-test)

Tablet : Elixir > 0.5
Tablet : Stabilisation <0.05> 0.02
Elixir : Stabilisation <0.05> 0.02

There was no significant difference in the percentage of patients experiencing side effects when on the tablets or the elixir. The most common side effect was transient drowsiness. Constipation was experienced in 71%, with nausea, vomiting and dizziness being the other toxicities encountered.

The intensity of side effects is as shown in Table 3.

Table 3. Intensity of side effects n = 15

		Tablet (mean score)		Elixir (mean score)
A	Drowsiness	10.54	A	9.3
B	Constipation	7.0	B	7.9
C	Nausea	4.7	C	6.5
D	Vomiting	3.5	D	2.9
E	Dizziness	1.5	E	2.0

$P > 0.5$ for A:A ; B:B etc.

Scoring was by means of a zero to three scale with maximum intensity of three for each side effect per 24 hours or twenty one over seven days.

Five patients withdrew from the study (including one who died) during the stabilisation period. One of those five was unable to complete the evaluation form, two had unacceptable nausea and vomiting despite anti-emetics and one patient when randomised refused to continue with the elixir. One patient developed severe pain after randomisation to the active elixir and required hospitalisation for adequate pain control and accordingly was also withdrawn from the study.

5. CONCLUSIONS

To facilitate the cancer patient's endeavour to live his life as near as possible to the standard he "enjoyed" prior to the development of his illness must be one of the paramount aims of those involved in the care of cancer patients. The development of the chronic pain syndrome defeats this objective. Thus the importance of adequate pain relief cannot be overstressed. While it is admitted that no formal attempt was made to assess the effect of this study on the participant's psychological state and its relationship to the pain experience, it was the impression that those recruited were well adjusted to, and coping reasonably well with, their disease.

No significant difference in V.A.S. score for pain was recorded at the end of seven days stabilisation (on active tablets) after seven days active elixir or after seven days active M.S.T. Continus 30mg tablets. From this we conclude that the formulation of M.S.T. Continus tablets is as efficacious as morphine sulphate solution on a milligram equivalent basis per unit time, providing that the pain process is not altering over the assessment period. Description of pain or its assessment is notoriously difficult, hence the wide S.D. in Table 1. We chose the V.A.S. as one of the most efficient means of quantifying this purely subjective phenomenon (8). The order of incidence of side-effects encountered in this study is much as recorded by Kantor (9). Drowsiness was transient over forty-eight to seventy-two hours and nausea controllable in all but two of the twenty-two patients. Use of a sustained release formulation might reasonably be expected to reduce the intensity and incidence of side effects, if the latter are related to large plasma fluctuations or high peak concentrations of the drug. However, this was not the case and there was no significant difference between the two presentations with respect to side effects.

In conclusion morphine sulphate formulated as M.S.T. Continus 30mg tablets is a generally acceptable preparation which sustains plasma morphine levels (10) and in a mg equivalent dose provides equivalent analgesia to morphine sulphate solution B.P. with a similar intensity and incidence of side effects. The tablet form is more convenient for carriage, and the twice or thrice daily dosage regime may lead to greater patient compliance.

5. ACKNOWLEDGEMENTS

Gratitude is expressed to Miss M. Richardson, Principal Pharmacist and Mrs. Jane Shaw, Pharmacist, and other members of the Pharmacy Department, Gartnavel General Hospital, Glasgow and to Miss L. Mills for her help in co-ordinating patients in the trial and also to Mrs. E. Singleton for her assistance with co-ordination and gathering of data. Thank you to Mrs. S. Cochrane for her timely secretarial help. Finally mention should be made of Napp Laboratories, Cambridge, who kindly supplied the M.S.T. Continus and placebo tablets and to Miss V. Woods and Dr. J. Dewhurst who helped in mobilising the study. The Cancer Research Campaign is also acknowledged for partial funding. Grant No. SP L429/P2.

REFERENCES

1. Cartwright A, Hockey L and Anderson ABM: Life Before Death. Routledge and Kegan Paul, London. 1973.
2. Foley KM: Pain syndromes in patients with cancer. In: Bonica JJ and Ventafridda V (eds) Advances in Pain Research and Therapy, Vol 2. Raven Press, New York, 1979, pp 59-75.
3. Parkes CM: Home or hospital? Terminal care as seen by surviving spouse. J R Coll Gen Pract (d28): 19-30, 1978.
4. Twycross RG: Clinical management with diamorphine in advanced malignant disease. Int J Clin Pharmacol (93): 184-198, 1974.
5. Emboden J: Narcotic Plants. Steedia Vista, London. 1972.
6. Wootton AC: Wootton's Chronicles of Pharmacy III. MacMillan & Co Ltd, London. 1910.
7. Brunk SF and Delle M: Morphine Metabolism in Men. Clin Pharmac Ther (16): 51-57, 1974.
8. Huskisson EC: Measurement of pain. Lancet 1127-1131, 1974.
9. Kantor TG, Hopper M and Laska E: Adverse effects of commonly ordered oral narcotics. J Clin Pharmacol (21): 1-8, 1981.
10. Welsh J, Stuart JFB, Haveshaw T, Blackie RGG, Whitehill D, Setanoians A, Milsted RAV and Calman KC: A comparative pharmacokinetic study of morphine sulphate solution and MST Continus 30mg tablets in conditions expected to allow steady-state drug levels. Roy Soc Med 2nd Congress and Symposium (58): 9-12, 1983.

NON-NARCOTICS AND CO-ANALGESICS

G.W. HANKS

NON-NARCOTIC ANALGESICS

Aspirin and Paracetamol

Aspirin and other non-steroidal antiinflammatory drugs (NSAIDs) and paracetamol are the most important of the non-narcotic analgesics. As simple analgesics they have equal potency but paracetamol is generally better tolerated, particularly with regard to gastrointestinal side-effects[1]. Paracetamol is preferable for use where no antiinflammatory action is required and the usual dose is 1g four hourly, or as required.

In recent years much has been made of the analgesic as opposed to the antiinflammatory effect of various NSAIDs. All members of this group of drugs have analgesic properties and there is no pharmacological or clinical evidence that drugs such as zomepirac (now withdrawn) or ibuprofen differ significantly from other NSAIDs. Nor do they appear to be more potent than aspirin or paracetamol. Paracetamol has no effect on prostaglandin synthetase (PS) in peripheral tissues, though it is a potent PS inhibitor within the CNS. Whilst there is some evidence that it has antiinflammatory activity in acute inflammatory conditions it is in no way comparable in this respect with the NSAIDs.

Benorylate

Benorylate is a lipid soluble ester of acetylsalicylic acid and para-cetamol which is well absorbed from the stomach and causes less gastric irritation and blood loss than aspirin. It is de-esterified to produce approximately 600mg of aspirin and 400mg of paracetamol from each gram and is a useful alternative to aspirin or other NSAIDs. The usual dose is 5 - 10mls (2-4g) b.i.d.; tablets (of 750mg) are also available.

159

Nefopam

Nefopam is chemically related to the antihistamine diphenhydramine and was originally investigated as a muscle relaxant. It has neither anti-inflammatory or opioid activity; the mode of action of its analgesic effect is unknown. Estimates of its potency vary from one third to one half that of morphine when given by intramuscular injection. After oral administration it appears to be no more potent than aspirin[2]. Clinical experience with nefopam is limited and it does not appear to have any particular advantages over more conventional analgesics for routine use. It may however have a place (used parenterally) in the treatment of moderate to severe pain in the rare patient who is unable to tolerate opioids.

CO-ANALGESICS

A co-analgesic is any drug (or device) which may not have intrinsic analgesic activity but which when used in conjunction with a conventional analgesic will contribute significantly to pain relief.

Psychotropics

Anxiety, depression, fear, restlessness and sleeplessness may all significantly reduce a patient's pain threshold and exacerbate pain complaints. All of these symptoms will respond to psychotropic medication with a consequent reduction in pain or a greater ability to tolerate it or cope with it. The benzodiazepines are the most useful group of drugs for the management of these symptoms in cancer patients because of their wide therapeutic index and small potential for interacting with other agents. Diazepam remains the first choice sedative anxiolytic (used in a single night-time dose of 5 to 20mg or in divided doses) and clobazam is a suitable alternative which produces less impairment of psychomotor performance and cognitive function (10mg being equivalent in anxiolytic activity to 5mg of diazepam). Short-acting benzodiazepine hypnotics such as temazepam (10-40mg nocte) are preferable to long-acting drugs such as nitrazepam and flurazepam, which are potent hangover producing medications.

The phenothiazines have traditionally been used as adjuncts to narcotics in cancer patients because of their antiemetic and sedative effects and because it has been widely believed that they have a specific analgesic potentiating action. A critical review of the literature indicates that the evidence for any analgesic or analgesic potentiating effect of these drugs has been exaggerated and is unconvincing[3]. Phenothiazines often produce excessive sedation, are associated with anticholinergic and cardiovascular side-effects, and lower seizure threshold. The benzodiazepines are not associated with these side-effects and thus have significant advantages in cancer patients where an anxiolytic or sedative effect is desired. Phenothiazines should be reserved for situations where their specific antiemetic or antipsychotic properties are required. Even then haloperidol may be a better alternative because of its relative lack of sedative, anticholinergic and cardiovascular effects and its long duration of action which permits single or twice daily dosing[3] (1.5-5mg nocte or bd as an antiemetic).

Antidepressants are widely used in the management of chronic non-cancer pain. As with the phenothiazines the evidence that they possess intrinsic analgesic activity is lacking, though there are grounds for believing that they may enhance or reduce the effects of narcotic analgesics depending on their action on central monoamine neurotransmitters[3]. Drugs which enhance serotoninergic mechanisms appear to potentiate opioid analgesics whereas antidepressants with noradrenergic activity may attenuate opioid analgesia. The clinical relevance of these interactions has yet to be elucidated.

Sadness and depressed mood are common in patients with cancer and are a normal emotional response to the illness: they are unlikely to respond to pharmacological measures. The diagnosis of morbid depression which will be amenable to drug therapy in such patients is difficult. The somatic symptoms which usually provide the indicators of a depressive illness are also common symptoms of cancer itself: sleep disturbance, anorexia, weight loss, loss of libido. A trial of antidepressants is indicated where the diagnosis is in doubt. In this circumstance it is particularly important to use drugs which will not themselves produce unpleasant symptoms. Mianserin (30-60mg nocte) and nomifensine (100mg daily or bd) are preferable to the tricyclics because of their relative lack of anticholinergic and cardiovascular effects. Mianserin is sedative, whereas nomifensine is non-sedative and should not be given late in the day.

The place of psychostimulants, such as the amphetamines, as co-analgesics remains unclear. Cocaine is not helpful but other related drugs may be[3]. Psychodysleptics drugs, cannabinoids and LSD, have no useful place in this area.

Non-steroidal antiinflammatory drugs (NSAIDs)

Prostaglandin synthetase inhibitors reduce tumour mediated osteolysis in vitro and this has prompted their use in patients with metastatic bone disease both to relieve pain and to inhibit tumour growth. NSAIDs do not appear to have a significant effect on the progress of bony metastases, nor is their pain relieving effect consistent in patients with skeletal metastases[4]. Response, in terms of significant pain relief, does not appear to depend on either the nature of the malignant process or on the in vitro potency of the anti-prostaglandin effect. In patients with bone pain it is generally always worth trying an NSAID but the response should be closely monitored and the drug discontinued in the absence of clear cut benefit. NSAIDs have a considerable potential for producing adverse effects (gastro-intestinal upsets and fluid retention) and their usefulness in cancer patients has been exaggerated.

Other conditions which may respond to NSAIDs as co-analgesics are pain from soft tissue infiltration or retroperitoneal tumour. Soluble aspirin (600mg four hourly) remains high on the list of NSAIDs in these indications and flurbiprofen (100mg bd) is a useful alternative.

Corticosteroids

Corticoids have an important role in the management of cancer patients, particularly those with advanced disease[5]. Their most common application as co-analgesics is in the treatment of pain due to raised intracranial pressure and nerve compression, and also pain associated with visceral distension such as hepatomegaly. Pain associated with head and neck malignancy and intrapelvic tumours are also indications for a trial of steroids. Dexamethasone appears to be more effective than prednisolone in these situations. It is also more potent (4mg = 30mg prednisolone) which means that less tablets are required, and is less likely to cause oedema, weight gain and dyspepsia. Whilst dexamethasone is associated with a greater tendency to cause psychological disturbance and hyperactivity, these problems are rare and the benefits outweigh this drawback in day to day use.

Other Coanalgesics

Anticonvulsants may be helpful in the management of lancinating or stabbing dysaesthetic pains associated with nerve infiltration, post-herpetic or post-traumatic (surgical) neuralgias, or nerve compression. Clonazepam

(0.5 - 2 mg nocte or bd) sodium valproate (200mg tid) and carbamazepine (100mg tid) seem to be equally effective (or ineffective) in this indication; doses tend to be somewhat lower than when they are being used for their anticonvulsant effect.

Muscle spasm is an important mechanism of pain in cancer, often occurring in association with skeletal deposits. Baclofen 5-10mg tid is preferable to diazepam if sedation is undesirable.

The pain of lymphoedema often responds to the combined use of an intermittent pneumatic compression sleeve (such as a Flowpulse machine) and a diuretic. The machine must be used regularly for at least an hour twice a day at the maximum tolerated pressure (usually around 60mm Hg) which should be worked up to over the course of a few days. The reduction in tissue turgor and limb circumference must be maintained by means of an elasticated bandage in between applications of the sleeve.

SUMMARY

Of the non-narcotic analgesics paracetamol is preferable to aspirin and other NSAIDs where no antiinflammatory activity is required because of its greater tolerability. Nefopam (given parenterally) may be useful in patients unable to tolerate opioids.

Psychotropics, corticosteroids, NSAIDs, muscle relaxants and anticonvulsants may all have an important part to play as co-analgesics in the management of cancer pain. Indications for their use and the choice of specific drugs are discussed.

REFERENCES

1. Editorial: Aspirin or paracetamol? Lancet (2):287-9,1981
2. Anonymous: Nefopam - a new analgesic. Drug Ther Bull (17):59-60,1979
3. Hanks GW: Psychotropic Drugs. In Twycross RG (ed) The Relief of Cancer Pain. Clinics in Oncology (3),No 1, 1984.In press
4. Coombes RC, Munro Nevill A, Gazet J-C, Ford HT, Nash AG, Baker JW, Powles TJ: Agents affecting osteolysis in patients with breast cancer. Cancer Chemother Pharmacol (3):41-4,1979.
5. Hanks GW, Trueman T, Twycross RG: Corticosteroids in terminal cancer - a prospective analysis of current practice. Postgrad med J (59):28-32, 1983

ADVANCED CANCER: ONCOLOGIST, FAMILY DOCTOR, OR HOSPICE?

F. RANDALL

Many of us began our medical career thinking that our work was to be directed towards the cure of our patients, and the prolongation of their lives. As one gains more experience it becomes apparent that this idea is rather naive. The number of illnesses which can be completely cured, that is totally eradicated from the body, is relatively small compared with those which are chronic. As our patients are now living longer, an increasing proportion of our time will be spent trying to ensure a comfortable and fulfilling life for those who have a chronic disease.

In the past it was sometimes thought that our task as Doctors ceased when the diagnosis of cancer was made. Now, as a result of advances in the field of oncology, we know that much more can be done by radiotherapy and chemotherapy to cure some malignancies, and palliate others. However, many patients still die of cancer. It is time that we came to appreciate that our work continues when a cure is not expected and active treatment has been stopped.

Since the opening of St. Christopher's Hospice in London there has been, among the medical and nursing professions, a steadily increasing awareness of the needs of the dying. As a result of this interest great advances have been made in the field of symptom control, and it is now possible to offer patients a much better quality of life during the last few months. As our expertise in therapeutics has grown, so has our ability to counsel and support patients and their families during the terminal phase of their illness.

Fortunately, through the media and medical press, and the

work of Hospices and Home Care Teams in the community, this knowledge is spreading steadily and it is THEORETICALLY possible for a patient to benefit from a very high standard of care either at home, attended by his Family Doctor, or in the Oncology Ward of his District General Hospital, or under the supervision of his local Hospice Team. During this discussion I would like to illustrate why, in this case, what is possible in theory is not so in practice.

As the general public has become aware of the need for specialist care for those terminally ill so the Hospice movement has developed very rapidly, and in many parts of the United Kingdom Home Care Teams with in-patient Hospice facilities are available. At the same time many General Practitioners and Oncologists, as a result of the Hospice example, have become much more enthusiastic about caring for their own patients until the time of their death.

Therefore, we must now consider how and where the best care can be provided for those patients whom we do not expect to be cured. Obviously there are many factors to be considered for every patient and there are advantages and disadvantages to care by the General Practitioner and Community Nurses, the Oncologist, and the Hospice Team.

I propose that the best standard of care can be provided for the majority of patients by the Hospice Team, regardless of whether the patient remains at home or is admitted to hospital. To support this view I would like to consider those particular skills which they use in caring for the dying and their families.

Firstly, good symptom control is more often achieved by the Hospice Team than by the General Practitioner or Oncologist alone. This applies not only to pain but also to anorexia, nausea, vomiting, weakness, confusion, etc.

The first requirement for success in this field is the belief that something can always be done to alleviate the patient's discomfort and that pain and other symptoms should never be accepted as an inevitable consequence of the disease. It is necessary to develop the habit of constant striving for patient comfort in order to achieve it.

Initially, daily adjustment of treatment is often required. This is based on assessment of symptoms by the patient, and on observations and suggestions from several members of the Hospice Team so that ideas and plans can be shared. The emphasis here must be on the Team approach. Constant observation by day and particularly by night is required. Moreover, since the perception of all symptoms is affected by the personality of the patient and by his psychological state, assessment which is based on the opinions of several different members of the Team usually proves more reliable than that which is made by the Doctor alone. Some staff are more sympathetic to a particular patient than others, and a good relationship with at least one member of the Team is essential if the severity of the symptoms is to be gauged accurately.

Once some assessment of the cause of the symptom has been made specialist knowledge is needed to relieve it using drugs and other measures, but without causing adverse side-effects. In this way pain and other symptoms can be completely controlled in the majority of cases and minimised in all cases by the appropriate use of drugs, radiotherapy and adjuvant treatments. By attention to every detail the patients can be kept comfortable so that they can continue to live a full life until they die.

In order that this can be achieved, time, Team work, specialist knowledge, and the discipline of continued striving for freedom from physical discomfort are essential. The average Family Doctor who cares for only a few patients per annum with a terminal malignancy is unlikely to be able to acquire the specialist knowledge necessary, and very unlikely to have sufficient time for frequent reassessment of the patient. The Oncologist has the opposite problem of having so many patients with a malignancy in his care that although he has the opportunity to acquire sufficient experience in symptom control, there is very rarely time to devote to this subject in the busy out-patient clinic.

Once the patient's consciousness is not dominated by unpleasant symptoms he becomes free to deal with the emotional work associated with dying. We know from the studies of

Dr. Kubler Ross that a person passes through many emotional phases whilst working towards acceptance of death. When this stage of acceptance is reached the patient is able to "put his house in order" with regard to relationships with his family and friends. All of us injure ourselves and those close to us during our lives, but very little damage, if any, is irreparable, and many wounds can be healed even at the eleventh hour thus giving peace to the patient and some lasting consolation to the family.

Most patients need help, to come to terms with the diagnosis, to support their families, and to salvage unhappy relationships. Compassionate but detached counselling and spiritual guidance, usually from several people, is required. The Hospice staff recognise this need and work as a team to help patients to solve their problems so that their last weeks are not haunted by regrets. Besides the Doctors and Nurses, the Social Worker and Chaplain are essential to this work in a Hospice. How many Family Doctors and Oncologists have the time and necessary skills to provide this kind of support? Even given unlimited time, the patient requires help from several different people and the General Practitioner and Oncologist do not have the clinical resources to organise an experienced and united team. Surely our patients deserve the help they need from skilled individuals working together in order to approach death with peace of mind.

And after death - how can we help relatives to cope then? The caring General Practitioner who has known the family for several years can do much to support the bereaved. Unfortunately, the Oncologist is not in a position to give any such help. The Hospice Team can offer bereavement counselling to those families who are most at risk of experiencing prolonged and abnormal grief reactions. This additional service is often of great benefit to bereaved relatives, who through social meetings at the Hospice can share their problems and receive support from others.

These considerations all apply whether the patient remains at home or is admitted to hospital. We should also look at the particular advantages of involvement of the Hospice Team in the patient's home. In this situation, visits by Home Care Nurses are an additional support to the family, often enabling them to continue carrying the emotional strain of caring for the patient at home much longer than they might otherwise be able. Where the patient is ambulant they may be able to attend a Day Centre at the Hospice if this is available. This enables the patient to meet others, to enjoy diversional therapy, and to talk to staff about his problems in a supervised and supportive setting, so that hope is restored and fears can be dispelled. It also provides a much needed break for the family for one or two days a week. Where a relative may be spending twenty-four hours a day in a caring role for many months this sort of relief is extremely valuable, and frequently essential, if the patient is to remain at home.

When the Home Care Team is backed by an in-patient Hospice facility they bring to the patient and family the assurance that admission to hospital is possible without delay if they cannot cope either emotionally or physically. This knowledge often helps them to continue at home. If, however, admission to hospital is needed the Hospice can provide a much more appropriate environment than the Oncology Ward of the District General Hospital. Peace and quiet are essential to the exhausted patient and this cannot be ensured in a busy Oncology Ward.

However, there is a more subtle difference between the Hospice and the general Ward which is probably much more important. The Hospice staff can assure the patient of his value as an individual even though he is no longer a fit member of society and cannot be restored to health. Although we tend to want all our patients to die reconciled and peaceful, it is essential that we recognise their individuality and that we are flexible enough to accept them, and to allow them to be themselves until they die. In order to do this there has to be time for listening, and a great deal of understanding from the staff. This is rarely available in a busy Ward with a high patient turnover, and unusual behaviour by patients in such a setting is disruptive, and therefore cannot be accepted.

On a general Ward patients may develop feelings of rejection as staff devote less time and enthusiasm to their care because they can no longer be cured. They may also become isolated if the emotional burden proves too great for inexperienced staff who therefore avoid them in order to escape personal trauma by spending time with them. Compassion is needed, not pity. The Hospice staff, who have apparently chosen to work with the dying, are usually more able to come close to the patients and so give them the support and contact which they need.

It is sometimes said that radiotherapy or chemotherapy are frequently necessary, even when the disease is very advanced, for the palliation of symptoms. However, this is not an argument for the patient to remain in the Oncology Ward. With good co-operation between the Hospice Physician and local Oncologists, such treatment can still be given from the Hospice environment so that the patient benefits in both respects.

Finally, with health care increasingly coming under the scrutiny of cost-conscious Administrators, the economical case for Hospice care should be considered. Although the staff: patient ratio is somewhat higher in the Hospice than in the general Ward, our use of expensive technology and facilities is minimal. This is because it is inappropriate to carry out investigations unless the results actually enable us to make the patient more comfortable, so that operations, scans, X-rays and blood tests are often unnecessary. Therefore, a bed in a National Health Service Hospice is no more expensive than one in a general Ward. In many respects the cost to the National Health Service is frequently less when a Home Care Team is involved with the General Practitioner in the care of the patient. Since additional support is provided for the family as I described earlier, admission to hospital may be avoided completely or be delayed. Therefore, the expense of in-patient treatment is reduced.

To sum up, I propose that the best standard of care can be given to the majority of patients by the Hospice Team. They provide good symptom control so that the patient is free to enjoy life without fear, either at home with maximum support, or in the Hospice setting. Rather than being a pipe dream, this is an attainable ideal.

If this view is generally accepted then there are widespread implications for the further development of the Hospice movement.

We have two alternatives. Either we can regard the Hospices we have as centres of excellence where a few priviledged patients enjoy a high standard of care, whilst the majority continue as before with less effective symptom control and considerably less emotional support, hoping that all Doctors will eventually learn from the Hospice example; or we can continue to work towards the provision of a higher standard of care for everyone by ensuring that the Hospice service is available throughout the United Kingdom. I believe that the latter approach is the right way to work towards the best care for all our patients.

WHY DO CANCER PATIENTS VOMIT?

G.W. HANKS

Nausea and vomiting are common in cancer patients whatever the stage of their disease. The management of these symptoms is often unsatisfactory. Emesis associated with some types of cytotoxic chemotherapy remains a particularly difficult and sometimes intractable problem, but there is no doubt that in general the treatment of nausea and vomiting in cancer could be improved by a systematic approach. It is important to try and identify the cause, or more specifically the mechanism, in each patient. The pathophysiology of these symptoms and the mode of action of antiemetic drugs are still poorly understood but sufficient is known to allow a rational treatment strategy. There is a need to be selective about antiemetic drugs: their relative efficacy in specific circumstances varies and they all have the potential to produce unpleasant side effects such as drowsiness, dry mouth, blurring of vision and urinary hesitancy. When combinations of antiemetics are required a knowledge of their site of action is relevant.

Physiology

The idea that there may be more than one centre in the brain involved in the control of nausea and vomiting dates from the early part of this century. However the suggestion that there is a chemoreceptor trigger zone (CTZ) responding to noxious substances in the body and separate from the emetic centre which is responsible for coordinating the reflex activity involved in vomiting is relatively recent[1]. The CTZ lies superficially in the area postrema of the medulla in the floor of the fourth ventricle and is bathed by CSF and blood. Emetic substances and antiemetic drugs can therefore reach the CTZ without crossing the blood brain barrier. The vomiting centre (VC) lies more deeply in the dorsal portion of the lateral reticular formation and receives input from the CTZ, and from other central and peripheral sites (Figure). It lies close to the salivary, vasomotor

173

and respiratory centres which may all contribute to the reflex activity
resulting in vomiting.

Figure: The sites of action of antiemetic drugs

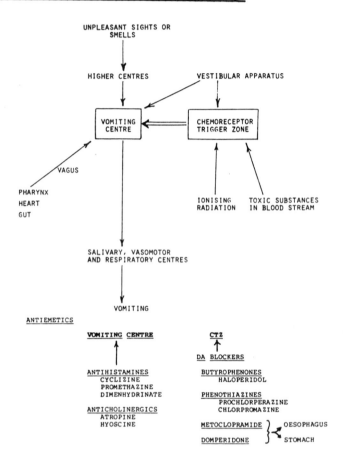

ANTIEMETICS

Antiemetic drugs

Antiemetics can be broadly divided according to their predominant site
of action (Figure), though there is some, perhaps considerable, overlap.
This may be to some extent dose dependent. The major groups are the neuroleptics, anticholinergics and antihistamines; their antiemetic effects are
probably dependent on their ability to block specific receptors. The neuro-

transmitter receptors which have been identified in the CTZ, are dopamine D_2, and in the vomiting centre, muscarinic cholinergic and histamine H_1[2].

Causes of nausea and vomiting in cancer

Cancer patients may vomit because of their disease, because of their drugs or other treatment, or because of their 'distress'. This is a facile approach: often it is not possible to be sure of the cause of nausea and vomiting in these patients. However where the underlying problem is obvious or where specific central or peripheral factors can be defined (Table) treatment can be directed in a rational way.

Vomiting related to the disease

CTZ mediated:

1. Cancer
2. Hypercalcaemia, uraemia, infection.

VC mediated:

1. Raised intracranial pressure
2. Vestibular disorders
3. G-I obstruction (tumour, constipation, ileus)
4. Pharyngeal stimulation
5. Small stomach syndrome

VC/CTZ:

1. Gastric irritation (blood, sputum)
2. Gastric stasis

Vomiting related to treatment

CTZ mediated:

1. Drugs (chemotherapy, opioids, oestrogens, others)
2. Radiotherapy

VC mediated:

1. Drugs (opioids, gastric irritants - NSAIDs, steroids)
2. Surgery

Vomiting related to distress

VC mediated:

fear, anxiety, offensive sights

Choice of antiemetic

Once the cause of nausea and vomiting has been determined a suitable antiemetic should be chosen according to whether the CTZ or the VC is the primary target. If gastric stasis or compression, or oesophageal reflux are significant factors in the cause of these symptoms then drugs with additional peripheral sites of action should be employed (metoclopramide or domperidone). Receptor binding studies have shown that the phenothiazine antiemetics prochlorperazine and chlorpromazine have the least specific central sites of action. It has been suggested that drugs or combinations which will interact with all of the three main receptor types involved in the central control of emesis may be more effective than drugs having a narrower spectrum of activity[2]. However there is some evidence that the use of more specific drugs, such as haloperidol, may not only be more effective in particular indications[3] but may also result in fewer unwanted effects.

In some cases a single antiemetic will fail and combination therapy will then be indicated. The choice of drugs should take into account both the cause of the symptoms and the specific pharmacological properties of the antiemetics. Two neuroleptics used together, for example, are unlikely to be more effective than one, whereas a neuroleptic plus an antihistamine are more likely to have complementary actions. If an antiemetic appears to be ineffective the cause of the problem should be reviewed and a change in antiemetic considered before an additional drug is prescribed, or the use of psychotropics or corticosteroids should be considered.

SUMMARY

It is important to attempt to identify the cause or mechanism of nausea and vomiting in individual cancer patients. Antiemetics can be classified according to their predominant central site of action or additional peripheral effects. Antiemetics can thus be used in a selective and rational manner according to the specific problem in individual patients. This should result in more effective control of these symptoms and a smaller incidence of unwanted effects.

REFERENCES

1. Borison HL, Wang SC: Physiology and pharmacology of vomiting. Pharmacol Rev (5) :193-230,1953.
2. Peroutka SJ, Snyder SH : Antiemetics: neurotransmitter receptor binding predicts therapeutic actions. Lancet (1) :658-9,1982.
3. Hanks GW: Antiemetics for terminal cancer patients. Lancet (1) :1410,1982.

CANCER, VOMITING, AND GUT MOTILITY

C. L. Smith

Vomiting is a violent ejection of stomach contents which is
usually preceded by two other phases.   In considering the
features of vomiting in relation to cancer patients with
possible changes in gastrointestinal motility, I feel it is
important that we review the modalities normally associated
with vomiting, both psychic and physical.
The activity of vomiting can be divided into three phases.
1) Nausea.   A psychic experience which is associated with
a variety of stimuli, including labyrinthine stimuli, visual
pain, mid-brain stimulation, from a variety of sources,
including higher centres and drugs.   Physically, nausea is
associated with a decreased tone in the stomach together
with an increased tone in the duodenum.   In most instances,
vomiting is preceded by nausea, though not always.   There
are episodes of vomiting which are unexpected and in which
the next two phases only are evidenced.
2) The next phase in the vomiting sequence is retching,
which is associated with spasmodic, abortive respiratory
movements in which the diaphragm moves down very sharply
with the mouth and glottis closed and the pyloric end of the
stomach contracts while the body of the stomach relaxes.
However, in this phase there is no ejection of material from
within the stomach.
3) The next and final phase of vomiting is forceful ejection
of stomach contents retrogradely, and is associated with
sharp, downward movement of the diaphragm against the con-
tracted abdominal wall.   At the same time, the cardia of

177

the stomach dilates and is usually found just within the chest. This upward movement of the oesophagogastric junction allows the lower oesophageal sphincter to be above the area of raised pressure which is generated by the downward contraction of the diaphragm and the abdominal muscles. At the same time, the oesophagus relaxes.

It has always been believed that antiperistalsis occurs, and although this can be demonstrated in some animals,there has been no confirmatory evidence produced in man to demonstrate this phenomenon. It is probable, however, that the pyloric and antral contraction seen during retching is once again evident in the process of vomiting.

Although on many occasions faecal contents can be found in the vomitus, it is not a pre-requisite that there is retrograde movement of small bowel contents during vomiting. Certainly in animals the duodenum and small bowel can be resected without interfering with the vomiting mechanism.

What mechanisms, therefore, are involved in the production of vomiting? These can be divided into two areas. Firstly, a central neurological control of vomiting and the peripheral control. In the central control it has been well demonstrated that there is a centre in the medulla which, when stimulated, produces vomiting and is central to the mediation of the act of vomiting whatever the stimulus or higher centre control. A chemoreceptor trigger-zone has also been demonstrated in the medulla, which is responsive to a variety of stimulants but which appears to require an intact vomiting centre for mediation of its effects.

In addition, there may well be higher centres which are responsive particularly to drugs. It has been demonstrated that the vomiting associated with Pilocarpine is mediated through a frontal lobe centre, but again it requires the medullary vomiting centre for its action.

As well as these central control mechanisms, there is the peripheral control which is manifest by the response of

stomach and small bowel to irritants and distension.Clearly,
if the gastrointestinal tract is going to respond to noxious
agents, there is a pre-requisite for receptors within the
GI tract to mediate the need for ejection of these materials
This control system is mediated through the vagus, since
transection of the vagus abolishes this response. It is
clear, therefore, that there are a number of mechanisms by
which patients with cancer may have vomiting produced.
It would seem that they may well affect the higher centres
and the centres of the medulla directly, either through the
chemotherapy they are being given or by some product of the
tumour or by direct involvement within the cerebral hemi-
spheres by the tumour.

In terms of gastrointestinal motility, the relationship
between neural control and gastrointestinal activity has
been well demonstrated, and it is clear that the central
control is mediated through psychic influences, feedback
mechanisms from the gastrointestinal tract and can be
affected by drugs. The psychic influences were first
demonstrated clearly by a Pavlovian-type experiment, and
all of us are aware of the changes in our gastrointestinal
activity when we are anxious. The feedback mechanisms
have already been alluded to in that the reflex arcs from
the gastrointestinal tract respond to mucosal stimulation
and distension.

Local factors involved in changing gastrointestinal
motility are the luminal contents in the form of food,
hormones stimulated by the intraluminal contents or by
direct vagal activity and drugs. There are also reflex
arcs within the gastrointestinal tract which modulate the
activity, depending on the form and site of the contents.
Let us look, therefore, at some of the agents which are
involved in the neural mechanisms related to gastrointestinal
motility.

Within the latter, the cholinergic activity is mediated
by the vagus, and we all know that interruption of the

vagus results, in particular, in relaxation of the gastrointestinal tract and certainly initially abolition of peristaltic activity.   As well as this cholinergic innervation
there is adrenergic involvement via the splanchnic nerves,
but also a second adrenergic system, namely the dopaminergic
innovation, which is also mediated via the vagus.   The
dopaminergic system is the control mechanism for relaxation
of the gastrointestinal tract and is usually the modulator
of the cholinergic activity.

In addition to these external neural influences, there
are intragastric reflex arcs, particularly between the
duodenum, pylorus and stomach, which regulate the initiation
and progression of peristaltic waves.   As well as these
neural influences, there are local neurotransmitters and
hormones which modulate gastrointestinal motility.   These
are predominantly cholecystikinin, which though chiefly
affecting gall-bladder activity and pancreatic secretion,
does influence oesophageal and gastric tone.   There are
also gastrointestinal polypeptide and vasoactive-inhibitory
polypeptide, which have a direct inhibitory effect on gastro
intestinal function,   In particular, vasoactive-inhibitory
polypeptide is a local neurotransmitter which is directly
involved in gut motility.

As well as these well recognised agents, there are
possibly other locally active neurotransmitters, such as
neurotensin and enkaphalin.   These are the neurotensin and
enkaphalin agents which have been shown to alter radically
the phase of activity, particularly the small bowel.

We come, therefore, to the possible cause of vomiting in
cancer, and this has already been dealt with in part by the
previous speaker.   However, looking at the factors which
might influence it, those which may be mediated by changes
in gastrointestinal motility involve the psychological
factors, direct influence on and interference in the GI tract
local hormonal and central hormonal agents and products of
the tumour.   In the context of psychological factors, we

are all well aware that stress produces changes in gastrointestinal motility, as witnessed by all people taking
examinations who find the frequent visits for excess bowel
action a predominant feature of the pre-examination phase.
These activities are probably mediated through the vagus
with a discoordination of the relationship between cholinergic and dopaminergic activity. There is also evidence
from studies on patients with irritable bowel syndrome that
they have abnormal gastrointestinal motility which can be
demonstrated either in the upper or lower gastrointestinal
tract. In this context, we have shown that patients with
irritable bowel have disorders of oesophageal function in
that they have a reduced lower oesophageal sphincter
pressure and increased frequency of spontaneous activity,
variable amplitudes of contractions, simultaneous activity
and repetitive contractions. Also, patients with irritable
bowel without any structural defect of their gastrointestinal
have a much higher frequency of nausea and vomiting than
do a control population. In connection with direct interference with the GI tract, this could either be from tumour
spread or from products of the tumour acting directly on the
musculature or the neuronal parts of the GI tract. However,
there is no evidence to suggest that this is present. Within
the context of the hormones, many tumours do produce hormones and these will affect the GI tract, but there is no
evidence that in general tumour products have a direct
influence on gastrointestinal motility. It would seem that
the most likely route of effect in GI motility is through
the centrally-mediated mechanisms.

In this context, therefore, we undertook a study in two
parts. The first part was to confirm that patients with
cancer had an increase in gastrointestinal symptoms, in
particular nausea and vomiting, over a matched control
population. For simplicity, we took, after a preliminary
study of a random group of patients with a variety of neoplastic disorders, a group of 17 patients with breast
cancer who were attending an out-patient department and

who were demonstrated to have no gastrointestinal involvement from their disease. Nor were they undergoing specific therapy at the time, either chemotherapy or radiotherapy. All the patients were aware of their disease and had been followed for not less than 3 years. These patients were matched against 17 control subjects who were matched for age ± 5 years and who were also undergoing hospital outpatient management, but again without disorders affecting the GI tract.

The results of this study demonstrated that while only 6 of 17 control subjects had symptoms referable to their GI tracts, 12 of 17 patients with breast cancer had GI symptoms, and these were predominantly nausea and vomiting. This indicates that there is a relative risk of having GI symptoms four times greater in the patients than in their controls. However, because of the small numbers the confidence limits for this study are wide and clearly need to be extended to include more patients.

On the basis of this study, we decided to look at GI function, and on the basis that nausea and vomiting are predominantly disturbances of gastric function we looked at gastric emptying in patients with breast cancer. For this purpose, 15 patients with breast cancer, aged 44 to 78 in whom there was no evidence of gastrointestinal involvement, undertook a study of gastric emptying using a radio-isotope-labelled mixed meal with Technicion added to the mashed potato part of the meal. These subjects were again matched with 15 controls in the same age range in whom again there was no evidence for GI disorder. The study was carried out using a gamma camera detection system with an on-line computer and comalysis based on 70 one-minute frames during the gastric emptying.

The result of this study showed that there was no difference in the emptying time between controls and cancer patients. This would suggest, therefore, that disturbance of gastric emptying is not a feature of the nausea and vomiting in cancer patients.

THE MEDICAL MANAGEMENT OF MALIGNANT BOWEL OBSTRUCTION

M. J. BAINES

ABSTRACT
    A study was made of 18 consecutive patients at St.
Christopher's Hospice suffering with intestinal obstruction
from advanced abdominal or pelvic malignancy. The majority
were managed medically, without using the traditional conservative
treatment of intravenous fluids and nasogastric suction. Good
control of obstructive symptoms such as intestinal colic,
vomiting and diarrhoea was obtained with the use of drugs and
details of medication are described. The place of further
surgery is discussed and a series of post mortems on obstructed
patients presented.

INTRODUCTION
    Intestinal obstruction is a relatively common complication
in patients with advanced abdominal or pelvic malignancy. We
monitored cases over an eight month period at St. Christopher's
Hospice and found that one in twenty-three patients died with
obstruction. Tunca, in a series of 518 patients with ovarian
cancer, found that intestinal obstruction developed in twenty-
five per cent.
    While surgery must remain the treatment of choice for the
majority of obstructed patients there will be many with recurrent
obstruction after one or more surgical procedure, those who are
too ill or have too extensive abdominal disease or who refuse an
operation which they know can only be palliative. All these
need skilful medical management to minimize the symptoms of
abdominal pain and vomiting which would otherwise characterise
their final days and weeks.
    The purposes of this paper are to illustrate the type of
183

patient who would benefit from intensive medical treatment of intestinal obstruction and to describe details of effective drug therapy.

PATIENTS AND METHODS

Patients   A study was made of 18 consecutive patients who died with intestinal obstruction between October 1981 and May 1982 and were under the care of St. Christopher's Hospice. Patients were omitted from the study if the final obstructive phase lasted less than 24 hours. The diagnosis and sex incidence are shown in Table 1.

TABLE 1. Diagnosis of Obstructed Patients

SITE OF PRIMARY	NUMBER	SEX
Ovary	7	7F
Rectum	3	2M, 1F
Caecum	2	1M, 1F
Unknown	2	1M, 1F
Endometrium	1	1F
Stomach	1	1F
Pelvic colon	1	1M
Peritoneal mesothelioma	1	1F

There was a M : F ratio of 5 : 13, the difference being caused entirely by gynaecological malignancy, predominantly ovarian. The age range was from 26 to 94, with a mean of 60 years.
Diagnosis of obstruction   This was made on clinical grounds in patients known to have malignancy involving the bowel. Abdominal X-rays were only done if surgery was contemplated.
Previous surgical treatment   All, except the 94 year old had received abdominal surgery, some on several occasions. 7 had already had palliative procedures for intestinal obstruction, their mean survival was 4 months, but 4 continued to have obstructive symptoms. 3 had had laparotomies at which no bypass was possible.
Clinical findings   11 patients had palpable abdominal tumours, 3 had marked hepatomegaly, 2 had ascites, 10 had a very distended abdomen.

<u>Pathology</u> Consent for 8 post-mortem examinations was obtained and one patient underwent a laparotomy. Therefore in 9 of our patients the pathology was known. The findings are shown in Table 2.

TABLE 2 POST-MORTEM FINDINGS

Age/sex		Primary	Macroscopic findings		Microscopic findings	
			Main Tumour Mass	Narrowed Bowel	Serosal Deposits	Muscle Infiltration
53	F	Stomach	Central omental	Ileum++	Minimal	Ileum & colon
62	F	Ovary	Malignant adhesions	Ileum++	Minimal	Minimal
62	F	Ovary	Central omental	Ileum & transverse colon	Extensive	None
70	F	Ovary	Central omental	Ileum, transverse & splenic colon	Extensive	None
76	F	Ovary	Pelvic	Ileum++	None	Ileum
80	F	Endometrium	Malignant adhesions	Ileum++	Extensive	None
51	M	Rectum	Multiple		Extensive	Ileum
34	F	Ovary	Malignant recto-sigmoid adhesion	Recto-sigmoid junction	Minimal	None
62	F	Caecum	Pelvic	Sigmoid colon	Extensive	Minimal

Although the series is small some conclusions can be reached:-
- No patient was suffering from a benign obstruction or simple constipation.
- Multiple sites of obstruction are usually found.
- Extensive infiltration of gut muscle was present in about half the cases, this is known to cause motility problems which will aggravate or even cause intestinal obstruction (Tunca).

RESULTS

<u>Surgery</u> Surgical relief of obstruction was considered for each patient, the criterion being "Good evidence of a single block in

a relatively fit patient" (Howard). However, 17 out of 18 were
managed medically for the following reasons:-
- previous laparotomy for obstruction - no procedure possible - 3
- previous surgeon's opinion e.g. "she remained in obstruction
after surgery" - 5
- extensive intra-abdominal tumour(s) - 6
- too old or ill - 2
- did not want surgery - 1
One patient was considered suitable for surgery following
abdominal X-rays. A defunctioning left colostomy was performed
for sigmoid obstruction but there was widespread peritoneal
carcinomatosis and death occurred the following day.

Symptom control

Intestinal colic This was a problem in 13 out of 18 patients,
in 11 it was intermittent. 7 developed increased colic in the
final days needing increased medication for control. The
following drugs were used:-

Loperamide (imodium) or diphenoxylate with atropine (Lomotil),
orally 1 - 2 tablets 6 hourly for persistent colic.

Hyoscine (Scopolamine) 0.3 - 0.6 mg given sublingually if
colic is anticipated e.g. before food. An injection of 0.4 mg
for rapid relief or 0.8 - 2 mg/24 hours given subcutaneously in
the syringe driver for the terminal management of a patient with
severe colic.

A coeliac axis block has been increasingly used in the management of colic due to obstruction as we have an anaesthetist who
can carry out the procedure on the ward, with the minimum of delay
or disturbance to patients who are already very ill. About half
report pain relief though the increased peristalsis and borborygmi
continue.

With a combination of these methods colic was satisfactorily
relieved in all 13 patients.

Other abdominal pain 16 patients had pain other than colic
due to hepatomegaly, tumour masses or abdominal distension. These
pains were invariably constant and required continuous medication,
the dose being adequate to control pain until the next dose had
been given and became effective.

Morphine solution 4 hourly, Morphine Sulphate Continus (MST) 12 hourly and oxycodone pectinate (Proladone) suppositories 8 hourly were used, also diamorphine 4 hourly by injection or subcutaneously over the 24 hours in the syringe driver. A coeliac axis block was also used and satisfactory pain control achieved in all patients.

Nausea and vomiting   16 patients suffered with vomiting and in 7 it was reported as severe. The vomiting from intestinal obstruction is probably due to a combination of reverse peristalsis and toxic absorption, its severity depends on the level of obstruction and it may at first be intermittent. The vomiting is accompanied by considerable nausea and may become faeculent. It is difficult to control fully, the most that can be offered is some improvement; a considerable lessening of nausea (which patients find worse than vomiting) and a diminution of vomits to once or twice a day. In this series good control was achieved in 4, moderate control in 9 and poor control in 3. However, during the course of our study the subcutaneous syringe driver became easily available and its use greatly improved our management.

The following drugs were used:-

Prochlorperazine (Stemetil) 15 - 30 mg/24 hours

Chlorpromazine (Largactil) 50 - 150 mg/24 hours

Methotrimeprazine (Veractil or Nozinan) 50 - 150 mg/24 hours

Cyclizine (Valoid) 100 - 150 mg/24 hours

These can all be given orally or by injection, prochlorperazine and chlorpromazine are available as suppositories. Methotrimeprazine is well tolerated when given subcutaneously in the syringe driver and 4 patients had severe terminal vomiting only controlled on this drug. It will give considerable sedation, though this may also be of value.

Diarrhoea   This was a major problem for 8 patients with subacute (or partial) obstruction, 5 of whom went into a final phase of complete obstruction. Loperamide, diphenoxylate with atropine and codeine were all used, moderate or good control was achieved in 6, poor control in 2.

Constipation   Only 2 patients complained of constipation and it was treated with faecal softening aperients. We consider that once the diagnosis of malignant obstruction has been made there is no place for stimulant purgatives or high enemas.

DISCUSSION

The traditional first-line treatment of patients presenting with intestinal obstruction from recurrent carcinoma is conservative, using intravenous fluids and nasogastric suction. If no improvement occurs a laparotomy is performed with ileostomy or colostomy or a bypass procedure.

However, a review of the literature shows how poor the results are. Papers by Aranha and Glass and Le Duc showed a 1 per cent and 15 per cent sustained response to conservative treatment. Piver, in a series of 60 patients with ovarian carcinoma showed a median survival of 2.5 months following palliative surgery. Aranha in a study of 73 patients (71 male) had an operative mortality of 35 per cent, a mean survival of 6 months in those who survived the 30th post operative day and 10 per cent developed faecal fistulae.

Presumably it is the fear that a death from intestinal obstruction is to be avoided, at any cost, that sometimes drives both doctors and patients into further surgery. We believe that such a death need not be distressing. Symptoms of colic, pain and vomiting can be well controlled by correct medication without using intravenous fluids or nasogastric suction. The patient is therefore free to move about the ward as strength allows or be cared for at home until death occurs.

REFERENCES

1. Tunca, J.C., Buchler, D.A., Mack, E.A., Ruzicka, F.F., Crowley, J.J. and Carr, W.F. (1981). The management of ovarian-cancer caused bowel obstruction. Gynecologic Oncology 12, 186.
2. Howard, E.R. (1982). Personal communication.
3. Aranha, G., Folk, F., Greenlee, H. (1981). Surgical palliation of small bowel obstruction due to metastatic carcinoma. American Surgeon 47, 99.
4. Glass, R.L., and LeDuc, R.J. (1973). Small intestinal obstruction from peritoneal carcinomatosis. Am. J. Surg. 125,316
5. Piver, M.S., Barlow, J.J., Lele, S.B., and Frank, A. (1982). Survival after ovarian cancer induced intestinal obstruction. Gynecologic Oncology 13, 44.

ETIOLOGY OF CHEMOTHERAPY-INDUCED VOMITING

A.L. HARRIS

CLASSICAL STUDIES

Borison and Wang showed that many emetics did not act directly on the emetic centre in the medulla, but acted via a chemoreceptor trigger zone (CTZ) in the floor of the 4th ventricle. Somatic afferents and vagal fibres via the nodose ganglion from the gastrointestinal tract acted directly on the vomiting centre.[1]

However, not all emetic drugs act via the CTZ.[2] Thus pilocarpine acts via a cortical effect and veratrum acts via the nodose ganglion. A suitable animal model has been developed and cats, dogs and ferrets have been used. There are species differences (e.g. mustine acts via the CTZ in dogs, but upper abdominal de-afferentation is necessary in cats).

ANTI-EMETIC CENTRE AND OPIATES

More recently investigations on opiates have shown that there is probably an anti-emetic centre as well as an emetic centre.[3] In cats, opiates are both emetic and anti-emetic to most other stimuli. The anti-emetic effect is blocked by naloxone but not the emetic effect.

Drug	Mode of Administration	Blocking Effects
MORPHINE) LEVORPHANOL) FENTANYL) METHADONE)	into cerebral ventricles	APOMORPHINE EMESIS
NALOXONE	intravenous	ANTIEMETIC EFFECTS OF MORPHINE
NALOXONE	into cerebral ventricles	EMETIC EFFECT OF MORPHINE
NALOXONE	intravenous	ANTIEMETIC EFFECTS OF CANNABINOIDS

These studies suggest that opiates may be acting at different sites to produce emesis and anti-emesis. μ receptors are blocked by naloxone and may be the mechanism for anti-emesis, but delta receptors are not blocked by naloxone and may be the receptors for emesis. The anti-emetic effect of cannabinoids may be mediated by this centre and can be blocked by naloxone.[4]

NEURO-TRANSMITTERS INVOLVED IN EMETIC PATHWAYS

Afferent pathways to the vomiting centre pass via the tractus solitarius and its nucleus and efferent pathways exit via the nucleus ambiguus and the dorsal motor nuclei of the vagus. Receptors for various different neuro-transmitters are present in these pathways, e.g. muscarinic cholinergic receptors for the tractus solitarius and the nucleus ambiguus; histamine H_1 receptors for the nucleus of the tractus solitarius and the dorsal motor nucleus of the vagus, opioid receptors are also present in these two nuclei; dopamine D_2 receptors for the chemoreceptor trigger zone[5,6]. Anti-emetic drugs acting on different neuro-transmitter systems may be synergistic in blocking emetic effects.[7]

Drug group	Dopamine D_2	Muscarinic cholinergic K_i n molar	Histamine H_1
H_1 antihistamines			
diphenhydramine	10,000	120	17
Neuroleptics			
prochlorperazine	15	2,100	100
chlorpromazine	25	130	28
metoclopramide	270	10,000	1,100
Tricyclics			
amitryptiline	290	10	3.2

Thus amitryptiline blocks both H_1 and muscarinic cholinergic receptors, chlorpromazine blocks all 3 types of receptors and nearly ten times more metoclopramide is necessary to block the D_2 receptor compared with chlorpromazine. Combinations acting at different sites may be more effective than even high doses of single agents and this approach needs to be tested in randomised studies.

CYTOTOXIC DRUGS AND NEUROPHARMACOLOGICAL INTERACTIONS

Although most cytotoxic drugs that have been investigated do act via the CTZ, the mechanism is unknown. Most chemotherapy has a latent phase before emesis and onset of vomiting starts several hours after the peak drug levels.[8] Drugs with different modes of action, chemical structures and lipid solubilities produce similar end effects.

(i) Emetic capacity and time frame of cytotoxic drug induced vomiting   Drugs with greater emetic capacity (e.g. producing vomiting in greater than 90% of patients, cis-platinum) produce a more rapid onset of vomiting, 1-2 hours, than those with a lower emetic capacity (onset over 4-6 hours, adriamycin).

(ii) Possible mechanisms

Since all the drugs ultimately effect protein synthesis it is possible that neurotransmitter mechanisms are affected by their action. Possible mechanisms include; inhibition of degradation of neurotransmitters near the CTZ leading to

increased effect (e.g. enkephalins); inhibition of synthesis
of neurotransmitters in the antiemetic centre with decreased
anti-emetic effects (e.g. enkephalins); inhibition of uptake of an inhibitory transmitter in the antiemetic centre
leading to decreased effect (e.g. GABA) of antiemetic centre.

(iii) <u>Relationship of mode of action of drug to emetic
effect</u>

Emetic ranking	Biochemical effects on neurotransmitters or degrading enzymes
1 heavy metal (cisplatinum) methylating agents (DTIC, streptozotocin) inhibitors of protein synthesis (cycloheximide)	Direct effects on proteins
2 bifunctional crosslinking agents intercalators (adriamycin) RNA inhibitors (actinomycin D)	Inhibition of mRNA production
3 antimetabolites	Inhibition of de novo DNA synthesis (also have RNA effects)
4 vinca alkaloids	Inhibition of mitosis

It can be seen that drugs acting on protein synthesis may
have a more rapid onset and be more emetic than those
acting earlier on the biosynthetic pathway. Since the cells
affected have a very slow turnover, antimetabolites and
drugs inhibiting mitosis may be expected to have very little
effect compared to those that affect RNA synthesis.

ENKEPHALINS AS CANDIDATE NEUROTRANSMITTERS FOR EMETIC
PATHWAYS

Although numerous neurotransmitter systems are involved
enkephalins may be of particular importance. Receptors
are present in the chemoreceptor trigger zone and in both
the afferent and the efferent pathways for emesis.[9]
Enkephalins are present in the CSF and could therefore
potentially be active at the CTZ.[10] Inhibition of their
degradation would lead to local high concentrations. Opiates
are directly emetic on the chemoreceptor trigger zone.[11]
There are close links of the enkephalin system with dopaminergic systems and enkephalins may produce dopamine release.[12,13] This may explain the effectiveness of some
anti-dopaminergic drugs. There is a suitable enzyme de-
grading system - enkephalinase that could be inhibited by
drugs.[14] There is fairly rapid turnover in enkephalins
and maximum labelling occurs 1 hr after an intracerebral
injection of tritiated tyrosine.[15] Cytotoxic drugs such as
cycloheximide, in animal models can produce marked inhib-

ition of enkephalin synthesis.[16] Recently butorphanol has
been shown to be a potent anti-emetic in the ferret model
blocking cisplatinum, adriamycin and cyclophosphamide induced
emesis.[17] Naloxone blocks the anti-emetic effects of opiates
but not the emetic effects.

This evidence suggests that further investigation of
enkephalin pathways may produce an alternative approach to
treatment.

THE ROLE OF GLIAL CELLS

Most synapses in the area of the CTZ and in the CNS are
surrounded by glial cells. These cells have many metabolic
roles and may be able to modulate neurotransmitters. Their
metabolic pathways can be stimulated by prostaglandins.
Glial cells can take up and release potassium and also take up
and release GABA.[18] They are electrically coupled with gap
junctions that can transfer low molecular weight molecules.[19]
GABA is an inhibitory neurotransmitter and its analogues
cause vomiting in man. Benzodiazepines interact with the
GABA receptor. Steroids also affect the functioning of
glial cells, apart from their effects on the blood brain
barrier (protection of anti-emetic centre) and dexamethasone
reduces the release of enkephalins.[20] Thus some of the
effects of chemotherapy may be mediated via metabolic pathways in the glial cells surrounding the synapses.

CONCLUSIONS

1. Although empirical trials have improved control of
emesis, further progress depends on better understanding of
the mechanisms. Current screens for antiemetics only detect
dopamine-blocking drugs.

2. Combinations of drugs acting on different receptors may
be more active.

3. Further investigation of enkephalin pathways is
necessary (e.g. blocker).

4. Application of current techniques to a suitable animal
model, using cytotoxic drugs is possible and should lead to
new approaches (lesioned animals, blocking agents, immuno-
fluorescence, receptor assays, isotope labelling).

1. Borison H L, Wang S C. Pharmacol Rev 1953; 5, 192-230
2. Wang S C. Physiological pharmacology vol II. N Y Academic Press 1965; 255-328
3. Costello D J, Borison H L. J Pharmacol Exp Ther 1977; 203, 222-230
4. McCarthy L E, Borison H L. Pharmacologist 1977; 19, 230
5. Stefanini E, Clement-Cormier Y. Eur J Pharmacol 1981; 74, 257-260
6. Palacios J M, Wamsley J K, Kuhar M J. Neuroscience 1981; 6, 15-17
7. Peroutka S J, Snyder S H. Lancet 1982; i, 658-659
8. **Fetting J H, Grochow L B, Folstein M F, Ettinger D S, Colvin M. Cancer Chemother Rep 1982; 66, 1487-1494**
9. Atweh S F, Kuhar M J. Br. Med. Bull. 1983; 39, 47-52
10. Dupont A, Villeneuve A, Bouchard J P, Bouchard R, Merand Y, Rouleau D, Labrie F. Lancet 1978; ii, 1107
11. Borison H L, Fishburn B R, Bhide N K, McCarthy L E. J Pharmacol Exp Ther 1962; 138, 229-235
12. Kuschinsky K. Arzneim-Forsch (Drug Res) 1976; 26, 563-567
13. Chenslet M F, Cheramy A, Reisine T D, Glowinski J. Nature 1981; 291, 320-322
14. Patey G, De la Baume S, Schwartz J-C, Gros C, Roques B, Fourne-Zaluski M C, Soroca-Lucas E. Science 1981; 212, 1153-1155
15. Hughes J. Br Med Bull 1983; 39, 17-24
16. Gros C, Malfory B, Swerts J P, Dray F, Schwartz J C. Eur J Pharmacol 1978; 5, 317-318
17. Schurig J E, Florczyk A P, Spencer S M, Bradner W T. Assoc Cancer Res 1982; 18, 889
18. Varon S S, Somjen G G. Neurosciences Res Prog Bull 1981; 17, 131-204
19. Smith B H. Neurosurgery 1978; 2, 175-178
20. Herz A, Hollt V, Gramsch C, Seizinger B R. In: Costa E & Trabucchi M ed. Regulatory peptides, from molecular biology to function, 1982; 51-59

THE MANAGEMENT OF NAUSEA AND VOMITING CAUSED BY ANTICANCER CHEMOTHERAPY

Christopher J. WILLIAMS

1. INTRODUCTION Although other side effects of cytotoxic therapy are potentially more serious and can be life threatening, nausea and vomiting is by far the most unpleasant toxicity from the patients' perspective. It may be severe enough to cause some patients to default treatment, even when they have a potentially curable tumour. However, the neuropharmacology of emesis is extremely complicated and not fully understood. The way the cytotoxic drugs induce emesis is variable and different antiemetics have different modes of action. When it is also remembered that cytotoxics are commonly used in combinations of 3 or 4 drugs and that studies of antiemetics to prevent chemotherapy associated emesis are a recent phenomenon (table 1), it is not surprising that no definitive statements can be made about the best ways to manage it. This chapter reviews the current state of the art.

Table 1. Incidence of antiemetic studies reported from 1960-1982.

Year	No. studies	Year	No. studies
1960	1	1977	2
1961	1	1978	6
1963	1	1979	10
1969	1	1980	16
1973	2	1981	15
1975	1	1982	22
1976	1	Total	79

2. STUDIES OF 'CONVENTIONAL' ANTIEMETICS

2.1. Phenothazines

Phenothazines have , in the past twenty years, been the class of antiemetics most commonly used to try to prevent emesis caused by cytotoxic therapy. Although they have been shown to be more effective than placebo (1), many patients still have nausea and vomiting and in

12 of 25 studies it was rated as inactive (2). With the introduction
of more highly emetic cytotoxic agents, such as cisplatin, it is
clear that phenothazines alone are relatively ineffective. They act
through blockade of dopamine receptors and as well as suppressing the
chemoreceptor trigger zone (CTZ) cause sedation, orthostatic
hypotension and extrapyramidal symptoms. Other toxicities (Jaundice,
blood dyscrasias, skin reactions and photosensitivity) are uncommon.

2.2. Metoclopramide Metoclopramide is a procainamide derivative
which acts by blocking dopamine in the brain and as a cholinergic
stimulant on the gut. It is an attractive drug to study because it
blockades the dopamine receptors of the CTZ as well as preventing
gastric stasis and dilation by its peripheral cholinergic effects.
However trials using conventional doses have yielded conflicting
results (3,4), though it is now clear that in oral doses of 0.2 -
0.3mg/kg it is relatively ineffective.

2.3 Benzimadazoles Domperidone is the only member of this class
that has been tested so far. It is a dopamine antagonist which
penetrates the blood brain barrier poorly and because of this is
virtually devoid of CNS effects. Domperidone enhances emptying of
the stomach and inhibits the effect of dopamine on gastric motor
function. It has been tested in seven studies (5,6) and was found
effective in all, though it does not completely control vomiting in
patients receiving strongly emetic drugs. The side effects of this
drug are minimal and studies testing high doses are currently in
progress.

2.4. Butyrophenones Droperidol and haloperidol, which act as
dopamine antagonists suppressing the CTZ, have been tested as antiemetics in patients receiving cytotoxic therapy. Haloperidol has
been used in 3 studies and showed moderate activity without abolishing
vomiting in patients receiving strongly emetic agents (6). Droperidol
has also shown similar moderate activity in 4 studies (6). In one
study it was more effective than prochlorperazine and trimethobenzamide
when used in patients receiving cisplatin but was inferior in patients
receiving CYVADIC chemotherapy (7).

2.5. Antihistamines Various antihistamines, used for motion sickness,
have been tested with uniformly poor results.

2.6. Benzoquinolizines Benquinamide was less effective than prochlor-

perazine in a randomized study (8) though it has shown some activity
when used after moderately emetic cytotoxic therapy.

2.7. Benzamides Trimethobenzamide was similarly less effective than
prochlorperazine in a study by Moertel (1). In a controlled trial it
was more effective than placebo in reducing the emesis of potent
emetogenic drugs.

3. 'NEW' ANTIEMETIC REGIMES

3.1. Cannabinoids Following the observation that patients who
smoked cannabis during chemotherapy had less emesis there has been
much interest in this group of drugs. Those most studied (table 2)
are tetrahydrocannabinol (THC), Nabilone and Levonantradol. THC has
been shown to have useful antiemetic effects in placebo controlled
studies (9) and in comparison with prochloperazine and metoclopramide
(10). Despite this there is a high incidence of side effects and it
is less well tolerated in older patients. Frytak et al (11) have
reported that despite moderate antiemetic effect CNS toxicity was so
great in one study that many patients discontinued the drug. The
major toxicities are: ataxia, hypotension, hallucinations, blurred
vision, disorientation, paraesthesias, depression, anxiety, nightmares,
amnesia, slurred speech, tachycardia and syncope. Chang et al
(12) have confirmed the antiemetic activity of THC but have suggested
that this may be confined to certain emetic cytotoxics and that it is
ineffective against Adriamycin and Cyclophosphamide.

Nabilone, a synthetic cannabinoid, causes less 'highs' than THC
and has been shown to be effective (table 2). Several randomized
trials have shown that it is more effective than prochloperazine
(13,14) though it has more side effects. The most troublesome of
these are: somnolence, dry mouth, dizziness, hypotension and dysphoria.
Levonantradol has recently shown activity in 3 studies but has
similar side effects to the other cannabinoids and a recent double
blind trial has shown no difference in activity and side effects
between THC and Levonantradol (15).

3.2. High dose metoclopramide Although low doses of metoclopramide
have been relatively ineffective, some patients benefited and
preclinical studies suggested that the best effect would be achieved
at doses higher than those used. Phase 1 studies have shown minimal

Table 2   Clinical studies with cannabinoids (16,17)

Drug	No. of studies	No. regarded as showing anti emetic effect.
THC	12	11
Nabilone	7	7
Levonantradol	3	3

toxicity using doses up to 3.0 mg/kg I.V. given over 20 mins. Subsequent phase II studies have used high doses 30 mins before and 1.5, 3.5, 5.5 and 8.5 hours after cisplatin. The results of four studies using high doses of metoclopramide are shown in table 3.

Table 3.   Results of uncontrolled trials of high dose metoclopramide in patients receiving cisplatin (18).

Metoclopramide dose	No. of patient trials	Major anti-emetic effect (0-2 emetic episodes)	Minor anti-emetic effect (3-5 emetic episodes)
2.0 mg/kg	20	13	5
1.5 mg/kg	20	6	6
1.0 mg/kg *	75	55	11
1.0 mg/kg *	18	12	4

* Lower doses of cisplatin were used in these studies.

Following the encouraging results in these studies, controlled trials were undertaken and have shown high dose metoclopramide to be superior to placebo and prochlorperazine (table 4).

Table 4.   Results of double-blind trials of high dose metoclopramide in patients receiving cisplatin (18)

Antiemetic	No. of patients	Mean No. of emetic episodes	Significance
Metoclopramide 2.0 mg/kg IV	11	1.0	0.001
Placebo	10	10.5	
Metoclopramide 20 mg/kg IV	10	1.5	0.005
Prochlorperazine	10	12.0	

Side effects were minor and extrapyramidal reactions have been rare (3%) in the series reported by Gralla et al, though other institutions (19) have reported them in up to 60% of patients. They are promptly reversed by diphenhydramine or valium. Kris et al. (20) has suggested that these reactions are more common in younger patients (table 5).

Table 5.   Incidence of extrapyramidal reactions in patients treated with high dose metoclopramide by age (20).

	Age of patient (yrs)	
	15-29	30-72
No. of patients treated	22	430
No. of extra pyramidal reactions	6 (27.3%)	8 (1.8%) (P = 0.00005)

3.3. Corticosteroids Both Dexamethasone and methyl prednisolone have been shown to have antiemetic effects (21) and have been used in combination with other drugs with some benefit.

3.4. Benzodiazepines Lorazepam (22) has been shown to have some antiemetic effect and also reduces patient recall.

4. COMBINATIONS OF ANTIEMETICS

No single antiemetic is uniformly successful and the use of combinations of antiemetics is of potential interest as emesis may be blocked at various points. This may be important as most cytotoxic regimes include several drugs causing emesis in different ways. Some trials of antiemetics have reported that activity was restricted to particular chemotherapy regimes (7,12) and it may be necessary to design the 'ideal' antiemetic therapy for each type of cytotoxic treatment. Studies of combinations of antiemetics will need to test drugs in a stepwise fashion and must be randomized. The use of multidrug antiemetic regimes, such as the 5 drug regime reported by Plezia (23), is hard to justify without controlled studies. Randomized trials of the type reported by Artim (24) and Tyson (25) (Table 6) are essential to demonstrate increasing benefit from additional drugs.

Combinations of antiemetics of known efficacy can be tried and useful agents with different patterns of toxicity and modes of action, for example dexamethasone and lorazepam, are of interest.

Table 6. Studies of combinations of antiemetics.

| Author | Antiemetic | Patients | % with | |
			no emesis	good relief
Artim	THC + Prochlorperazine	20	-	90
	Placebo + Prochlorperazine	20	-	15
Tyson	HD Metoclopramide (MCP)	36	39	64
	MCP + Dexamethasone (Dex)	25	60	88
	MCP + Dex + Diphenhydramine (50mg)	15	66	93

Combinations may also include drugs which reduce the potential for
toxicity of the primary agent.

5. ANTICIPATORY VOMITING

Once a patient has experienced nausea and vomiting after chemotherapy it is likely that they will become conditioned and this may
result in failure of subsequent antiemetic drug therapy. Adequate
antiemetic therapy should be striven for from the start and every
attempt be made to reduce anxiety at the time of chemotherapy
administration. Studies of progressive muscular relaxation training
and other techniques have shown that some patients have reduced
vomiting, and eat better (26). These techniques need further
evaluation but may well be useful together with conventional
antiemetics and have the added benefit that they include the patients
in their own treatment. Other social factors may affect the incidence
of emesis and one study has reported reduced emesis in 'heavy'
drinkers (27) Table 7.

Table 7. Relationship between cis-platin induced emesis and daily
alcohol intake.

| No. of patients | No. with uncontrolled nausea and vomiting | | | P value |
	<20g.alc/d	20-80g.alc/d	>80g.alc/d	
157	34/51	43/65	4/41	<0.001

6. RECOMMENDATIONS

Before considering currently recommended approaches to the
control of cancer chemotherapy induced emesis, it is worth defining
an "ideal" antimetic. Ideal properties would include:

- An antiemetic effect against a wide variety of cytotoxic drugs.
- A very high degree of activity against potent emetic drugs.
- Minimal side effects especially sedation, extrapyramidal reactions and dysphoria.
- Effective with repeated use.
- Available and effective in oral, injectable and suppository formulation.
- Prolonged half-life with dosage every 6-12 hours.
- Low potential for abuse.
- No interactions with cytotoxic drugs.
- Reasonable cost.

Currently no antiemetic, alone or in combination, comes close to that ideal. However, if patients are being treated with powerful emetic drugs such as cisplatin or nitrogen mustard recommendations can be made which will control and lessen vomiting in many patients. These include:

- Ensuring that the chemotherapy is given in such a way as to try to reduce the patient's anxiety as much as possible. Where available, training in relaxation may help the patient to deal with the stress of chemotherapy and may help avoid conditioning. Continuity of staff and the administration of cytotoxics by a chemotherapy nurse helps reduce stress.
- Try to ensure adequate antiemetic therapy from the beginning.
- When dealing with potent emetic drugs consider a) high dose metoclopramide (18) or a cannabinoid (9-13) as first line treatment. b) If this does not control the emesis try adding a second or third drug to the regime (24, 25). Drugs that may be considered include prochlorperazine, dexamethasone and lorazepam. Combinations of multiple antiemetics may have many more side effects of their own and sedation may be severe. This may be acceptable to some patients, though others will feel that it is worse than the emesis. These sorts of antiemetic regime generally require hospital admission and parenteral administration.
- If mild or moderately emetic cytotoxics are to be used then antiemetic therapy may be started with simpler oral agents (prochlo-

rperazine, cannabinoids, haloperidol etc) or drugs that can be used in suppository form. More complex antiemetic regimes need only be considered if the emesis is not controlled.

- If emesis is severe careful attention to fluid and electrolyte balance is important (28).

7. CONCLUSION

The multiplicity of available agents and complex nature of the problem make the evaluation of antiemetics a difficult task. Improved control of emesis will come but trials need to build systematically on current knowledge, must be randomized and data collected with scrupulous care. Combinations of antiemetics may well be the most effective approach, though this remains to be proven.

References

1) Moertel CG, Reitemeier RS and Gage RP. Controlled clinical evaluation of antiemetic drugs. JAMA 186: 116–118, 1963.
2) Lucas VS. Phenothiazines as antiemetics. In: Laszlo J (ED). Antiemetics and cancer chemotherapy. Williams and Wilkins. Baltimore. 1983 p 93–107.
3) Kahn T, Elias E, Mason G. Single dose of metoclopramide in the control of vomiting from cisdichlorodiammineplatinum in man. Cancer Treat. Rep. 62: 1106–1107, 1978.
4) Williams CJ, Bolton A, de Pemberton R, Whitehouse J. Antiemetics for patients treated with antitumour chemotherapy. Cancer Clin Trials 3: 363–367, 1980.
5) D'Souza DP, Reyntjens A and Thornes R. Domperidone in the prevention of nausea and vomiting induced by antineoplastic agents : a three-fold evaluation. Curr. Ther. Res. Clin Exp. 27: 384–387, 1980.
6) Penta J, Poster D, Bruno S. The pharmacologic treatment of nausea and vomiting caused by cancer chemotherapy : a review. In Laszlo J (ED). Antiemetics and cancer chemotherapy. Williams and Wilkins. Baltimore 1983 p 53–92.
7) Mehrotta S, Rosenthal C, Barile B. A comparison between Droperidol and prochlorperozine in combination with Trimethobenzamide as antiemetics for antineoplastic combination chemotherapy (Abstract). Proc. ASCO 22: C-335, 1981.
8) Moertel C, Schitt A, Hahn R, Oral benzquinamide in the treatment of nausea and vomiting. Clin. Pharmacol. Ther. 18: 554–557, 1976.
9) Sallan S, Zinberg N, Frei E. Antiemetic effect of delta-9-tetra-hydrocannabinol in patients receiving cancer chemotherapy. N. Engl. J. Med. 293: 795–797, 1975.
10) Ekert HW, Waters K, Jurk I. Amelioration of cancer chemotherapy – induced nausea and vomiting by delta-9-tetrahydrocannabinol. Med. J. Aust. 2: 657–659, 1979.

11) Frytak S, Moertel C, O'Fallon J, Delta-9-tetrahydrocannabinol as an antiemetic for patients receiving cancer chemotherapy. Ann. Intern. Med. 91: 825-830, 1979.

12) Chang A, Shiling D, Stillman R. A prospective evaluation of delta-9-tetrahydrocannabin or as an antiemetic in patients receiving adriamycin and cytoxan chemotherapy. Cancer 47: 1746-1751, 1981.

13) Herman T, Einhorn L, Jones S. Superiority of nabilone over prochlorperazine as an antiemetic in patients receiving cancer chemotherapy. N. Engl. J. Med 300, 1295-1297, 1979.

14) Steele N, Gralla R, Braun W. Double-blind comparison of the antiemetic effects of nabilone and prochlor perazine on chemotherapy-induced emesis. Cancer Treat. Rev. 64: 219-224, 1980.

15) Citran M, Herman T, Fossieck B. Double lined, randomized, cross over study of the antiemetic effect of levonantradol versus Tetrahydrocannabinol (Abstract) Proc. AACR 24: 652, 1983.

16) Cronin C, Sallan S. Delta-9-THC and Marijuana in : Laszlo 5 (ED) Antiemetics and cancer chemotherapy. Williams and Wilkins, Baltimore 1983. p 108-115.

17) Laszlo J, Lucas V. Synthetic cannabinoids in : Laszlo J (ED) Antiemetics and Cancer Chemotherapy. Williams and Wilkins, Baltimore 1983, p 116-128.

18) Gralla R. Antiemetic studies with metochlopramide in chemotherapy-induced nausea and vomiting. In: Laszlo J (ED) Antiemetics and Cancer Chemotherapy. Williams and Wilkins, Baltimore 1983. p 129-141.

19) Ellerton J, Myers A, Graze P. Control of frequent extrapyramidol effects of high dose metoclopramide by anticholinergics (Abstract) Proc. ASCO 2: C-328, 1983.

20) Kris M, Tyson L, Gralla R. Extrapyramidal reactions with high-dose. Metoclopramide. New. Engl. J. Med 309: 309-310, 1983.

21) Aapro M, Plezia P. Alberts D. Double-blind cross-overstudy of the antiemetic efficacy of high dose dexamethasone vs. high dose metoclopramide (Abstract) Proc. ASCO 2: C-364, 1983.

22) Laszlo J, Hanson D, Lucas V. Lorazepam as an antiemetic against cisplatin (Abstract) Proc. ASCO 2: C-369, 1983.

23) Plezia P, Alberts D, Aapro M. Immediate termination of intractable cisplatin induced vomiting with an intensive 5-drug antiemetic regime (Abstract). Proc. ASCO 2: C-363, 1983.

24) Artim R, DiBella N. Tetrahydrocannabinol plusprochlorperazine for refractory nausea and vomiting (Abstract) Proc. ASCO 2: C-330, 1983.

25) Tyson L, Gralla R, Clark R. Combination antiemetic trials with metoclopramide (Abstract) Proc. ASCO 2: C-356, 1983.

26) Cotanch P. Relaxation training for control of nausea and vomiting in patients recieving chemotherapy. Cancer Nursing 4: 277-283, 1983.

27) Sullivan JR, Leyden MJ, Bell R. Decreased cisplatin-induced nausea and vomiting with chronic alcohol ingestion. New Engl. J. Med. 309: 796, 1983.

28) Dennis V. Fluid and electrolyte changes after vomiting. in Laszlo J (ED) Antiemeics and cancer chemotherapy, Williams and Vilkins, Baltimore 1983 p 34-42.

CHAPTER III

PERSPECTIVES IN NEW DRUG DEVELOPMENT

1. PROBLEMS IN ACHIEVING DRUG SELECTIVITY

EXPERIMENTAL MODELS AND THEIR PREDICTIVE VALUE IN NEW DRUG DEVELOPMENT: A CRITICAL APPRAISAL: I. TOXICITY MODELS.

ABRAHAM GOLDIN AND PHILIP S. SCHEIN

The toxicity of antitumor agents for the host constitutes a prime limiting factor in clinical chemotherapy and it is essential that models be employed which will predict for both the quantitative and qualitative toxicity of new drugs undergoing development (1-4). The potential risks for the patient are significant: a) in order to maximize therapeutic efficacy and with the goal of cure, doses of drug in a moderately toxic range are generally employed; b) the testing of new compounds in the clinic is frequently accomplished with patients who have received prior therapy or are in an advanced stage of disease, so that the ability to withstand drug toxicity is diminished; c) the patients are usually treated for an extended period of time with repeated regimens. Further, many of the antitumor agents act via cytotoxicity for the host, increasing the risk of mutagenesis, carcinogenesis and teratogenesis.

The National Cancer Institute USA (NCI) developed a standardized pre-clinical toxicologic protocol (5) as part of the flow of drugs in development for the clinic. Large animals including the rhesus monkey and beagle dog were employed in order to meet the requirements of the Food and Drug Administration of the USA. More recently on the basis of retrospective analyses indicating correlations with clinical findings, emphasis has been placed on the utilization of mice for the determination of lethality, and dogs for the determination of the nature of toxicity.

PREDICTION OF STARTING DOSE FOR PHASE I CLINICAL TRIALS

Pinkel (6) reported on the use of body surface as a criterion of drug dosage in cancer therapy, and in an extension of these studies Freireich and colleagues (7) conducted a detailed investigation in which a comparison was made of the toxicity of a total of 18 antitumor agents in 5 animal species including mouse, rat, hamster, dog and monkey, with the results obtained in man. The analysis was based on a schedule of single treatments on 5 consecutive days. An important conclusion was that the experimental systems that were utilized in an attempt to predict the toxicity of antitumor agents were quite successful in correlating with the findings in patients. In mg per square meter of body surface area (mg/M^2) the maximum tolerated dose (MTD) was essentially the same in the various animal species and in humans. Thus, mouse, rat, hamster, dog or monkey could be employed with equal relevancy for the prediction of the MTD in patients. In terms of mg/kg, the maximum tolerated dose in humans was found to be approximately 1/12 the LD_{10} in mice, 1/7 the LD_{10} in rats, 1/2 the MTD in dogs, 1/3 the MTD in rhesus monkeys, and 1/9 the LD_{10} in hamsters. For the series of anticancer agents, on a mg/M^2 basis, there was a linear relationship (1:1) between the MTD in humans and the LD_{10} in mice. This was in similarity to the 1:1 linear relationship for the MTD of humans with dogs and monkeys. On a mg/kg basis the linear relationships remained demonstrable, with the values for the mouse approximately 12 times higher than those in man.

Goldsmith, *et. al.*, (8) conducted a retrospective analysis of a safe dose for Phase I clinical trials; 1/3 of the LD_{10} (mg/M^2) in the mouse appeared quite useful in quantitative prediction for human toxicity, comparing favorably with 1/3 Toxic Dose Low (TDL) in the monkey and the dog. Rozencweig, *et. al.*, (9) extended this evaluation, including 21 drugs, and found that the safe starting dose was equally predicted by mice as by dogs. The analysis indicated that the safe starting dose for Phase I clinical trials could be based safely on 1/10 of the LD_{10} (mg/M^2) in the mouse.

There is at present a general consensus that the mouse is an acceptable predictive model for estimation of a safe starting dose for Phase I trials; the MTD (mg/M^2) in man corresponds in general to the LD_{10} in mouse as well as to the MTD in dog and monkey. Also, it was considered that in the selection of a safe starting dose the incidence of dangerous toxicity could be essentially eliminated by further reduction of the dosage fraction employed (3, 4).

On the basis of the above and related investigations, the toxicology program of the NCI now utilizes mouse lethality as the primary indicator of a safe starting dose in man. The dose employed clinically is generally 1/10 of the mouse LD_{10} in mg/M^2 on single or 5 daily treatments. The clinical starting dose should be reduced further if unacceptable toxicity is observed in the dog at 1/10 of the LD_{10} on a mg/M^2 basis, using either a single or 5 daily treatment schedule.

Additional advantages may accrue with the mouse as the primary model for quantitative toxicologic evaluation. It is possible to conduct careful quantitative studies of dose-responsive relationships requiring a large number of animals, including routes and schedules and other pertinent parameters in both normal and tumorous animals. The mice provide a ready subject for detailed toxicologic, pharmacologic and other biological investigations. They may be utilized for the determination of combined drug toxicity and drug interactions of pertinence to the choice of drugs and safe starting dose and the relevance to therapeutic outcome. The toxicologic and related investigations in mice may provide leads with individual drugs, drug combinations and combined modalities of therapy. The principal limitation of the murine system is the inability to provide serial analyses of clinical chemistries. This impediment is now being overcome with the development of micro-analyses.

EXPERIMENTAL MODELS FOR PREDICTION OF QUALITATIVE DRUG TOXICITY FOR MAN

Schein, *et. al.*, (3) utilizing 25 anticancer drugs with diverse functional characteristics conducted a retrospective analysis comparing the ability of dog and monkey to predict for qualitative human organ system toxicity, and this led to the decision at the NCI to utilize the dog as the primary indicator of qualitative toxicity. No advantage was identified for the monkey as compared with the dog, and for specific adverse reactions, the dog appeared to be superior. The dog and the monkey were equally effective in the prediction of leucopenia (60% and 61% true positives and 20% and 17% false negatives, respectively). The dog was more accurate for prediction of anemia, since this species had a higher percentage of true positives and fewer false positives and false negatives as compared with the monkey. The dog data provided a distinct advantage over the monkey for the determination of thrombocytopenia, with only 19% false negative predictions, as compared with 56% underprediction for the monkey. The dog also tended to provide an advantage in the prediction of gastrointestinal toxicity, resulting in 92% true positives and no false negatives as compared with 74% true positives and 19% false negatives with the monkey. The monkey proved quite resistant to the emetogenic properties of most anticancer drugs. For both the dog and the monkey there was an important overprediction for liver toxicity,

with 44% and 35% false positives for the dog and monkey, respectively.
Overprediction also occurred in the case of renal toxicity, with the dog
yielding 56% false positives and 20% false negatives and the monkey 48%
false positives and 10% false negatives.

Overall, the dog and monkey provided reasonable models for the prediction of qualitative toxicities. This occurred, however, at the expense
of a high percentage of overprediction (false positives), most applicable
to hepatic, renal, neurologic and hematologic toxicity. This may be attributable, at least in part, to the utilization of high dosage levels in the
animal testing in order to evoke the entire spectrum of qualitative toxicities for each of the compounds (3, 4). This is in contrast to the Phase I
clinical trials in which treatment is discontinued at the point where dose-
limiting toxicity is demonstrated.

A number of features are worthy of note pertaining to prediction of
qualitative toxicity from dogs, as well as monkeys, for man: a) despite
the finding that there is a correspondence in susceptability to toxicity
of specific organ systems in animals and in humans, the toxicity may be
manifested for different specific clinical or chemical parameters; b) the
toxic manifestations in the clinic may be observed at a lower or a higher
dose than in the animal; c) there may be a difference in the order of
appearance of the various qualitative toxicities elicited by a compound;
d) the testing in the animals may provide false negatives, failing to predict toxicologic responses that may be subsequently observed in clinical
testing. Historically this occurred for cardiac toxicity on treatment
with daunomycin and for pancreatitis on clinical trials with L-asparaginase.
It should be pointed out, however, that in later studies, the cardiotoxicity
of anthracyclines has clearly been demonstrated in animal test models.
This raises important questions about the adequacy of observations using
current methodologies, and the potential need for the development of more
sophisticated techniques for future studies involving preclinical prediction;
e) the preclinical evaluation is conducted in healthy animals, whereas in
patients undergoing treatment, there may be organ specific damage resulting
from progression of the disease or from prior therapy, complicating attempts
at definitive correlations; f) furthermore, the administration of other drugs
such as analgesics, antiemetics and hypnotics may have an impact on the
extent of specific toxicities.

The utilization of the mouse for the prediction of qualitative toxicity

213

has not been evaluated in extenso. However, such investigations should
indeed be encouraged particularly in view of the increased availability
of micromethods for hematologic and biochemical determination of the action
of potential antitumor agents (3, 4).

FURTHER PROSPECTUS FOR TOXICITY MODELS IN NEW DRUG DEVELOPMENT

Taking into account the triad of the host, tumor and drug, the acute
and chronic toxicity of antitumor agents constitutes a critical limitation
to therapy. There are clearly a number of directions that may be exploited
that may have an important impact on the clinic. Some of these may be
outlined as follows: a) prediction of diminished limiting toxicity for
new agents and analogs of known antitumor agents. The preclinical toxicologic models have already been demonstrated to be successful in the
identification of drugs, such as streptozotocin and bleomycin, that do
not manifest limiting bone marrow toxicity. Anthracycline analogs and
liposome preparations of anthracyclines have shown reduced cardiotoxicity
in experimental models as compared with the parent drugs doxorubicin and
daunorubicin, and it is indicated that these studies may have clinical
applicability; b) prediction of optimal routes, and in some instances
schedule, of drug administration to avoid limiting drug toxicity and to
maximize therapeutic effectiveness. Routes and schedules of drugs may have
important impact on the nature and extent of clinical toxicity; c) prediction
of delayed toxicity such as for chloroethylnitrosoureas and imidazolecarboxa-
mides; d) prediction for carcinogenic and teratogenic activity; e) prediction
of specific organ toxicities which may in turn lead to the identification of
drugs that are useful in the treatment of tumors arising in these organs.
Streptozotocin is an example in which the diabetogenic activity of the
compound has been exploited for the treatment of malignant insulinoma;
f) the importance of a drug's pharmacokinetic profile, its extent of
binding to cell membrane and macromolecules, and its metabolism and excretion
has been abundantly demonstrated; g) the utilization of protective agents,
such as in leucovorin "rescue" with methotrexate, may provide selective
protection against drug toxicity for the host with retention of antitumor
effectiveness. Thus, there is a wide array of investigations that may be
undertaken with the current and new experimental models that may be employed
to further characterize drugs in development in a predictive manner for
the clinic.

The results of the preclinical quantitative and qualitative toxicologic evaluation of a new drug currently serve as the basis for determination of dosage and evaluation of risk. While preclinical toxicology data can never be discounted, it must be emphasized that the final decision to enter a new drug into Phase I trial must be heavily weighted toward the expectation of therapeutic activity, rather than toxicity in a drug-sensitive organ of an animal.

REFERENCES

1. Schein, PS: Preclinical toxicology of antitumor agents: Cancer Res (37): 1934-1937, 1977.
2. Schein PS, Winokur SH: Immunosuppressive and cytotoxic chemotherapy: Long-term complications. Ann Intern Med (82) 84-95, 1975.
3. Schein PS, Davis RD, Carter SK, Newman J, Schein DR, Rall DP: The evaluation of anticancer drugs in dogs and monkeys for the prediction of qualitative toxicities in man. Clin Pharmacol Therap (11) No 1, 3-40, 1970.
4. Goldin, A, Rozencweig M, Guarino AM, Schein P: Quantitative and qualitative prediction of toxicity from animals to human. In Tagnon HJ, Staquet, MJ. Controversies in cancer. Design of trials and treatment. Masson Pub USA Inc, 83-104, 1979.
5. Prieur DJ, Young DM, Davis RD, Cooney DA, Homan ER, Dixon RL, Guarino AM: Procedures for preclinical toxicologic evaluation of cancer chemotherapeutic agents. Protocols of the Laboratory of Toxicology. Cancer Chemother Rep (4) No 1, 1-30, 1973.
6. Pinkel D: The use of body surface as a criterion of drug dosage in cancer chemotherapy. Cancer Res (18): 853-856, 1956.
7. Freireich EJ, Gehan EA, Rall DP, Schmidt LH, Skipper HE: Quantitative comparison of toxicity of anticancer agents in mouse, rat, hamster, dog, monkey and man. Cancer Chemother Rep (50): 219-244, 1966.
8. Goldsmith MA, Slavik M, Carter SK: Quantitative prediction of drug toxicity in humans from toxicology in small and large animals. Cancer Res (25): 1354-1364, 1975.
9. Rozencweig M, Von Hoff DD, Staquet MJ, Schein PS, Penta JS, Goldin A, Muggia FM, Freireich EJ, DeVita VT Jr: Animal toxicology for early clinical trials with anticancer agents. Cancer Clin Trials (4): 21-28, 1981.

IN VIVO ANTITUMOR MODELS AND DRUG DEVELOPMENT

A.E. BOGDEN, J.M. VENDITTI AND W.R. COBB

The objective of this report is to suggest alternatives directed to resolving a growing need for more predictive tumor models in drug development as visualized in the context defined by the title of this symposium, "Cancer Chemotherapy and Selective Drug Development". The term "selective" excludes from consideration models used in large scale drug screening programs such as that sponsored by the Division of Cancer Treatment of the United States National Cancer Institute. The rationale and methods which form the basis for such drug screening programs, with an objective analysis of the requirements of a large scale primary screen, have been discussed in-depth by Venditti (1). Therefore, for purposes of this discussion, we assume that the developmental agents to be evaluated have successfully passed large scale primary screens and have exhibited a desired level of activity that warrants additional and more stringent preclinical evaluation. The increasing effectiveness of chemotherapy as a modality for cancer treatment, and the resultant demand for new and more effective antitumor agents, has awakened the private sector to the profitability of developing and marketing anticancer drugs, including the biological response modifiers (BRM) such as monoclonal antibody conjugates, interferons, interleukins, etc. As a result, there is an increasing expenditure of money and effort on anticancer drug development. An unexpected problem arising because of this concentration of resources by individual companies is a plethora of developmental agents having similar activity against standard test systems. There is an urgent need, therefore, for tumor models that can be inserted as an additional selective step for ranking drugs for further progression to preclinical or clinical toxicology. Our focus, then, is on this level of drug development and will include a potpourri of suggested practical modifications to existing tumor models, as well as alternatives, that will assist in identifying those developmental chemotherapeutic agents with greatest clinical potential.

215

Experimental and clinical evidence suggests that any tumor, either animal or human, is sensitive to a finite number of chemotherapeutic agents (1,2). No one tumor can model for cancer in man. There is a restriction, therefore, that is imposed on the search for new compounds when a single tumor is used as a test system. Logically, increasing the number of tumors in a drug development program increases the chances of not only detecting new agents but provides a more stringent basis for comparing the spectrum of activity of agents under development. The practicability of carrying human tumors in serial transplantation in genetically immunodeficient athymic nude mice, or in the immunocompromised conventional rodent, has spurred the use of antitumor assays in which human neoplasms are grown as xenografts. As an in vivo test system utilizing human tumors, the xenograft model is a potential candidate for the ideal predictive test system. What could be more predictive of a human tumor response than a human tumor? The attributes of validity, selectivity and predictability are desirable in model tumor systems at all levels of drug development, as are those that relate to cost and time efficiency. Attempts to broaden panels of human tumors for testing and measuring activity by percentage responders, and yet live within the aforementioned constraints, prompted the following modifications to the human tumor xenograft model.

In adapting the human tumor xenograft-athymic nude mouse model to drug testing, experimental oncologists have mimicked the transplantation technology developed with transplantable, solid, animal tumor systems. Human tumors are routinely carried in serial transplantation by subcutaneous implantation, and procedures for drug evaluation are based upon treating subcutaneously growing human tumors. There are certain disadvantages in the use of subcutaneously implanted human tumor xenografts for drug testing that impinge significantly on time and cost efficiencies. Evaluation of drug efficacy requires 1-2 months of effort measuring tumors and weighing animals. This effort plus the need to maintain large numbers of athymic mice for long periods is costly and hampers the ability to test materials at projected rates (1). There are, however, two basic test procedures which can effectively substitute for the long term Subcutaneous (SC) Assay, using the same transplantable human tumors, at a significant savings in time and costs. These are (a) the Subrenal Capsule (SRC) Assay and (b) the Tumored Ear (TE) Assay.

The SRC Assay has all the advantages of an in vivo test system in terms of metabolic activation mechanisms and pharmokinetics. The subcapsular site provides a naturally rich vascular bed which permits unrestricted nutrient as well as drug and antibody delivery. A tumor fragment is implanted as a xenograft rather than a cell suspension in consideration of the need to maintain cell membrane integrity and cell-to-cell contact, thus retaining normal permeability barriers and representative microarchitecture of the donor tumor intact within the fragment. Furthermore, tumor fragments in which the heterogeneous cell populations maintain an undisturbed spatial relationship provide a more realistic sampling of antigen distribution as well as availability to BRM that is representative of the tumor of origin. Details of SRC Assay methodology have been published in detail (3).

There are several variations to the SRC Assay method which are identified by assay duration. The 11-day SRC Assay utilizes the same transplantable human tumors as does the SC Assay, with the tumors propagated by serial passage in athymic nudes and tested as subcapsular xenografts in athymic nudes. This assay of 11-days duration utilizes change in tumor size or weight as a parameter of drug activity. The 6-day SRC Assay utilizes the same transplantable human tumor systems as does the 11-day SRC Assay. Propagation of tumor lines is also the same. However, for drug testing, the normal immunocompetent mouse rather than athymic nude is implanted subcapsularly for a 6-day period, a significant saving in time and animal costs.

The subcapsular site is not immunologically privileged. In earlier studies it was found that the growth rates of transplantation established human tumor xenograft systems were essentially the same, whether tumors were implanted for six days in immunodeficient athymic nude mice or in normal immunocompetent mice, and that immunosuppression of the immunocompetent animal did not appear to affect growth rate but permitted tumors to grow larger by extending the time before the onset of rejection (4). These observations have been recently corroborated and extended by Aamdal et al (5). Microscopic and ultrastructural examinations showed that after six days under the renal capsule of normal mice, transplantable human tumor xenografts retained the morphology of the parent subcutaneously passaged tumor. When such xenografts were removed from the subcapsular site and transplanted subcutaneously into athymic mice, they were capable of forming tumors having growth rates similar to those of the original tumors. When subcapsular xenografts were dispersed and cultivated in soft agar, the tumor cells proved to be clonogenic with plating efficiencies similar to those of the original subcutaneous xenografts. When the response of subcapsular xenografts to drug treatment was compared with that of tumors growing subcutaneously in athymic mice good agreement between the two assays was found. In our own laboratory, using identical activity criteria and data computation methods, the overall correlation of drug responsiveness between 6-day SRC Assays in normal and athymic nude mice was 83%.

The 3-day SRC Assay, using the same human tumor/animal systems as the 6-day assay, is especially suitable for testing BRM such as monoclonal antibodies and interferons. In an assay of this duration, monoclonal antibodies are tagged with a radioisotope and their localization in the tumor easily quantitated (6). Interferon effects on protein and/or DNA synthesis of tumors is quantitated by measuring tumor uptake of ^{3}H-leucine and/or ^{3}H-thymidine on day 3. It is stressed that the inherent qualities of the tumor fragment implant and the subcapsular site, found advantageous for drug testing, also meet the requirements for evaluating BRM activity.

The more novel alternative to the SC and SRC Assays is the less labor intensive Tumored Ear (TE) Assay (7). The TE Assay is essentially a subcutaneous test system of 10 to 15 days duration using athymic nude mice both for carrying tumors in serial passage and for drug testing. Commonly, for intrapinnal implantation, the ear is grasped between thumb and forefinger with the forefinger providing support to the ear as the trocar or needle is inserted from above. Invariably, both the ear and finger are pierced. The innovative feature which makes this assay feasible and practicable is the method of implanting a tumor fragment or mince. A 16 gauge trocar is inserted through the skin dorsally between the scapulae and then easily slid subcutaneously toward the ear, then along the pinnal ridge, and the graft deposited in a well vascularized pinna. There is little residual trauma and a single technician can easily perform an implant with the animal under light anesthesia. Quantitation of tumor response to treatment is also relatively simple and precise with excision of exact and duplicate portions (1/4" diameter plugs) of tumor bearing and normal ears with a #3 cork borer of 1/4" ID. Since the tumors are essentially implanted subcutaneously in the TE Assay, drugs may be administered by any route. Endpoints are group body weights on days 1 and 10 to monitor systemic toxicity and group tumored ear and group normal ear weights measured directly on a balance at sacrifice. Indicator of therapeutic activity is average final tumor weight, i.e., group tumored ear plug weight minus normal ear plug weight divided by the number of animals in the test group. These data can then be used to calculate % Test/Control values.

Transplantation established human tumor xenografts are stable and reproducible test systems that can be used for comparing the relative activities of new agents and their analogs over prolonged drug development-al periods. Use of fresh surgical explants of human tumors as xenografts, in 3-day or 6-day SRC Assays, provides a more stringent, and perhaps a more clinically predictive model, for advanced drug activity evaluation. As in the clinic, drugs tested against fresh surgical explants are evalu-ated on the basis of "response rate". Feasibility of such testing has been demonstrated (5,8). If new and more effective anticancer drugs are to be developed, the time-worn murine tumor systems will need to be re-placed or modified. The human tumor xenograft model, with all of its practicable modifications, is a viable alternative.

REFERENCES

1. Venditti JM: Pre-clinical drug development: Rationale and Methods. Sem Oncol (8): 349-361, 1981.
2. Bellet RE, Danna V, Mastrangelo MJ, Berd D. Evaluation of a "nude" mouse-human tumor panel as a predictive secondary screen for cancer chemotherapeutic agents. J Natl Cancer Inst (63): 1185-1188, 1979.
3. Bogden AE, Haskell PM, LePage DJ, Kelton DE, Cobb WR, Esber HJ: A rapid screening method for testing of chemotherapeutic agents against human tumor xenografts. In: Houchens DP and Ovejera AA (ed) Proc Sym-posium on the Use of Athymic (Nude) Mice in Cancer Research. Gustav Fischer, New York, 1978, pp. 231-250.
4. Bogden AE, Haskell PM, LePage DJ, Kelton DE, Cobb WR, Esber HJ: Growth of human tumor xenografts implanted under the renal capsule of normal immunocompetent mice. Exp Cell Biol (47): 281-293, 1979.
5. Aamdal S, Fodstad O, Johanessen JV, Pihl A: Chemosensitivity testing in vivo. Comparison of the Subrenal Capsule Assay in immunocompetent mice with the subcutaneous nude mouse model. Proc 13th Intern Cong Chemother, Vienna, 1983.
6. Bogden AE, Hnatowich DJ, Doherty PW, Griffin TW: In vivo localization of monoclonal antibody in fresh surgical explants of human tumors: 3-day Subrenal Capsule (SRC) Assay. Proc Am Assoc Cancer Res (24): 218, 1983.
7. Bogden AE, Cobb WR, LePage DE, Speropoulos S: A rapid method for screen-ing drugs against subcutaneously implanted human tumor xenografts: Tumored Ear (TE) Assay. Proc Am Assoc Cancer Res (23): 222, 1982.
8. Bogden AE, Cobb WR, LePage DJ, Haskell PM, Gulkin TA, Ward A, Kelton DE, Esber HJ: Chemotherapy responsiveness of human tumors as first trans-plant generation xenografts in the normal mouse: Six-day Subrenal Capsule Assay. Cancer (48): 10-20, 1981.

ASSAYS FOR CLONOGENIC HUMAN TUMOUR CELLS IN EXPERIMENTAL AND CLINICAL
CHEMOTHERAPY

G.G. STEEL, V.D. COURTENAY AND R.R. SANDHU

The population of cells that make up a tumour is invariably complex
and heterogeneous, including neoplastic cells in various states of
proliferation, degeneration, and differentiation, as well as a variety
of non-neoplastic host cells.

Among the many ways of evaluating the response of such a cell
population to chemotherapy, a widely-held view is that attention should
be directed at neoplastic stem cells, i.e. the primitive cells that
basically are responsible for growth and for regrowth after treatment.
Stem cells cannot be identified in situ within the tumour; what one
must do is to remove the cells, prepare a single-cell suspension, and
investigate colony formation in artificial environments. Although a
range of *in vitro* and *in vivo* techniques have been developed for this
purpose (1), work with human tumour cells has concentrated on the growth
of colonies in semi-solid culture media (soft agar or methylcellulose).
The main purpose of the gelling agent is, by removing the opportunities
for cell anchorage, to make it difficult for normal (non-neoplastic)
cells to grow, although it is increasingly being appreciated that it may
be a minority of tumour cells that can grow in the total absence of
anchorage. Furthermore, some classes of host cells (particularly
haemopoietic and macrophage precursors) do grow in soft agar and sometimes may appear as a contaminant of clonogenic assays (2).

The disaggregation of 'solid' human tumours for clonogenic assays
often presents considerable problems. Some tumours, such as melanomas,
are easily made into single-cell suspensions by mechanical or enzyme
treatments; others, such as many breast or colon tumours, are extremely
difficult to disaggregate without irreparable damage to the cells.
There is evidence that failure to exclude the presence of small cell
clumps has seriously complicated published studies using cloning assays
(3,4). In order to distinguish a growing colony from the clusters of

221

cells that may result from limited post-treatment division of damaged cells, it is necessary to fix a criterion of growth to at least 50 cells. When the plating efficiency is low it is difficult to avoid the possibility that for every 1000 cells plated there may have been a few clumps which, with a degree of post-treatment enlargement, might be mistaken for colonies. The effect of this will be a background of colonies that persist even at high drug doses, thus giving the impression of a resistant component in the cell population (5).

The Courtenay assay

   The development of this assay (6,7) took account of the relatively slow growth in tissue culture of human tumour cells. The tumour cells are suspended in 1.0 ml of Ham's F12 medium with serum in 0.3% agar in the bottom of a plastic test tube. After an initial culture period of 5 days, fresh liquid medium is placed on top of the agar and this is replenished as necessary to keep the culture in good condition. The method incorporates two factors often found to improve the plating efficiency: the use of low (3-5%) oxygen concentrations, and the addition to the agar of rat red blood cells that lyse during the early part of the culture period.

   This assay has been found to be successful in a wide range of studies on the sensitivity of human tumour cells to cytotoxic drugs or radiation. In an independent investigation (8) it has been compared with the Salmon-Hamburger assay (5) and found to be superior.

   The Courtenay assay has so far mainly been applied to studies of the drug and radiation sensitivity of human tumours grown as xenografts (9,10). A significant observation has been that in the majority of cases the dose-response curves for drug treatment have been exponential. With the exception of melanomas treated with DTIC (11), it has invariably been found that agents producing multi-decade cell kill give cell survival curves that are close to exponential (Fig. 1). The implication is that the inherent sensitivity of clonogenic cells to drug treatment is relatively uniform in the cases studied: there is no prima facie evidence for heterogeneity. Studies of radiation sensitivity of xenografted human tumours have demonstrated shouldered (often continuously-bending) survival curves for irradiation *in vitro* and the presence of a hypoxic component when irradiations are *in vivo*.

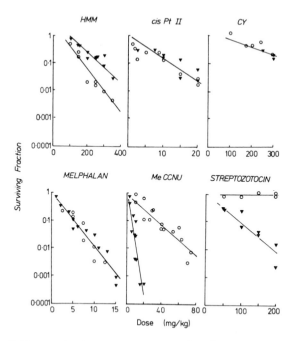

FIGURE 1. Cell survival curves for the *in vivo* treatment of two human tumour xenografts: O a pancreatic carcinoma, and ▼ a melanoma. Cell survival was measured (11) by the soft agar assay and in each case the drug dose scales extend up to the approximate LD_{10} dose in mice.

Table 1 summarises our experience of the drug sensitivity of xeno-grafted human tumour cells, given in terms of the number of logs of cell kill observed at an LD_{10} drug dose to the mouse. Each of these values was read from a cell survival curve defined by repeated experiments. The work has concentrated on tumours that give high plating efficiencies. It will be seen that insensitivity to chemotherapy has been common: the maximum cell kill often does not exceed 1 decade. However, even in diseases that clinically do not respond well to chemotherapy, we have sometimes seen up to 4 decades of cell kill by this type of assay. The only examples of clinically responsive disease in Table 1 are the small-cell lung cancers treated with methotrexate + cyclophosphamide + CCNU combination. The donor of one of these (HX72) was known to have been treated and become resistant before the xenograft was taken. The other line (HX81) had not been previously treated; it

TABLE 1. Cell survival following *in vivo* treatment (Decades of cell kill at LD_{10} dose)*

	PE**	CY	Mel	MNU	Adr	DTIC	HMM	Pt	MCC
Pancreatic ca.:									
HX32	25-30	0.4	3.0	1.0			2.3	0.7	
HX58	7-18	1.0	3.0	1.0			0.2	0.7	
Melanomas:									
HX34	10-40	0.4	2.2	7	0.1	2.6†	1.5	0.9	
HX40	2-13		2.1	3.0	0.1				
HX41	10-75	0.3	0.9	0.3	0	0.1			
HX46	2-6		3.0	2.0	0.1				
HX47	3-18		2.0	4.5	0	2.2†			
Colon ca.:									
HX18	1.0	0.6							
Small cell lung tumours:									
HX72	3								4.3
HX81	3-6								21
Lung Adenocarcinoma:									
HX70	2-5	0.7			0.5				

*Values in excess of 3.0 were obtained by extrapolation. See reference (13) for abbreviations and sources.
**Plating Efficiency (%).
†Non-exponential survival curves.

gave a steep exponential cell survival curve down to 10^{-3}, which extrapolated to 21 decades of cell kill at the LD_{10} dose.

A further significant observation has been that the two pancreatic carcinoma xenografts (HX32 and HX58) showed remarkable similarity in sensitivity to 4 of the drugs used, a slight difference in response to cyclophosphamide, and a large difference in response to hexamethylmelamine. This is one of the best examples so far described of differences between similar tumours in their spectrum of drug response.

REFERENCES

1. Steel GG: The Growth Kinetics of Tumours. Oxford University Press, Oxford, England, 1977.
2. Stephens TC, Currie GA, Peacock J: Repopulation of γ-irradiated Lewis lung carcinoma by malignant cells and host macrophage progenitors. Br J Cancer (38): 573-582, 1978.
3. Clonogenic assays for the chemotherapeutic sensitivity of human tumours. The Lancet, 780-781, April 3 1982.
4. Selby P, Buick RN, Tannock I: A critical appraisal of the "human tumor stem-cell assay". New Engl J Med (308): 129-134, 1983.

5. Salmon SE (ed): Cloning of Human Tumor Stem Cells. Alan Liss Inc., New York, 1980.
6. Courtenay VD, Mills J: An *in vitro* colony assay for human tumours grown in immune-suppressed mice and treated *in vivo* with cytotoxic agents. Br J Cancer (37): 261-268, 1978.
7. Courtenay D: The Courtenay clonogenic assay. In: Dendy PP, Hill BT (eds) Human Tumour Drug Sensitivity Testing *in vitro*: Techniques and Clinical Applications. Academic Press (in press) 1983.
8. Tveit KM, Fodstad O, Lotsberg J, Vaage, S, Pihl A: Colony growth and chemosensitivity *in vitro* of human melanoma biopsies. Relationship to clinical parameters. Int J Cancer (29): 533-538, 1982.
9. Smith IE. Courtenay VD, Mills J, Peckham MJ: *In vitro* radiation response of cells from four human tumors propagated in immune-suppressed mice. Cancer Research (38): 390-392, 1978.
10. Courtenay VD, Mills J, Steel GG: The spectrum of chemosensitivity of two human pancreatic carcinoma xenografts. Br J Cancer (46): 436-439, 1982.
11. Selby PJ, Courtenay VD, McElwain TJ, Peckham MJ, Steel GG: Colony growth and clonogenic cell survival in human melanoma xenografts treated with chemotherapy. Br J Cancer (42): 438-447, 1980.
12. Steel GG, Courtenay VD, Peckham MJ: The immune-suppressed mouse as an alternative host for heterotransplantation. In: The Nude Mouse in Experimental and Clinical Research, Vol.2. Academic Press, 1982, pp.207-227.
13. Steel, GG, Courtenay VD, Peckham MJ: The response to chemotherapy of a variety of human tumour xenografts. Br J Cancer (47): 1-13, 1983.

MECHANISMS OF RESISTANCE TO ANTICANCER AGENTS

B.W. FOX

Resistance to antitumour agents has been known to occur within tumour tissue since its discovery by Burchenal and his colleagues in 1950. Its meaning in the experimental laboratory may differ from that in the clinic in several important ways, stemming from the difference in the parameters with which it is possible to identify and measure it in each situation. The clinical experience is that of the patient who, following an initial success after treatment with an anticancer drug, relapses in spite of continued treatment with the same initially active drug. The clinician is then faced with the problem of trying to identify another anticancer drug to which he can turn, in order, hopefully, to effect a suitable regression which would benefit the patient at least as much as the first dose of the earlier drug.

The "resistance" which has apparently developed may not, of course, involve the tumour itself, but may result from an increasing inability of the patient to activate the drug in vivo. Alternatively, the patient may not be able to catabolise the drug due to progressive liver damage, and a lowered dosage may appear to be associated with a "resistance" of the tumour. In any case the patient would appear no longer to tolerate the drug and is said to have become "resistant" to further treatment.

The usual methods of overcoming this form of increasing intolerance towards the drug is to use different treatment schedules, additional protective agents (e.g. MESNA) or to change to a different anticancer drug.

The experimental view of resistance usually concerns only the tumour tissue itself divorced from any host based changes, and can be measured by direct transfer of pieces of tumour tissue into cell culture. In such cases the property of resistance continues to be seen.

The subcellular structure of tumour tissue has been studied for many years but the apparently daunting task of studying the individual cell biochemistry has generally been avoided due to lack of suitable technology. It is however, clear that true tumour resistance is a property of a single

227

cell and that in a mixed population of cells of varying sensitivity to a drug, a shift in the relative proportion of the cell present may give the illusion of increasing resistance. Thus the methods devised to overcome the resistance property of the whole tumour must take this concept into account.

In order to rationalise the interpretation of the origin of resistance, it is necessary to apply the term "resistance" more accurately to reflect its origin. It seems that "resistance" can only justifiably be applied to the property of a single cell, and could be defined as the ability of a single tumour cell to survive a local concentration of a damaging drug, that would otherwise have been expected to kill it. This could be an innate property of the cell ("intrinsic resistance") or could have been acquired by a rapid adaptive response ("adaptive resistance"). If a cell were to survive a low concentration of a damaging agent and divide, probably in the face of a loss of many similar cells within the population of which it is a part, it could give rise to a new population of resistant cells. These may be further selected for reduced sensitivity or actively become adapted by expressing alternative biochemical pathways, on a more permanent basis, e.g. by enhanced protective group synthesis, gene amplification of key enzymes, permeability changes in membranes, etc. ("acquired resistance"). In all these cases the type of "resistance" would describe the property of a single cell within the system being studied.

The tumour mass includes not only tumour cells but also many other non-tumour cell types which make up the matrix of the mass itself. A change in the total volume resulting from an effect of the drug treatment could be due to killing of matrix cells with or without any effect on the tumour cells associated with them, so that a change in tumour volume may not be associated with the antitumour effectiveness of the drug. The basic tumour sensitivity could be described as a "population resistance" or "population tolerance".

However, in those cases where the bulk of the tumour cells can be shown to be reduced by the effects of the antitumour agent, a difference in the growth pattern of the tumour resulting from repeated or continuous treatment could result simply from a shift in the relative proportion of intrinsically sensitive and resistant cells. Such a form of tumour resistance could be described as a "selected resistance" or "selected tolerance". A measurement of a biochemical change in such a tumour would thus represent the mean of the biochemical change within each individual cell of which it is made up.

There are clearly other forms of resistance with which a cell can be associated, such as that derived from a change in the genetic make-up of the cell, arising from either a mutational event or from other less random changes in the genome. Many of the long term and apparently permanent forms of selected or intrinsic resistance may be of this type and there appears to be little justification at this stage in distinguishing the genetic from epigenetic forms of resistance. We need more evidence with respect to these latter types, if indeed they differ in principle, before they can be considered in detail.

The advent of flow cytometric techniques has contributed a valuable tool for understanding the changes which occur in mixed populations of cells, possesing individual differences which can in turn be studied by fluorochrome-labelled substrates and products. This technique has been used to study the effects of a drug on the subpopulation structures of mixtures of drug sensitive and resistant cells at different times during the development of resistance. An important prerequisite of such an investigation is the selection of a suitable fluorochrome, related to the level of the drug within the cell (e.g. fluoresceinated methotrexate, daunorubicin, etc.), and to the level of a key enzyme which may be a receptor for the drug (e.g. dihydrofolate reductase for methotrexate). The availability of such fluorochromes is still limited, but it may be possible to undertake rapid testing of tumour populations to indicate possible overall sensitivities provided the number of cell types present is not great. Specific fluorochrome detection of resistant cells could be applied to histopathological material in sections and assist, not only in the interpretation of the section but also in indicating differences in drug sensitivity of different cell types.

Gene amplification has been shown to be an important mechanism by which a cell becomes adpated to drug cytotoxicity. In general, at low levels of resistance, double minutes may be present which, as the higher levels of amplification are developed, may revert to homogeneously staining regions of chromosomes. Although the phenomenon has been most extensively studied in methotrexate resistant cell lines, it is apparent that this may be a more general phenomenon especially associated with those antitumour agents like the antimetabolites in which a key enzyme is involved. So far, no gene amplification has been associated with alkylating agent resistance, but the observed increase in DNA repair capacity of alkylating agent treated cells may be the result of such activity.

Membrane permeability changes have been clearly associated with some forms of resistance, especially where active transport processes have been demonstrated to occur. The future of this area of work must inevitably take into consideration some of the interesting findings of Peterson et al (1) and Juliano and Ling (2). The close relationship of glycoprotein changes in the membrane with the changes in cell sensitivity during the development of resistance, and the concomitant changes in metastasising ability and malignancy will provide material for many interesting studies in the future.

REFERENCES

1. Peterson RHF, Meyex MB, Spengler A, Biedler JL: Alteration of plasma membrane glycopeptides and gangliosides of Chinese hamster cells accompanying development of resistance to Daunorubicin and Vincristine. Cancer Res (43): 222-228, 1983.
2. Juliano RL, Ling VA: A surface glycoprotein modulating drug permeability in Chinese hamster ovary cell mutants. Biochim Biophys Acta (455): 152-162, 1976.

THE ROLE OF PHARMACOKINETICS IN DRUG DESIGN AND USE

J.G. McVie

Pharmacokinetics is now standard in the early evaluation of a new drug
in vivo. Preclinical pharmacology aims to determine the range of peak plasma
concentrations achieved after different doses, given often in various
vehicles or carriers, by assorted routes of administration. The speed and
direction of clearance is usually obtained along with degree of protein
binding. This is of direct consequence in the eventual   choice of patients
for clinical phase I study. Thus n-methyl formamide was known to be metabolised in liver and excreted in low amounts in urine prior to clinical
trial. It was also predictable and indeed confirmed by pharmacokinetics
in the eventual patient study that bioavailability was high, thus
indicating that an oral preparation would be worth-while.[1]

Distribution studies are also useful in the preclinical phase,
particularly if the drug, as is the case for aziridynyl benzoquinone
(AZQ), is intended for treatment of an intracerebral tumour. The brain
is the best example of a priviliged site, where tumor cells can harbour
safe from non-lipophilic cytostatics. Thus the measurement of active drug
(or metabolite) in the mouse brain can be used as a baseline requirement
for development of such a group of drugs. Ftorafur is a more lipophilic
5-fluorouracil and indeed gives higher brain levels (and more central
nervous toxicity). Doxifluridine takes up a median place in both brain
levels and neurotoxicity.

Screening of analogues which may replace known active compounds is
simpler than for new molecules, because a database of pharmacokinetics
usually exists for the parent of the family. So metabolism of 4-epidoxo-
rubicin will probably differ little from that of doxorubicin. The eventual
finding of a difference in turn as may be the case for this drug, gives
rise to further evaluation of the new metabolites as potential new drugs.[2]
The uptake of anthracyclines in tumour cells and heart cells is only

possible in wide scale in animals, so this part of the preclinical work up is of increased importance.

Another example of analogues and application of pharmacokinetics, is the cisplatin family. Considerable variations have been seen in the clinical evaluation which may lead to decisions on the appropriate analogue for a given clinical role. Carboplatin is excreted fast and as intact active non-protein bound drug (80% of the dose within 48 hours). TNO 6 (1.1-diamminomethylcyclohexane (sulphato) platinum II) on the other hand is more slowly cleared from plasma though the half life is shorter than the parent cisplatin ($T\frac{1}{2}\beta$ 3.7 $\pm$ 1.3 v 5.4 $\pm$ 1.0 days). The area under the time concentration curves was however greater for TNO 6 (644 $\pm$ 171 v 332 $\pm$ 66/mg Pt/m^2). A third platinum compound JM40 (ethylene-diaminoplatinum II malonate) has given yet another spectrum viz long delay in excretion (65.6% in 5 days) and measurable free platinum in plasma at the end of day 5 (0.075 µg/ml after a dose of 300 mg/m^2).[3]

The clinical need for pharmacokinetics is not restricted to analogue assessment. Patients with abnormal renal and liver function should receive particular attention if eventual delayed excretion is found and toxicity explained.

An example of the latter is the accumulation of carminomycinol (a metabolite of carminomycin) which was noted on giving the drug twice weekly in low dose, instead of once each three weeks in full dose. Remarkable myelosuppression was very quickly noted in the first schedule occurring at 50% of the planned dose. Carminomycinol has been proved to be cytotoxic and myelotoxic, so the fact that it circulates at detectable plasma levels for seven days, explains the cumulative effect of the schedule.[4]

It is of importance to measure metabolism of cytotoxic drugs in early clinical trial for one other reason - there exists a marked species difference in metabolism and this can explain failure to reproduce cytotoxic effect seen in mice in the clinical experiment-. Pentamethyl melamine is a good example of this problem. The drug is quickly converted in the mouse and slowly in man to the active n-methyloyl metabolites. This finding has in turn led to the development of prodrugs with an optimal metabolic potential in man.[5]

The application of drug measurement in plasma, urine and tissues is essential to check bioavailability, disposition and clearance of the drug.

Metabolism studies can explain toxicity or failure of effect and identification
of active metabolites may lead to their synthesis as new drugs. Further,
dose and schedule studies can be accelerated and drug interactions (in
the inevitable combination chemotherapy) better monitored and defined.

References
1. Brindley C, Geschner A, Harpur ES: Studies of the pharmacology of
   n-methylformamide in mice. Cancer Treat Rep (66): 1957-1965, 1982.
2. Weenen H, Lankelma J, Penders PGM, McVie JG, Ten Bokkel Huinink WW,
   de Planque MM, Pinedo HM: Pharmacokinetics of 4'-epi-doxorubicin in man.
   Invest New Drugs (1): 59-64, 1983.
3. Vermorken JB, Ten Bokkel Huinink WW, McVie JG, van der Vijgh WJF,
   Pinedo HM: Clinical pharmacology of cisplatin and some new platinum
   analogs. Proc. of 2nd World Conference on Pharmacology,1984 (in press).
4. de Planque MM, Ten Bokkel Huinink WW, Simonetti GPC, McVie JG: A phase
   II study of carminomycin in a twice weekly schedule for patients with
   advanced breast cancer. Europ J Cancer and Clin Oncol (in press).
5. Rutty CJ, Newell DR, Muindi JRF, Harrap KR: The comparative pharmacokinetics of pentamethylmelamine in man, rat and mouse. Cancer Chemother Pharmacol (8): 105-112, 1982.

NOVEL STRUCTURES IN DEVELOPMENT

V. L. NARAYANAN

Many novel anticancer leads have resulted from the screening of a large variety of structural types against murine tumor models. A few leads have originated through the synthesis of compounds designed on some sort of rational hypothesis. Comprehensive descriptions of the preclinical drug discovery and development program at the National Cancer Institute (NCI) have recently become available (1,2). The strategy for new lead discovery involves the following steps: (a) the acquisition phase; approximately 10,000 compounds are acquired annually for screening, primarily from industrial sources, under provisions of confidentiality; (b) the preselection phase; the compounds acquired are preselected from large lists of structures using a two-stage selection process, namely; i) novelty and activity rating based on a computerized model (3) and ii) structure-activity analysis and chemists' review; (c) the anticancer evaluation phase; compounds are prescreened using the mouse P388 leukemia model and active compounds are selected (5%) for detailed evaluation against a panel of four cancer models; L1210 leukemia, B_{16} melanoma, Lewis lung carcinoma and mammary xenograft. It should be pointed out that the only practical definition of an "active" lead must be in terms of available tumor systems.

235

Figures 1 through 3 illustrate several examples of novel synthetic compounds that are currently under active development at NCI. The spectrum of activity of each compound, as well as its stage of development is indicated. In particular, I would like to draw your attention to NSC 340847 whose activity against Lewis lung carcinoma is extraordinary.

Figure 1 **INVESTIGATIONAL NEW DRUGS IND — 1983**

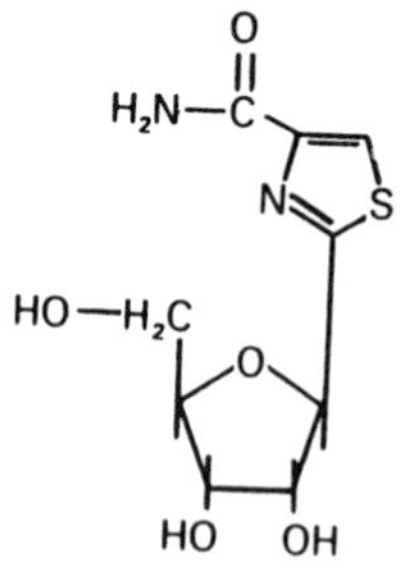

TCAR
NSC-286193

Tumor Model	Activity
P388	+ +
L1210	+ +
Lewis Lung	+ +

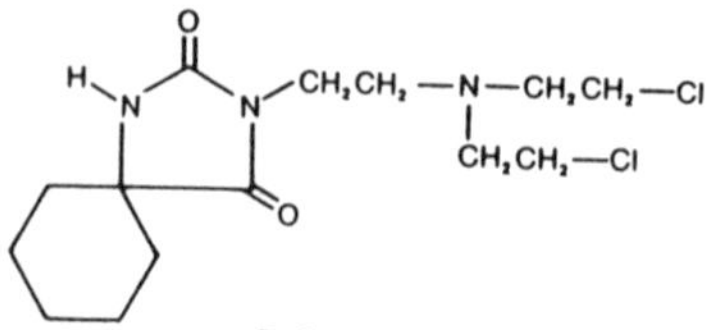

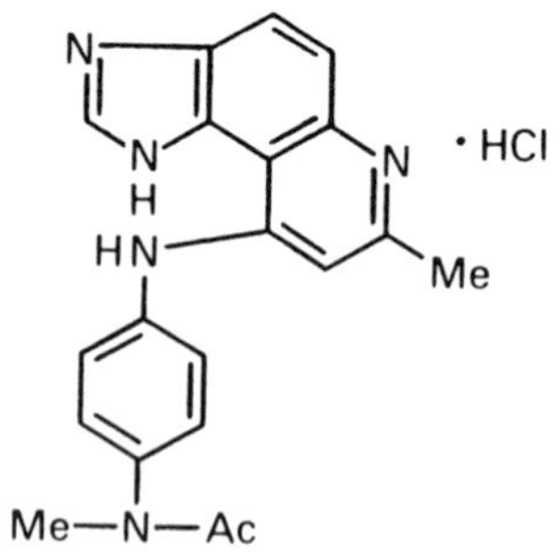

NSC-305884

Tumor Model	Activity
P388	+ +
B16	+ +

Spiromustine
NSC-172112*

Tumor Model	Activity
P388	+ +
B16	+ +
CD8F₁	+
Colon 38	+
L1210	+
MX1	+ +

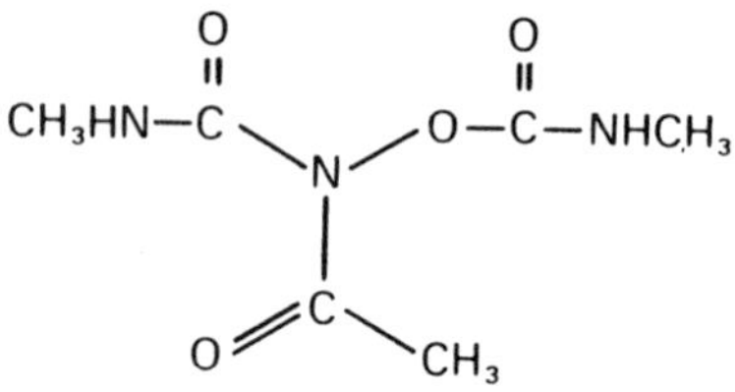

Caracemide
NSC-253272

Tumor Model	Activity
P388	+
CX1	+
MX1	+ +

Figure 2 **PROMISING NEW LEADS
SYNTHETIC COMPOUNDS IN TOXICOLOGY**

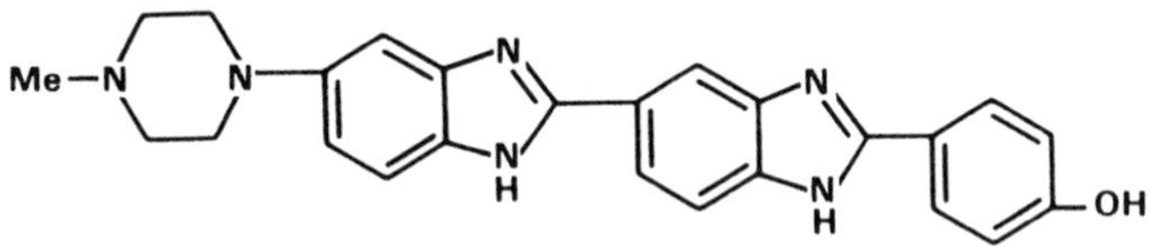

·3 HCl
NSC-322921

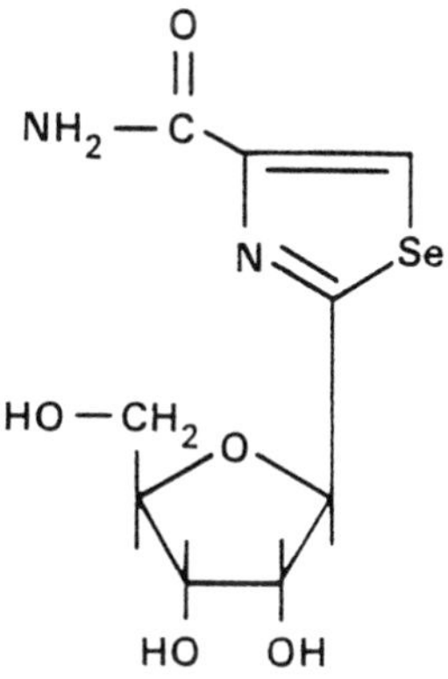

Tumor Model	Activity
P388	+
L1210	+ +
MX1	+ (?)

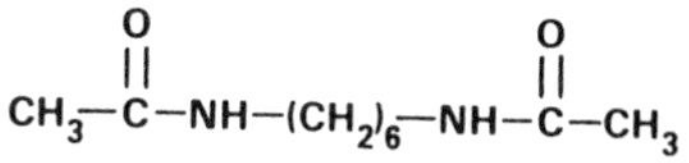

NSC-340847

HMBA
NSC-95580

**EFFECT OF NSC-340847 ON THE LIFE SPAN OF MICE INOCULATED
INTRAVENOUSLY WITH LEWIS LUNG CARCINOMA**

Drug	Dose, mg/kg	Median Life Span, Days	ILS, %	Cures
		Experiment 1		
untreated controls		16.9		0/40
6	200	10.7		0/10
	100	20.3	20	3/10
	50	60.0	255	6/10
	25	60.0	255	7/10
	12	60.0	255	8/10
		Experiment 2		
untreated controls		20.2		0/40
6	24	60	197	9/10
	12	60	197	9/10
	6	60	197	5/10
	3	31	53	0/10
	1.5	22	10	0/10

Figure 3 **PROMISING NEW LEADS**
SYNTHETIC COMPOUNDS — PRETOXICOLOGY

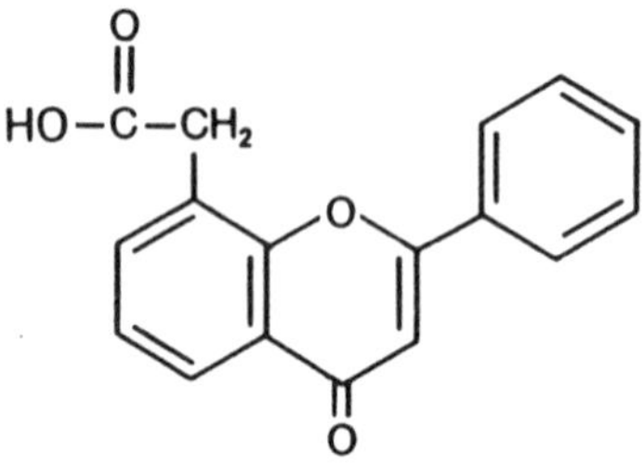

Flavoneacetic acid
NSC-347512

Tumor Model	Activity
P388	+
B16	+
Colon 38	+ +

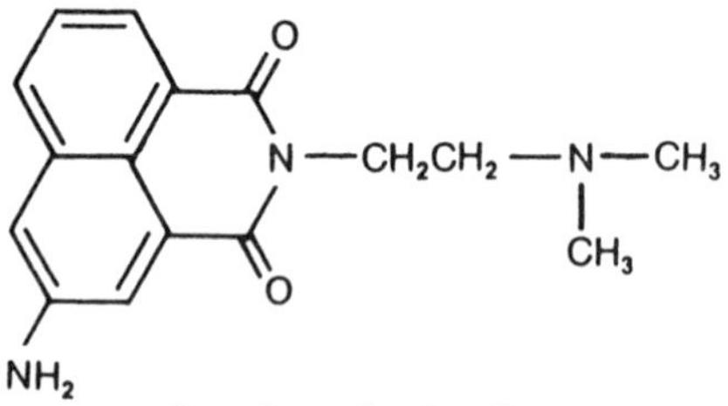

Benzisoquinolinedione
NSC-308847

Tumor Model	Activity
P388	+ +
B16	+
Colon 38	+
LE1210	+ +

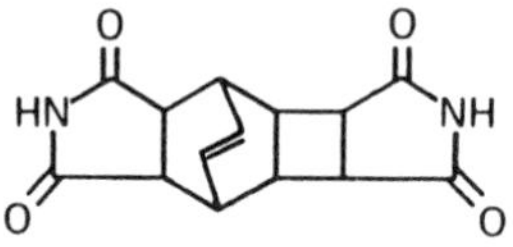

Mitindomide
NSC-284356

Tumor Model	Activity
P388	+ +
B16	+
CD8F$_1$	+ +
Colon 38	+
L1210	+ +

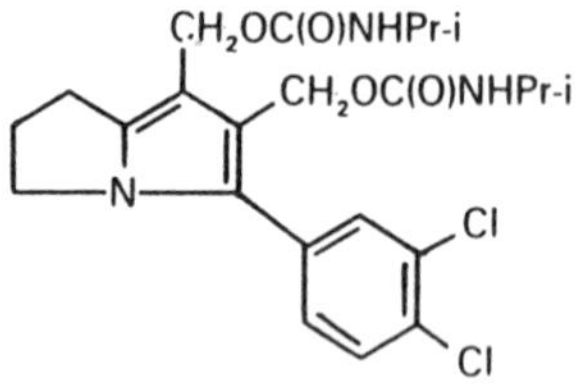

NSC-278214

Tumor Model	Activity
P388	+ +
B16	+ +
CD8F$_1$	+ +
Colon 38	+
L1210	+
MX1	+ +

Dihydrotriazine benzenesulfonyl fluoride
NSC-127755

Tumor Model	Activity
P388	+ +
B16	+ +
CD8F$_1$	+ +
Colon 38	+
L1210	+

Trimetrexate
NSC-352122

Tumor Model	Activity
CD8F$_1$	+

Azolastone
NSC-353451

Tumor Model	Activity
P388	+ +
B16	+ +
Colon 38	+ +
LE1210	+ +
LL39	+ +
LX1	+ +

Ara-AC
NSC-281272

Tumor Model	Activity
P388	+ +
B16	+
L1210	+ +
LL39	+ +
CX1	+ +
LX1	+ +
MX1	+ +

REFERENCES

1. Driscoll JS: The pre-clinical new drug research program of the National Cancer Institute. Cancer Treat. Rep., in press.
2. Narayanan VL: Strategy for the discovery and development of novel anticancer agents. In: Reinhoudt DH, Connors TA, Pinedo HM and Van de Pollkw (eds) Structure-activity relationships of anti-tumor agents. Martinus Nijhoff, Hague, 1983, pp 5-22.
3. Hodes L: Selection of molecular fragment features for structure-activity studies in antitumor screening. J. Chem Inf. Comput. Sci. (21): 132-136, 1981.

HYPOXIA-MEDIATED DRUGS FOR RADIO- AND CHEMOTHERAPY

G.E. ADAMS, I.J. STRATFORD AND P.W. SHELDON

1. INTRODUCTION

The relative radiation resistance of hypoxic tumour cells is believed to be a major limiting factor in the local control of some human tumours treated with fractionated radiotherapy. Hypoxic cells, which are present in most solid tumours arise as a result of tumour-cell proliferation essentially outstripping the development of the vascular supply of the tumour. They occur in and around areas of tumour necrosis where oxygen access is poor. Cells may also become temporarily hypoxic by normal variations in capillary blood flow.

Some chemical agents act like oxygen in increasing the radiation sensitivity of hypoxic cells. Most compounds belong to the electron-affinic group, where sensitization efficiency correlates directly with the redox properties of the compounds. Usually the sensitization is confined to hypoxic cells and provides the basis for improved therapeutic efficacy in that increased tumour-radiation sensitivity occurs without increase in radiation damage to normal tissues.

This paper indicates some aspects of research aimed at overcoming hypoxic cell radiation resistance and also methods for exploiting tumour hypoxia for enhancing the activity of some anti-cancer drugs.

2. RADIATION SENSITIZERS

Of the many known chemical radiation sensitizers the nitroimidazoles show the most promise at the present time.

The generality of radiosensitization in experimental tumours shown by one compound, misonidazole, led to wide-spread clinical investigation and there is some evidence that modest radiosensitization can be achieved in some clnical situations. However the neurotoxicity of this drug is a severe restriction and it is generally accepted that this will prevent its use clinically at doses sufficient for complete eradication of hypoxic cell radioresistance. The search for a clinically superior drug has been aimed at both improving

241

sensitization efficiency and reducing toxicity. Progress has been achieved in
both directions.

2.1. Reduced neurotoxicity

Neurotoxicity of nitroimidazoles decreases with decreasing lipophilicity
(1). Further, i.v. administration of hydrophilic analogues gives higher
tumour/plasma ratios than can be achieved with misonidazole. One compound
that has emerged from such studies is SR 2508 (N-2-hydroxyethyl)-2-(2-nitro-1-
imidazoyl)acetamide) (2). It has been estimated that due to the more
favourable pharmacology and toxicology of this compound, levels of SR 2508
about 7 times greater than misonidazole should be achievable in human tumours
for equitoxicity. Clinical studies with this agent are in progress.

2.2. Increased potency

It has been well demonstrated that the electron-affinity is the major
determinant of sensitization efficiency. However, sensitizers exist where
efficiency is abnormally high. One such compound is CB 1954 where the
efficiency is much greater than that of misonidazole (3,4) although their one-
electron reduction potentials are similar. The increased sensitization is
likely to be associated with the multifunctionality in the molecule.

RSU1954   RSU1069

There is evidence that the aziridine group is important. The compound
RSU1069 is a nitroimidazole containing an aziridine moiety in the side chain
(5,6). Studies both in vitro and in vivo have shown that this compound can be
at least 10-fold more efficient than misonidazole.

Figure 1 compares radiosensitizing efficiency of RSU1069 and misonidazole
in V79 cells in vitro and in the MT tumour irradiated in vivo, assayed in
vitro by cell clonogenicity. The enhancement ratios were obtained from
relative slopes of cell survival plots and given as a function of i.p. dose.
RSU1069 is clearly more efficient than misonidazole in the tumour particularly
at higher doses. Similar studies with this tumour using a local cure endpoint

verified the superior efficiency (5). This substantial sensitization occurs at considerably less than the MTD. Toxicological studies with compounds of this type are in progress in order to make comparisons with misonidazole concerning therapeutic ratio.

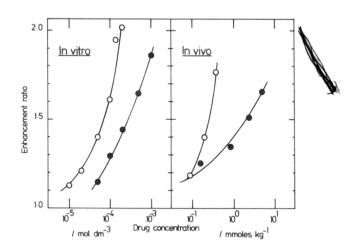

FIGURE 1. Comparison of the radiation sensitization efficiency of RSU1069 (O) and misonidazole (●) in hypoxic V79 cells in vitro and the MT tumour in vivo.

2.3. Modification of cellular thiol levels and radiation response

Reduction of intracellular GSH levels can enhance cellular radiation sensitivity. Interestingly this augments the radiation sensitizing efficiency of electron-affinic agents such as misonidazole both in vitro and in vivo. Reduction of intracellular GSH can be achieved in several ways. These include chemical binding by agents such as diethylmaleate (7) or phorone (8) and by inhibition of essential steps in GSH biosynthesis by agents such as buthionine sulfoximine (BSO) (9).

Table 1 shows suppression of GSH, by BSO and phorone either alone or incombination, in Lewis lung tumours and livers in C57 mice. In the MT tumour, reduction of GSH by such treatments increases radiosensitization by misonidazole (Table 2).

Table 1. Depletion of GSH in C57 mice bearing the Lewis lung tumour following treatment with BSO and phorone (8).

Treatment	% GSH	
	Liver	Tumour
Control	100	100
0.9mg BSO/g	22	57
0.2mg phorone/g	17	92
BSO + phorone	2	22

Table 2. Radiosensitization of the MT tumour by the combination of BSO, phorone and misonidazole (8).

Treatment	Do/Gy	ER
None	4.2	1
0.9mg BSO/g + 0.2mg phorone/g	4.4	0.95
0.2mg misonidazole/g	2.7	1.6
BSO + phorone + misonidazole	1.9	2.2

Further the high sensitizing efficiency of RSU1069 can also be increased. Figure 2 shows the influence of GSH suppression by diethylmaleate on the sensitizing efficiency of RSU1069 in hypoxic V79 cells irradiated in vitro.

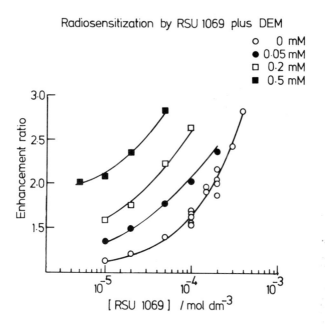

Radiosensitization by RSU 1069 plus DEM

○　　0 mM
●　0.05 mM
□　0.2 mM
■　0.5 mM

FIGURE 2.　Radiation sensitization of hypoxic cells by RSU 1069: The effect of pretreatment with various concentrations of diethylmaleate for 2hrs in air at 37°C.

3. CHEMOSENSITIZATION

Some chemical radiosensitizers including misonidazole increase or "sensitize" the anti-tumour activity of various drugs particularly agents such as cyclophosphamide, melphalan and nitrosoureas. While the overall mechanism is undoubtedly complex, there is convincing evidence that chemosensitization can be mediated through hypoxia (10,11).

Mammalian cells pre-incubated in hypoxia with misonidazole (12) and some other radiosensitizers including RSU1069, become much more sensitive to various alkylating agents. The effect is still observed even if the pre-treated cells are subsequently oxygenated before treatment with the alkylating agent (12).

The timescale for chemosensitization is much longer than that required for radiosensitization which occurs predominantly via fast free-radical processes. On the other hand, chemosensitization requires fairly long contact times and depends also upon drug concentration, cell type and other factors.

Figure 3 shows an example of chemosensitization by two sensitizers, Ro 03-8799 and RSU1069 in an experimental solid tumour (5). The sensitizers were administered at various times either before, or after, treatment of the MT tumour with a single dose of melphalan. Tumour response was assayed by clonogenic cell assay. The greater chemosensitization [enhancement of log kill from one (for melphalan alone) to almost four decades], is seen with RSU1069 in this system and appears to be optimal when the drug is given about 1 hour before treament with melphalan.

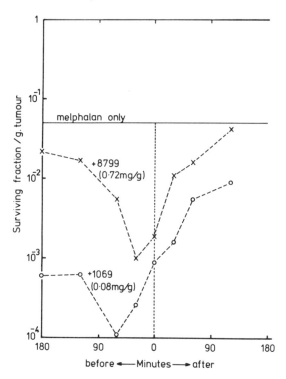

FIGURE 3. Potentiation of the cytotoxic effect of melphalan towards the MT tumour in WHT mice. The effects of Ro 03-8799 (X) or RSU 1069 (0) given at various times before and after 0.5mg/kg melphalan.

Chemosensitization by RSU1069 is greater than that seen with Ro 03-8799 and occurs at a 7-fold lower molar dose. Space precludes further discussion of the mechanisms of this effect. However the evidence is accumulating that anerobic reduction of the sensitizer occurs in the hypoxic region of the tumour to produce a toxic substance that makes the cells in the tumour more susceptible to the cytotoxic action of the alkylating agent. Since hypoxia is a physiological abnormality of tumours rather than normal tissues, chemosensitization is a differential anti-tumour phenomenon. Whether or not this approach will find a place in cancer chemotherapy remains to be seen. At this stage, the experimental evidence is encouraging.

REFERENCES

1. Brown JM and Workman P: Partition coefficient as a guide to the development of radiosensitizers which are less toxic than misonidazole. Radiat Res (82): 171-190, 1980.
2. Brown JM, Yu NY, Brown DM and Lee W: SR 2508: A 2-nitroimidazole amide which should be superior to misonidazole as a radiosensitizer for clinical use. Int J Radiat Oncol Biol Phys (7): 695-703, 1981.
3. Chapman JD, Raleigh JA, Pedersen JE, Ngan J, Shum FY, Meeker BE and Urtason RC: Potentially three distinct roles for hypoxic cell sensitizers in the clinic. In: Okada S, Imamura M, Terashima T and Yamaguchi H (eds) Proc 6th Int Congress Radiat Res, May 13-19, 1979, Tokyo. JARR, Tokyo, 1979, pp 885-892.
4. Stratford IJ, Williamson C, Hoe S and Adams GE: Radiosensitizing and cytotoxicity studies with CB 1954 (2,4-dinitro-5-aziridinylbenzamide). Radiat Res (88): 502-509, 1981.
5. Adams GE, Ahmed I, Sheldon PW and Stratford IJ: Radiation sensitization and chemopoentiation: RSU1069, a compound more efficient thatn misonidazole in vitro and in vivo. Br J Cancer, 1984 (in press).
6. Adams GE, Ahmed I, Sheldon PW and Stratford IJ: RSU1069, or 2-nitroimidaozle containing an alkylating group: High efficiency as a radio- and chemosensitizer in vitro and in vivo. Int J Radiat Oncol Biol Phys, 1984 (in press).
7. Bump EA, Yu NN and Brown JM: The use of drugs which deplete intracellular glutathione as radiosensitizers of hypoxic tumour cells in vivo. Int J Radiat Oncol Biol Phys (8): 439-442, 1982.
8. Stratford IJ, Sheldon PW and Adams GE: Hypoxic cell sensitizers. In: Steel GG, Peckham MJ and Adams GE (eds) The Biological Basis of Radiotherapy. Elsevier Science Publishers, 1983.
9. Griffith OW and Meister A: Potent and specific inhibition of glutathione synthesis by buthionine sulphoximine (s-n-butyl homocysteine sulphoximine). J Biol Chem (254): 7558-7560, 1979.
10. Sutherlands RL: Conference on Chemical Modification: Radiation and Cytotoxic Drugs. Int J Radiat Oncol Biol Phys (8): 323-815, 1982.
11. Wheeler KT, Wallen CA, Wolf KL and Siemann D: Hypoxic cells: an in situ chemopotentiation of nitrosoureas by misonidazole. Br J Cancer (in press).
12. Stratford IJ, Adams GE, Horsman MR, Kandaiya S, Rajaratnam S, Smith E and Williamson C: The interaction of misonidazole with radiation, chemotherapeutic agents, or heat: A preliminary report. Cancer Clinical Trials (3): 231-236, 1980.

2.   TARGETTED CHEMOTHERAPY

INDUCTION OF CELL DIFFERENTIATION AS A TARGET FOR CANCER THERAPY

A. BLOCH

The clinically effective anticancer agents are characterized by their ability to specifically inhibit the synthesis and/or function of DNA (1). Agents that primarily interfere with the synthesis of RNA, protein or other cell constituents lack such antitumor selectivity.

If cytotoxicity alone were a sufficient condition for providing selective antitumor action, then a multitude of cytotoxic agents that inhibit the synthesis or function of cell constituents other than DNA should also be clinically effective. Since that is not the case, selectivity is indicated to derive from the inhibition of DNA-centered activity. Induction of tumor cell differentiation is suggested to be one mechanism by which this selectivity is expressed.

This suggestion derives from the notion that the cancer cell is arrested at stages of incomplete maturation, without cessation of its proliferative activity (2,3). Induction of its differentiation to more mature or to terminally mature forms offers a means for removing it from its uncontrolled proliferative state.

Support for this view is provided most persuasively by the hematologic neoplasms, which are classified according to the stages of differentiation at which the cells are arrested in their maturation sequence. Normally, hematopoietic proliferation and differentiation is sensitively controlled by exogenous protein factors that serve as growth (GF) or differentiation (DF) signals (4-6). The lack of cancer cell differentiation can be ascribed to various causes, including increased sensitivity to GFs, decreased responsiveness to DFs, lowered elaboration of competent DFs by the host and endogenous production of GF-related products by the cancer cell itself.

Whichever the case, the cancer cell has not lost its ability to differentiate. For instance, a variety of agents, including the clinically effective DNA-specific anticancer drugs (7-15), some membrane-reactive substances such as dimethylsulfoxide (16-18) and tetradecanoylphorbol acetate [TPA] (19-27), and natural effectors such as retinoic acid (28-30) and protein factors present in conditioned media (31-35) are capable of initiating leukemic cell differentiation in vitro. In contrast, agents that interfere with RNA or protein synthesis, including cordycepin, puromycin and cycloheximide are unable to induce this event (36). This inability is undoubtedly related to the fact that these agents prevent the formation of RNA and protein required for the expression of differentiated structure and function. While interference with RNA and protein synthesis leads to the inhibition of cell growth, it occurs only at cytotoxic drug concentrations that preclude antitumor selectivity. DNA-reactive agents, on the other hand, induce differentiation at concentrations that are limitedly cytotoxic, providing a means for the selective removal of tumor cells through induced maturation (37). Therapies based on maximally tolerated cytotoxic doses are destructive to tumor as well as host cells, without assuring the destruction of the last cancer cell. In contrast, minimally toxic or non-toxic doses of antineoplastic agents have the capacity to sensitize leukemic cells to the action of natural DFs (38,39), and this phenomenon may constitute a critical component of effective clinical drug therapy, particularly with low-dose drug regimens which have demonstrated significant clinical potential (40,41). Sensitization with drugs appears particularly useful where the leukemic state derives from a lowered responsiveness of the leukemic cells to DFs, or where inadequate levels of DFs are elaborated by the host.

Unlike the anticancer agents, which at differentiation-inducing doses are cytotoxic to a fraction of the (ML-1) myeloblastic leukemia cell population treated in vitro, DFs present in mitogen-stimulated human leukocyte-conditioned media induce differentiation at non-toxic doses (42). Combining the two categories of agents at essentially non-toxic concentrations provides for optimal differentiation-induction.

Whereas DNA-reactive agents cause a rapid decline of DNA synthesis prior to the appearance of differentiated morphology, DFs cause a gradual decline in DNA synthesis during the emergence of the mature cell population (43). A course of events similar to that initiated by DFs is followed upon treatment with retinoic acid, an agent that interferes with the mitogenic stimulation exerted by GF (44). Both retinoic acid and DFs permit continuation of some cell proliferation, likely at intermediate maturation stages as occurs in vivo. TPA, which interferes to some extent with DNA synthesis (43) and inhibits binding of GFs to specific receptors (45) displays characteristics of both classes of agents, causing a rapid decline in DNA synthesis simultaneous with the appearance of differentiation-associated characteristics (43). The DNA-reactive agents, TPA and the DFs present in conditioned medium induce ML-1 leukemic cell differentiation to monocyte/macrophages, whereas retinoic acid causes differentiation to proceed along the granulocyte path (15).

The differences in the maturation-inducing capacity of theses agents are also reflected in their effects on cell cycle progression. Drugs such as adriamycin and actinomycin D cause the rapid accumulation of leukemic ML-1 cells in G_1, from whence they enter the differentiation path. DF and retinoic acid give rise to a more gradual accumulation of the cell population in G_1, in keeping with the limited extent of cell proliferation that occurs during maturation induced with these agents (43).

These observations are compatible with a scheme (46) that has a proliferation-controlling factor as its central operant. It determines proliferation-associated cell cycle transition from G_1 to S, and entry into the differentiation path from the G_1 phase of the cell cycle. Inhibition of DNA synthesis/function by the antineoplastic agents interrupts formation of the RNA transcript specifying this factor, whereas interference with GF activity, by TPA or retinoic acid, causes its inactivation, possibly by the intervention of DF, which can overcome GF activity when provided at high enough concentrations.

These regulatory events may relate to the action of cellular oncogenes, which freeze the neoplastic cell in its proliferation mode. In human myeloplastic leukemia cells (ML-1), induction of differentiation is followed by a rapid decrease in c-myb expression, detectable after 3 hours and preceding the decline of DNA synthesis (47).

Taken together, these observations demonstrate that the oncogenic arrest of cell differentiation is not an irreversible event, and that the freeze of the cancer cell in its proliferation mode can be removed by stimulating its differentiation to a non-proliferating mature stage or to a stage where self-renewal yields cells that are sensitive to normal growth and differentiation controls.

The success of a differentiation-centered approach depends, of course, on numerous auxiliary parameters, among them the level of functioning DFs present in the host and the size of the tumor burden that can adversely affect the proliferation of normal precursor cells (48,49).

254

The balanced utilization of sensitizing DNA-reactive agents together with DFs, or with agents that stimulate their production or inhibit GF activity has, thus, the potential for making a meaningful contribution to the therapy of cancer.

REFERENCES

1. Bloch A. Purine and Pyrimidine Analogs in Cancer Chemotherapy In: Mihich E (ed) New Leads in Cancer Therapeutics. GK Hall and Co., Boston, 1981, pp 65-72.
2. Pierce G, Shiles R, Fink L: Cancer, a Problem of Developmental Biology. Prentice Hall, Englewood Cliffs, 1978.
3. Greaves MP. J Cell Physiol Suppl 1: 113-125, 1982.
4. Mak TW, McCulloch EA: Cellular and molecular biology of hemopoietic stem cell differentiation. AR Liss, New York, 1982.
5. Clarkson B, Marks PA, Till JE: Differentiation of normal and neoplastic hematipoietic cells. Cold Spring Harbor Laboratory, 1978.
6. Golde DW, Cline MJ, Metcalf D, Fox CF (eds): Hematopoietic Cell Differentiation. Academic Press, New York, 1978.
7. Schubert D, Jacob F: Proc Nat Acad Sci (USA) (67):247-254, 1970.
8. Silbert SW, Goldstein MN: Cancer Res (32):1422-1427, 1972.
9. Hozumi M, Honma V, Tomida M, Okabe J, Kasukabe T, Sugiyama K: Acta Haematol Jap (42):941-952, 1979.
10. Friedman SJ, Skehan P: Cancer Res (39):1960-1967, 1979.
11. Collins SJ, Bodner A, Ting R, Gallo RC: Int J Cancer (25):213-218, 1980.
12. Lotem J, Sachs L: Int J Cancer (25):561-564, 1980.
13. Papac RJ, Brown AW, Schwartz EL, Sartorelli AC: Cancer Letts (10):33-38, 1980.
14. Bodnar AJ, Ting RC, Gallo RC: J Nat Cancer Inst (67):1025-1030, 1981.
15. Takeda K, Minowada J, Bloch A: Cancer Res (42):5152-5158, 1982.
16. Friend C, Scher W, Holland JG, Sato T: Proc Nat Acad Sci (USA) (68):378-382, 1971.
17. Tanaka M, Levy J, Terada M, Breslow R, Rifkind RA, Marks PA: Proc Nat Acad Sci (USA) (72):1003-1006, 1975.
18. Collins SJ, Ruscetti FW, Gallagher RE, Gallo RC: Proc Nat Acad Sci (USA) (75):2458-2462, 1978.
19. Rovera G, O'Brien TG, Diamond L: Science (204):868-870, 1979.
20. Huberman E, Callaham MF: Proc Nat Acad Sci (76):1293-1297, 1979.
21. Lotem J, Sachs L: Proc Nat Acad Sci (USA) (76):5158-5162, 1979.
22. Koeffler HP, Bar-Eli M, Territo MC: Cancer Res (41):919-926, 1981.
23. Nagasawa K, Mak TW: Proc Nat Acad Sci (USA) (77):2965, 1980.
24. LeBien T, Kersey J, Nakazawa S, Minato K, Minowada J: Leukemia Res (6):299, 1982.
25. Nakao Y, Matsuda S, Fujita T, Watanabe S, Morikawa S, Saida T, Ito Y: Cancer Res (42):3843-3850, 1982.
26. Totterman TH, Nilsson K, Sundstrom C: Nature (288):176-178, 1980.
27. Sakagami H, Minowada J, Ozer H, Takeda K, Bloch A: Leukemia Res, in press.
28. Strickland S, Mahdani V: Cell (15):393-403, 1978.
29. Breitman TR, Selonick SE, Collins SJ: Proc Nat Acad Sci (USA) (77):2936-2940, 1980.

30. Honma Y, Takenaga K, Kasukabe T, Hozumi M: Biochem Biophys Res Commun (95):507-512, 1980.
31. Ichikawa Y: J Cell Physiol (74):223-234, 1969.
32. Hozumi MT, Takenaga K, Tornida M, Okabe J: Gann (39):5127-5131, 1979.
33. Metcalf D: J Cell Physiol Suppl 1, 175-183, 1982.
34. Moore MAS: Ibid 53-64, 1982.
35. Sachs L: Ibid 151-164, 1982.
36. Takeda K, Minowada J, Leasure JA, Bloch A: Proc Am Assoc Cancer Res (23):226, 1982.
37. Craig RW, Frankfurt O, Takeda K, Chneda GB, Bloch A: Proc Am Assoc Cancer Res (24):15, 1983.
38. Hayashi M, Okabe J, Hozumi M: Gann (70):235-238, 1979.
39. Okabe J, Honma Y, Hayashi M, Hozumi M: Int J Cancer (24):87-91, 1979.
40. Baccarani M, Tura S: Br J Haematol (42):485-490, 1979.
41. Castaigne S, Daniel MT, Tilly H, Herait P, Degos L: Blood (62):85-86, 1983.
42. Takeda K, Minowada J, Bloch A: Cell Immunol (79):288-297, 1983.
43. Craig RW, Frankfurt OS, Sakagami H, Bloch A: manuscript in preparation.
44. Jetten AM: J Cell Physiol (110):235-240, 1982.
45. Lee L-S, Weinstein IB: Science (202):314-315, 1978.
46. Bloch A: Cancer Treatm Repts, in press.
47. Craig RW, Bloch A: Cancer Research, in press.
48. Broxmeyer HE, Jacobsen N, Kurland J, Mendelsohn N, Moore MAS: J Nat Cancer Inst (60):497-510, 1978.
49. Okabe J, Hayashi M, Honma Y, Hozumi M: Int J Cancer (22): 570-575, 1978.

COMPLEMENT LYSIS OF TUMOUR CELLS INDUCED BY UNIVALENT ANTIBODIES

G. T. STEVENSON, V. M. COLE, M. J. GLENNIE and H. F. WATTS

Increasing knowledge of the mammalian cell surface and the advent
of monoclonal antibodies have revived interest in treating cancer by the
simple infusion of xenogeneic antibody. This approach can be monitored
with precision, partly at the molecular level, in contrast to the
popular immunotherapy of the 1970s in which attempts were made to invoke
immune responses to autochthonous tumours. Furthermore the antibody
infusion is relatively innocuous, with problems such as hypersensitivity
fairly well understood. A large question remains, however, about its
efficacy.

The idiotypic determinants (collectively the "idiotype") on surface
immunoglobulin of neoplastic B lymphoid cells represent highly specialized
and well characterized differentiation antigens. For all practical
purposes they are tumour-specific (1): to eliminate all cells expressing
them would eliminate, or considerably reduce, the lymphoma, at negligible
cost to the residual normal lymphoid tissue. Because of the great
variety of idiotypic structure a different anti-idiotype will in general
be required for each tumour.

Human B-lymphocytic tumours have been treated with both polyclonal
(2) and monoclonal (3) anti-idiotype. Both in published and current
cases better results have been obtained with monoclonal reagents,
although to date only one case (3) in which an indefinite remission has
been induced is known to us. One advantage of the monoclonal antibodies
is availability in indefinitely large amounts. This is particularly
desirable in the idiotype-anti-idiotype system, where frequently an
appreciable amount of extracellular idiotypic Ig (4) must be swamped by
the antibody.

It is not yet clear which adjunctive functions of anti-idiotype are
important in killing the neoplastic target cells. Activation of

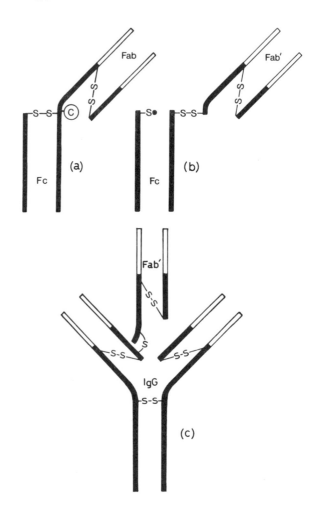

FIGURE 1. Some univalent antibody derivatives. (a) Fab/c obtained from rabbit IgG by limited proteolysis with papain (12). (b) FabFc hybrid derived by linking Fab'γ, from peptic digestion of antibody, with Fc from papain digestion of an arbitrary IgG (8). (c) FabIgG hybrid derived by linking antibody Fab'γ to host IgG by a thioether bond formed between a hinge region -SH of the Fab'γ and a maleimide group introduced into the IgG (14).

complement may well be effective against cells in the bloodstream, but its usefulness against cells in tissues is problematical. Studies in vitro with the guinea pig L₂C leukaemia have shown anti-idiotype to be able to invoke killing of the tumour cells by either complement or K cells (5). The antibody has invoked neither phagocytosis nor extra-

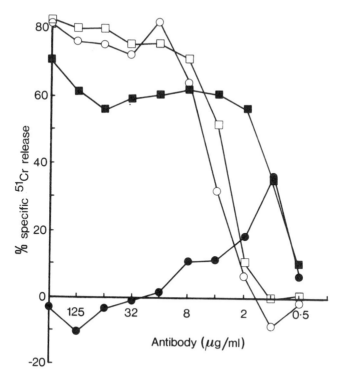

FIGURE 2. Complement lysis of L$_2$C cells invoked by Fab/c (O,□) or IgG (●,■); from rabbit antibody to the surface Ig λ chains. Washed, ^{51}Cr-labelled cells were incubated at 5 x 10^5 ml^{-1} with antibody derivates at the indicated concentrations at 37° for 15 minutes to permit modulation (O,●); control incubations were at 0° (□,■). All suspensions were then brought to 0°, 1·5 vol of 1:2 fresh rabbit serum was added as a source of complement, and the temperature was raised to 37° for 30 minutes to promote complement activity. Finally the suspensions were chilled and the supernatants assayed for released ^{51}Cr. From (12).

cellular killing by guinea pig peritoneal macrophages: instead the antibody-coated L$_2$C cells adhere to the macrophages, and undergo cytostasis as judged by an abrupt cessation of thymidine uptake (6).

An important mechanism of defence for mammalian cells confronted by antibody is provided by antigenic modulation (7). It probably yields an avenue of escape from K cells (8) and phagocytosis (9) as well as from complement. It depends - at least in the case of surface Ig - upon redistribution of surface antigen after cross-linking by bi- or multi-valent antibody, and can occur sufficiently swiftly to yield some

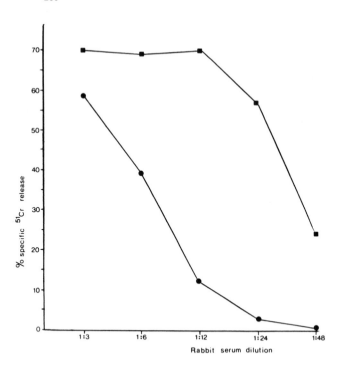

FIGURE 3. Complement lysis of L_2C cells invoked by Fab/c (■) or IgG (●) from rabbit antiserum to Fabμ of the surface Ig. First the cells were labelled with ^{51}Cr and washed. 100 μl of cells (1 x 10^6 ml^{-1}) were incubated for 15 minutes at 0° with 100 μl of antibody derivative (5μM). 300 μl of fresh rabbit serum was added as the complement source, at the dilutions shown above. After mixing, the temperature was raised to 37° for 30 minutes to promote complement activity. The suspensions were then chilled, spun, and the supernatants assayed for ^{51}Cr release.

protection to cells confronted simultaneously by antibody and complement (10). Complete clearing of antigen-antibody from the cell surface need not be required: resistance to complement lysis has been noted while the complexes persist on the surface in a patched configuration (10).

A variety of antibody derivatives are being investigated in the hope of enhancing the therapeutic efficacy of anti-idiotype (11). One type of derivative, the *univalent antibody* (12), avoids antigenic modulation by having only one antibody site, but retains an intact Fc for adjunctive functions such as complement activation. The loss of the "multiple binding bonus" - a lower rate of dissociation if two Fab arms instead of one engage antigen - could be serious when attacking a bacterium with immobile constituents in its cell wall. However a mammalian cell target, able to move its surface molecules actively in the plane of the membrane (13), could stress the bonds formed by two surface molecules with one bivalent antibody and thereby reduce the multiple binding effect.

The simplest univalent derivative available, Fab/c from rabbit IgG antibody (Fig. 1), has been investigated in the model anti-idiotype system provided by the L_2C leukaemia (12). It attaches to the L_2C cell and is seen by fluorescence microscopy and flow cytofluorimetry not to undergo redistribution. Typically it induces complement cytotoxicity at a higher level than does whole IgG, although not titrating out as far (Fig. 2). It can be seen also in Fig. 2 that incubation of the cells with Fab/c at 37° before adding the complement does not diminish the cytotoxicity achieved: that is, antigenic modulation has not occurred. In Fig. 3 the levels of cytotoxicity are examined as a function of *complement concentration*, with the concentrations of antibody IgG and Fab/c kept constant at levels found previously to yield maximum achievable lysis with conventional high levels of complement. It is apparent that the Fab/c antibody utilizes dilute concentrations of complement much more efficiently. Both the ability to avoid modulation and the more efficient utilization of complement may have contributed to the superiority of Fab/c over IgG antibody in the immunotherapy of L_2C leukaemia (12).

The prospect of using rabbit Fab/c for human therapy is logistically unattractive, and it is unlikely that it can be prepared from rat or mouse antibody. Two other univalent derivatives that could be prepared from rat or mouse IgG, and which have given results in vitro similar to Fab/c, are shown in Fig. 1. Both of these derivatives offer the advantage of being able to exploit host Fc for recruiting effector functions. Monoclonal technology also offers the possibility of harvesting, from genetically suitable cells, four-chain IgG molecules in which one of the light chains derives from the parent myeloma line; or, from hybrid hybridomas, molecules in which each heavy-light pair derives from a different parent cell (15).

1. Stevenson GT, Stevenson FK: Antibody to a molecularly defined antigen confined to a tumour cell surface. Nature(254):714-716,1975.
2. Hamblin TJ, Abdul-Ahad AK, Gordon J, Stevenson FK, Stevenson GT: Preliminary experience in treating lymphocytic leukaemia with

antibody to immunoglobulin idiotypes on the cell surfaces. Brit J Cancer(42):495-502, 1980.

3. Miller RA, Maloney DG, Warnke R, Levy R: Treatment of B-cell lymphoma with monoclonal anti-idiotype antibody.N Engl J Med(306):517-522,1982.

4. Stevenson FK, Hamblin TJ, Stevenson GT, Tutt AL: Extracellular idiotypic immunoglobulin arising from human leukemic B lymphocytes. J Exp Med(152):1484-1496,1980.

5. Stevenson FK, Elliott EV, Stevenson GT: Some effects on leukaemic B lymphocytes of antibodies to defined regions of their surface immuno-globulin. Immunology(32):549-557,1977.

6. Lawson ADG, Stevenson GT: Macrophages induce antibody-dependent cytostasis but not lysis in guinea pig leukaemic cells.Brit J Cancer (48):227-237, 1983.

7. Boyse EA, Old LJ: Some aspects of normal and abnormal cell surface genetics. Ann Rev Genetics(3):269-290, 1969.

8. Stevenson GT, Glennie MJ, Gordon J: The killing of lymphoma cells by univalent derivatives of tumor-specific antibody. UCLA Symp Molec Cell Biol(24):459-472, 1982.

9. Griffin FM, Griffin JA, Silverstein SC: Studies on the mechanism of phagocytosis. J Exp Med(144):788-809, 1976.

10. Gordon J, Stevenson GT: Antigenic modulation of surface immuno-globulin yielding resistance to complement-mediated lysis. Immunology (42):13-17, 1981.

11. Stevenson GT, Stevenson FK: Treatment of lymphoid tumours with anti-idiotype antibodies. Springer Semin Immunopathol(6):99-115, 1983.

12. Glennie MJ, Stevenson GT: Univalent antibodies kill tumour cells *in vitro* and *in vivo*. Nature(295):712-714, 1982.

13. Taylor RB, Duffus PH, Raff MC, de Petris S: Redistribution and pinocytosis of lymphocyte surface immunoglobulin molecules induced by anti-immunoglobulin antibody. Nature New Biol(233):225-227, 1971.

14. Yoshitake S, Yamada Y, Ishikawa E, Masseyeff R: Conjugation of glucose oxidase from Aspergillus niger and rabbit antibodies. Eur J Biochem(101):395-399, 1979.

15. Milstein C, Cuello AC: Hybrid hybridomas and their use in immuno-chemistry. Nature(305):537-540, 1983.

ANTIBODY-TOXIN CONJUGATES AS ANTI-CANCER AGENTS

PHILIP E THORPE

1. INTRODUCTION

A possible means of making anti-cancer agents that has excited much recent interest is to link highly potent toxins of bacterial or plant origin to monoclonal antibodies with specificity for tumour cells. Ricin, from castor beans, and abrin, from jequirity beans, have been the two plant toxins most widely used. The attraction of these toxins is their supremely powerful cytotoxic action. It has been calculated that just one molecule needs to penetrate a cell to kill it. This maximises the likelihood of killing malignant cells that do not have a high density of specific antigens on their surface or that reside in solid tumours not freely permeable to the conjugate.

2. MODE OF ACTION OF ABRIN AND RICIN

Abrin and ricin are glycoproteins of approximate Mr 65,000 that comprise two polypeptide chains, A & B, joined by a disulphide bond. They bind to virtually all nucleated eukaryotic cells with which they come in contact and kill them by essentially the same mechanism (in ref 1). The B-chain binds to galactose-containing glycoproteins and glycolipids on the cell surface and the A-chain, by a process which is not understood, traverses either the plasma membrane itself or the membrane of an endocytic vesicle and stops protein synthesis by catalysing a modification to the 60S subunit of the ribosomes that prevents the binding of the elongation factor, EF-2.

3. A-CHAIN CONJUGATES

The most widely adopted strategy for conferring specificity of cytotoxic action on a toxin is to remove the B-chain and couple the isolated A-chain by a disulphide bond directly to the antibody. This type of conjugate thus superficially resembles the native toxin in construction having a binding subunit and an inhibitory subunit in disulphide linkage, and is only capable of binding to cells with the appropriate antigens. The cytotoxic action that the conjugates elicit is sometimes outstandingly powerful and specific. For example, treatment of normal and leukaemic murine T-lymphocytes with a conjugate of monoclonal anti-Thy 1.1 antibody and ricin A-chain at the very low concentration of 10^{-12}M inhibited their rate of protein synthesis by 50%. Comparable toxicity to cells lacking the Thy 1.1 determinant was only seen when the conjugate was applied at 10^{-7}M, representing a 100,000 fold differential in potency between the specific and non-specific cytotoxic effects of the conjugate (Thorpe et al, unpublished results). Unfortunately, conjugates of some antibodies and ricin A-chain are weakly or non-cytotoxic towards the cells to which they bind and no clear patterns have yet emerged that allow the cytotoxic performance of a conjugate to be predicted. For instance, the W3/25 monoclonal antibody that recognises an antigen upon helper T-lymphocytes in the rat was not rendered cytotoxic to W3/25-expressing normal or leukaemic T-cells by its linkage to ricin A-chain. Even when capping and endocytosis of the conjugate was induced by treating conjugate-coated cells with polyclonal anti-mouse immunoglobulin antibodies, no toxicity ensued[2]. By contrast, as has been our experience with many conjugates made from intact toxins, W3/25 antibody linked to intact ricin was as powerful a cytotoxic agent as ricin itself[3]. The data support the view that the B-chain of the toxin can facilitate A-chain penetration. This is true not just for conjugates like W3/25-ricin A that are totally non-toxic without the B-chain, but also for highly effective A-chain conjugates such as anti-Thy 1.1-ricin A whose cytotoxic action has been shown by Youle and Neville to be markedly accelerated by the addition of free B-chain[4].

4.   BLOCKED RICIN CONJUGATES

The second strategy for preparing antibody-toxin conjugates is to couple the intact toxin to the antibody and to block the galactose-binding sites on the toxin B-chain to prevent the conjugate from binding to and killing cells non-specifically. This type of conjugate offers the potential advantage over the A-chain conjugate that the properties of the B-chain that facilitate A-chain penetration may be preserved so that the conjugates consistently display high toxicity. The method that we devised for blocking the galactose-binding sites in intact ricin conjugates involves three steps[5]. The N-hydroxysuccinimidyl ester of iodoacetic acid is used to introduce an average of 1.5 iodoacetyl groups into each molecule of ricin. Next an average of 1.7 thiol groups is incorporated into each molecule of antibody by pyridyldithiolation with the Pharmacia SPDP reagent and reduction with dithiothreitol. On mixing, the two derivatised proteins react to form a conjugate in which the linkage is a thioether bond. Approximately half of the conjugate molecules are assembled with their galactose-binding sites vacant and the other half with their sites hindered. The two forms are readily separated by affinity chromatography on Sepharose (matrix containing β-galactosyl residues) and on immobilised asialofetuin (a glycoprotein with complex carbohydrate side chains resembling those to which ricin would attach on cell surfaces). FACS analyses confirmed that the 'blocked' ricin conjugate does not bind detectably to cells lacking the appropriate antigens. No diminution in galactose binding was observed with iodoacetylated ricin: the blockade in the conjugate therefore appears to be a consequence of completing the linkage of the modified toxin to the antibody. The most plausible explanation is that a proportion of conjugate molecules initially forms with the galactose-binding sites orientated towards the antibody.

The 'blocked' form of a monoclonal anti-Thy 1.1-ricin conjugate was as powerful a cytotoxic agent for Thy 1.1-expressing AKR-A cells in tissue culture as the form that had retained Sepharose binding activity and was ten times more potent even than ricin. The concentration of conjugate needed to reduce the rate of protein synthesis of the AKR-A cells by half was 10^{-12}M as opposed to 10^{-8}M for EL4 cells which lack the Thy 1.1 determinant. This represents a 10,000 fold differential between the specific and non-specific cytotoxic effects. As was predicted from its column binding properties, the 'non-blocked' form of the conjugate substantially retained non-specific toxicity and this diminished the differential in its toxicity to AKR-A as opposed to EL4 to only fifty-fold. Similarly, the blocked form of a W3/25-ricin conjugate displayed impressive potency and selectivity in its cytotoxic action upon W3/25-expressing rat leukaemia cells. It was as toxic as the non-blocked form and ten-fold more so than ricin. This is an important result because W3/25 antibody is ineffective when directly linked to ricin A-chain, suggesting that the property of the B-chain that is needed for the A-chain to traverse cell membranes is independent of the recognition of galactose.

5. ANTI-TUMOUR EFFECTS

The experimental design was to inject 10^6 AKR-A lymphoma cells intraperitoneally into nude or T-cell deficient CBA mice and then to administer a single high dose (16 pmoles) of anti-Thy 1.1-ricin (blocked or non-blocked) intraperitoneally or intravenously one day later. The Thy 1.1 antigen expressed by the lymphoma cells is not found in nude or CBA mice and so it constituted a tumour-specific marker. The extension in the median survival time of the animals that received either the blocked or the non-blocked ricin conjugate intraperitoneally was ten to fifteen days. Experiments in which graded numbers of tumour cells were injected into mice suggested that a prolongation in survival time of this magnitude is that expected if the conjugates had destroyed 99.99% of the lymphoma cells in the peritoneum. The effect of the conjugates appears to be specific since antibody alone, ricin alone, antibody plus ricin, and control conjugates made with a monoclonal antibody of irrelevant specificity were all without protective effect. When the anti-Thy 1.1-blocked ricin conjugate was administered intravenously rather than intraperitoneally, then the prolongation in median survival time of the animals was reduced to eight to ten days and this corresponds to an elimination of 99.9% of the tumour cells in the peritoneum. The non-blocked conjugate was ineffective when injected intravenously, probably because it bound to galactose-containing glycoproteins and glycolipids that are in plasma or on blood cells and so was incapable of free diffusion into the peritoneum.

The blocked ricin conjugate was superior in protective effect to a conjugate of anti-Thy 1.1 antibody and ricin A-chain. An intravenous injection of 1.3 nmoles of the A-chain conjugate (i.e. a dose eighty-fold higher than of the blocked ricin conjugate) produced an extension in median survival time of the animals that corresponded to only 99% eradication of tumour cells. It is possible that the blocked ricin conjugate is more stable in animals than the A-chain conjugate because it is formed with a thioether linkage rather than with a disulphide linkage which conceivably could be cleaved by reduction by thiol-containing molecules such as glutathione.

ACKNOWLEDGEMENTS

The work described in this manuscript was performed in collaboration with Alex Brown, Simone Detre and Brian Foxwell of the Imperial Cancer Research Fund, London, and with Walter Ross, Alan Cumber and Tony Forrester of the Institute of Cancer Research, London.

REFERENCES
1   Olsnes, S & Pihl, A. Toxic lectins and related proteins. In: Cohen, P, Van Heyningen, S (eds) Molecular Action of Toxins and Viruses. Elsevier Biomed. Press, New York, 1982, pp 51-105.

2   Thorpe, P E & Ross, W C J.   The preparation and cytotoxic properties
     of antibody-toxin conjugates.   Immunol. Rev. <u>62</u>, 119-158, 1982.

3   Thorpe, P E, Mason, D W, Brown, A N F, Simmonds, S J, Ross W C J,
     Cumber, A J, & Forrester, J A.   Selective killing of malignant cells
     in a leukaemic rat bone marrow using an antibody-ricin conjugate.
     Nature <u>297</u>, 594-596, 1982.

4   Youle, R J & Neville D M.   Kinetics of protein synthesis inactivation
     by ricin-anti-Thy 1.1 monoclonal antibody hybrids.   J Biol. Chem.
     257, 1598-1601, 1982.

5   Thorpe, P E, Brown, A, Foxwell, B, Myers, C, Ross, W, Cumber, A, &
     Forrester, A. Blockade of the galactose-binding site of ricin by its
     linkage to antibody. <u>In</u>: Boss, D B, Langman, R E, Trowbridge I S
     & Dulbecco, R (eds) Monoclonal Antibodies in Cancer.   Proceedings of
     the IV Armand Hammer Cancer Symp. Acad. Press, New York, 1983, (in
     press).

3. REGULATORY MOLECULES IN CHEMOTHERAPY

BIOLOGICAL RESPONSE MODIFIERS AS ANTICANCER AGENTS

ROBERT K. OLDHAM

1. INTRODUCTION

Major technological advances have been made in the last five years
which give a strong basis for a fourth modality of cancer treatment (1).
First, advances in molecular biology have allowed scientists to clone
individual genes and thereby produce huge quantities of highly purified
products of the mammalian genome. A second major advance was the discovery
of hybridomas, where one can now make immunoglobulins at the same level of
molecular purity as for drugs and cloned gene products.

Biologicals are products of the mammalian genome. Biological response
modifiers (BRM) are agents and approaches utilizing the individual's own
biological responses (2).

How should these new molecules be tested in man? In opposition to the
historical dogma of immunotherapy, these molecules can have activity on
clinically apparent disease, and their testing is not restricted to situations
where the tumor cell mass is imperceptible (3,4). Thus, testing has been
initiated for the interferons, lymphokines/cytokines, growth and maturation
factors, monoclonal antibodies and immunoconjugates thereof and adoptive
cellular therapy (5).

2. INTERFERON

Interferon, as a prototypic biological molecule, has proven very useful
in advancing our understand of biologicals. Various interferons have greatly
different biological effects and the interferons can be active as anticancer
agents indirectly through the immune system and by direct effects on the
tumor cell (6,7).

The principles of Phase I clinical trials have been delineated during the
development of chemotherapy (8) and have been extended to the Phase I testing
of biologicals (1). As is shown in Table 1, Phase I clinical trials with alpha
interferons have delineated certain toxicologic and biologic effects in man.

271

Table 1. Biological effects of alpha interferons

Clinical and Toxic Effects		Biological/Immunological Effects
fever	hepatic/hematologic depression	↑ or ↓ NK activity
chills	CNS effects (confusion & EEG changes	↑ macrophage activity
headache	nausea/vomiting	alters antigen display
fatigue	myalgia	↑ or ↓ in ADCC
anorexia	weight loss	↓ lymphoproliferation
		antitumor activity

While it is recognized that these Phase I trials are not designed to measure therapeutic efficacy, approximately 10 percent of the patients demonstrated an objective response, most of which clearly fell into selected disease categories such as lymphoma, myeloma, Kaposi's sarcoma, melanoma, renal cancer and breast cancer (8). By contrast, very few responses have been seen in patients with the more common malignancies of colon, lung and the lower genitourinary system. Selected Phase II data, subdivided into the general categories of alpha Cantell, alpha lymphoblastoid and alpha recombinant, are summarized in Table 2.

Table 2. α interferon Phase II studies[1]

Tumor Type:	Interferon	Dose	CR & PR
Lung	α –Cantell	3 mu/d x 5	1/37
Breast	α –Cantell	3-9 mu daily	7/17
Breast	α2 –Recombinant	$50/mu/m^2$ 3 x wk	0/17
Breast	α –Cantell	3 mu daily	5/23
Colon	α –Cantell	3 mu/d x 5	0/19
Colon	α2 –Recombinant	5 mu tiw	1/18
Carcinoid	α –Cantell	3-6 mu/daily	6/9
Ovary	α –Cantell	1-6 mu daily	1/15
Renal	α –Cantell	3 mu daily	5/19
Renal	α2 –Recombinant	50 mu tiw	2/19
Renal	α2 –Recombinant	$2 mu/m^2$ daily	0/8
		$20 mu/m^2$ daily	2/8
Melanoma	α –Lymphoblastoid	$2.5 mu/m^2$ daily	1/17
Melanoma	α2 –Recombinant	$50 mu/m^2$ x 3 wk	7/31
Myeloma	α –Cantell	3-9 mu daily	6/10
Lymphoma	α –Cantell	3-9 mu daily	6/11
Kaposi	Various	Low Dose <10 mu/m^2 d	1/17
Hairy Cell Leukemia	α –Cantell	3 mu daily	7/7
CML	α –Cantell	9-15 mu daily	22/25

[1] Summarized from and referenced in (8).

3. MONOCLONAL ANTIBODY

The therapeutic use of murine-derived monoclonal antibodies in early Phase I trials in humans has recently been reviewed (9-11). Most of the responses have been transient, except for a lymphoma patient treated with an anti-idiotype monoclonal antibody (12). There have been few data regarding the precise in vivo localization of antibody, particularly in solid tumors (13-15). It is critical to demonstrate that monoclonal antibodies, when given intravenously, actually reach the tumor and show a degree of specificity for the tumor cells. While labeled antibodies can be used to image the tumor, sensitive immunological techniques, such as immunoperoxidase and flow cytometry, provide direct evidence for localization of the antibody on the tumor cell membrane.

Patients with malignant melanoma whose tumors reacted in vitro with the 9.2.27 monoclonal antibody were treated with escalating doses of antibody to demonstrate localization of antibody in skin nodules as determined by repeated biopsies after treatment (14). The 9.2.27 antimelanoma monoclonal antibody was selected since it recognizes a 250 Kd melanoma associated antigen on most (90%) melanomas and is relatively selective for the tumor cells. Patients with chronic lymphocytic leukemia (CLL) and cutaneous T-cell lymphomas (CTCL) have been treated with the T101 monoclonal antibody which binds a 65 Kd antigen on these tumors (15). All patients were monitored for clinical response and toxicity, antibody pharmacokinetics, antigenic modulation and antimurine antibody formation.

Table 3. In vitro and in vivo reactivity of 9.2.27 antibody with melanoma cells in cutaneous skin lesions

| | | | 9.2.27 Reactivity | | | |
| | | Days Post | Flow Cytometry (%) | | Immunoperoxidase | |
Patient	Dose 9.2.27	Treatment	In Vitro	In Vivo	In Vitro	In Vivo
#1	Pre-treatment		83	ND	++	−
	1 mg	1	0	0	+	−
	50 mg	1	72	0	++	+
	200 mg	1	ND	ND	++	+
#2	Pre-treatment		97	ND	++	−
	10 mg	1	98	2	+	−
	100 mg	1	72	50	+	+
	200 mg	4	98	91	+	+
#3	Pre-treatment		76	ND	++	−
	1 mg	1	91	0	++	−
	200 mg	1	41	35	++	+

In vivo localization of monoclonal antibody in melanoma: Biopsies were performed from 24 hours to 4 days following infusion of 9.2.27, and typical results are summarized in Table 3. The intensity and homogenity of tumor staining was increased with increasing dose as did the diffusion of antibody out into the tumor nodule. Flow cytometry demonstrated there was no antigenic modulation secondary to therapy with 9.2.27.

In vivo binding of T101 antibody and antigenic modulation of the T65 antigen: We compared in vivo versus in vitro staining in one representative patient from each treatment group (Figure 1). These data demonstrate the dose response curve for in vivo binding and the clear antigenic modulation with this antibody (15).

Bone marrow and lymph nodes were removed to assess the in vivo localization of T101 antibody. With infusions as little as 10 mg, 80% of the leukemic bone marrow cells demonstrated in vivo labeling followed by a antigenic modulation. As in the peripheral blood, the antigen returned within 24 hours in the absence of circulating antibody. When full antigenic modulation was induced in the peripheral blood and further T101 was rapidly infused, lymph node biopsies revealed the modulation of the T65 antigen as evidence that T101 reached the lymph node.

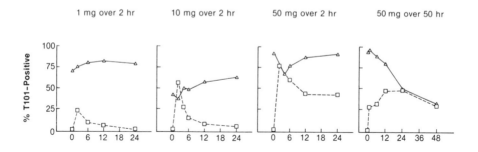

Hours After Start of Infusion

Legend: FIGURE 1 In vivo versus in vitro binding of T101 antibody by circulating chronic lymphocytic leukemia cells. Results from one patient at each dose level are shown. The lower curve (□) represents in vivo labeling of circulating leukemia cells with T101 antibody. The upper curve (△) represents the same circulating leukemia cells treated in vitro with excess T101 and then labeled with fluorescein-tagged goat antimurine antibody. The difference between these curves at each time point measured represents the number of cells that were not labeled in vivo with T101.

Pharmacokinetics and antiglobulin response: Circulating antibody levels were dose related, and higher, more prolonged levels of 9.2.27 were achieved with higher doses of antibody. Transient antiglobulin responses did not impede localization in cutaneous nodules.

Toxicity: Only mild toxicity consisting of fever to $103°$, mild nausea, anorexia, chills and headache was seen in a minority of the melanoma patients. One patient developed a syndrome consistent with serum sickness which responded to steroids. By contrast, T101 induced considerable toxicity with fever, chills and urticaria in over 50% of the patients. Pulmonary toxicity, consisting of sudden shortness of breath with chest tightness, followed rapid infusion of the antibody. With infusions of $1 - 2$ mg/hour, this toxicity was no longer seen (15).

Clinical responses: There were no measurable decreases in the size of the the melanoma skin lesions, lymph nodes, or visceral metastases, although some of the nodules softened during treatment. Circulating leukemia cell counts routinely dropped to approximately 50% of pretreatment levels immediately following a 2-hour infusion of T101. However, by 24 to 48 hours the cell count generally recovered to the pretreatable level. The circulating cell count cor-related inversely with the degree of antigenic modulation of the T65 antigen.

4. DISCUSSION

These data with the alpha interferons and with monoclonal antibodies indi-cate that highly purified biologicals can be prepared for clinical trials. The advantages inherent in the use of genetically engineered biologicals include access to highly purified material that can be available in large quantities for clinical testing to determine if the pharmacological administration of physiologically active biologicals can induce therapeutic responses in patients with cancer. Monoclonal antibodies may represent the prototype for specific antitumor therapy. These early studies indicate that patients with bulky disease can demonstrate clinical responses to biologicals. As these biologi-cals are further tested in Phase II trials, the clinical activity with respect to disease range can be precisely determined, and later trials can be initiated to determine their activity in less advanced disease. Like chemotherapy and radiotherapy, it is likely that biologicals, when active in bulky disease, will be more effective in the adjuvant setting. Finally, the advent of biologicals makes available a fourth modality which should enhance considerably the thera-peutic efficacy of surgery, radiotherapy and chemotherapy (1).

REFERENCES

1. Oldham RK. Biologicals and biological response modifiers: The fourth modality of cancer treatment. Cancer Treat Rpt , 1983. (In press) References

2. Oldham RK. Guest Editorial. Biological response modifiers. J Natl Cancer Inst (70):789-796, 1983.

3. Oldham RK, Smalley RV. Immunotherapy: The old and the new. J Biol Resp Modif (2):1-37, 1983.

4. Hanna, Jr MG, Key ME, Oldham RK. The biology of cancer therapy: Some insights into adjuvant treatment of metastatic solid tumors. J Biol Resp Modif (2):295-305, 1983.

5. Oldham RK. Biological response modifiers program. J Biol Resp Modif (1):81-100, 1982.

6. Smalley RV, Oldham RK. Interferon as a biological response modifying agent in clincial trials. J Biol Resp Modif (5):401-408, 1983.

7. Herberman RB, Thurman GB. Summary of approaches to the immunological monitoring of cancer patients treated with natural or recombinant interferons. J Biol Resp Modif (6):1983. (In press)

8. Oldham RK. The role of interferon in the treatment of cancer. In: Zoon KC, Liu D (ed) Proceedings of Workshop on Interferon. Elsevier Press, New York, 1983. (In press)

9. Foon KA, Bernhard MI, Oldham RK. Monoclonal antibody therapy: Assessment by animal tumor models. J Biol Resp Modif (1):277-304, 1983.

10. Ritz J, Schlossman SF. Utilization of monoclonal antibodies in the treatment of leukemia and lymphoma. Blood (59)1-11, 1982.

11. Oldham RK. Monoclonal antibodies in cancer therapy. J Clin Onc (9): 582-590, 1983.

12. Miller RA, Maloney DG, Warnke R, Levy R. Treatment of B cell lymphoma with monoclonal anti-idiotype antibody. N Eng J Med (306):517-522, 1982.

13. Moshakis V, McIlhinney RAJ, Neville AM. Cellular distribution of monoclonal antibody in human tumours after I.V. administration. Brit J Cancer (44):663-669, 1981.

14. Oldham RK, Foon KA, Morgan AC, Woodhouse CS, Schroff RW, Abrams PG, Fer M, Schoenberger CS, Farrell M, Kimball E, Sherwin SA. Monoclonal antibody therapy of malignant melanoma: In vivo localization in cutaneous metastatsis after intravenous administration, 1983. (Submitted)

15. Foon KA, Schroff RW, Bunn PA, Mayer D, ABrams PG, Fer M, Ochs J, Bottino GC, Sherwin SA, Herberman RB, Oldham RK. Effects of monoclonal antibody serotherapy on patients with chronic lymphocytic leukemia, 1983. (Submitted)

PROSTAGLANDINS AND CANCER - THERAPEUTIC POTENTIAL

T.J. POWLES

INTRODUCTION

Inhibition of tumour growth by prostaglandins (P.G.s) has been shown to occur in various in vitro and in vivo experimental tumour systems. For example division of B_{16} melanoma cells in vitro can be inhibited by a synthetic P.G.E.$_2$ derivative as can development of this tumour in mice (1,2). Similarly, P.G.A. will inhibit tumour growth in vitro and in vivo (3-6).

Inhibition of P.G. synthesis with agents such as non-steroidal anti-inflammatory drugs may also have potentially useful antitumour effects. For example P.G.s are probably involved in mechanisms of osteolysis necessary for development of bone metastases (7,8) and non-steroidal anti-inflammatory drugs can prevent this development in animals bearing osteolytic tumours.

Finally, there are experimental indications that P.G.s are involved in mechanisms of action of some anti-inflammatory drugs indomethacin and flurbiprofen have been shown to enhance the anti-tumour effects of cytotoxic agents such as chlorambucil on the Walker and other tumours in rats (9,10).

These experimental observations provide the scientific basis for various clincal trials aimed at testing for beneficial therapeutic effects of agents which affect P.G. synthesis in patients with cancer.

PROSTAGLANDIN STUDIES

To test for any direct anti-tumour activity of P.G.s in man, patients with refactory disseminated cancer or leukaemia were given PGE or PGA.

In the PGE study four patients had assessable disseminated breast cancer, two had acute myelogenous leukaemia and all had failed previous conventional treatment. PGE was initially administered to some patients by intravenous infusion at a rate of 0.05μg/kg per minute for 48 hours followed by sublingual administration of 1.5mg six times per day (dose adjustments according to tolerability). The other two patients received only oral medication and all patients continued medication until evidence of progression of disease or symptoms. The PGE infusions were tolerated satisfactorily, with mild diarrhoea occurring in two patients. Oral administation of 6 to 9mg/day was associated with diarrhoea in two patients, nausea and vomiting in one patient, and headache with arthralgia in another patient. The patients received PGE for between 7 and 60 days with total dosage of 127 to 540mg. During this period, we noted no change in pulse rate, blood pressure, respiration rate, renal function, serum calcium or blood count. None of the six patients showed evidence of tumour regression.

In the PGA study seven patients with clinically assessable disseminated breast cancer who had previously failed conventional therapy were given PGA_1 or PGA_2. Pure crystalline PGA_1 and liquid PGA_2 (kindly supplied by Ono Pharmaceutical Company, Japan) were dissolved in ethanol and diluted in 5% dextrose for administration at 1 to 3µg/kg per minute for 6 hours once per week. Patients were assessed for toxicity and tumour response, and all continued with dose modification according to toxicity until evidence of progression of disease. Patients received between 2 and 11 infusions at rates varying between 1 and 3µg/kg per minute to a total dose of 40 to 380mg. Generally, PGA_1 was better tolerated than PGA_2 at dose rates between 2 and 4 µg/kg per minute. Otherwise facial flushing, pyrexia, tachycardia, nausea, vomiting, headache and hypertension occurred in some patients but did not necessitate cessation of infusion.

Blood count, serum calcium, phosphorus, electrolytes, blood urea, liver or lung function tests did not significantly alter during PGA infusions. One of the seven patients showed evidence of tumour regression.

NON-STEROIDAL ANTI-INFLAMMATORY DRUG STUDIES

To test whether anti-inflammatory drugs had a beneficial effect on development of bone metastases, patients with primary poor risk breast cancer were given the aspirin/paracetamol conjugate benorylate (Benoral, Winthrop) which had been shown to prevent bone metastases in rats (11). From January 1975 to August 1977, 160 patients with primary breast cancer were stratified according to prognostic criteria and then randomised to receive either Benoral 10ml (4g) twice per day or placebo for 18 months. All patients were clinically assessed and investigated for evidence of metastases at the time of primary treatment. Following this, patients have been regularly staged and clinically assessed, and none have been lost to follow up. The relapse rate in bone, other sites or overall survival for the two groups is the same.

To test whether anti-inflammatory drugs had any effect on established bone metastases, 26 patients with histologically confirmed breast cancer and radiological evidence of oesteolytic bone metastases were studied for periods ranging from 5 to 51 days. Eight patients received soluble aspirin, 2,700mg/day and indomethacin 75mg/day; 2 received indomethacin 300mg/day; 9 received flurbiprofen 300mg/day; and 7 received benoxaprofen 300mg/day.

Serum calcium and urinary hydroxyproline excretion were estimated before and at weekly intervals during the studies. Pain and analgesic requirements were assessed weekly by an independent observer. All patients had previously received endocrine or chemotherapy but not for at least 4 weeks before these studies commenced. Paracetamol or opiates were used for pain control and these analgesic requirements were taken into consideration for assessment of pain relief by the agents under study.

Although aspirin/indomethacin, flurbiprofen and benoxaprofen relieved bone pain in some patients, they generally were unable to influence osteolysis. Serum calcium was significantly, but not markedly, reduced in two patients who had flurbiprofen and in one who had benoxaprofen. Growth of soft tissue metastases remained clinically unaffected by these agents.

To test whether there was any interaction between anti-inflammatory drugs and cytotoxic agents, we added flurbiprofen or placebo to the standard breast unit adriamycin/vinca alkaloid combination chemotherapy schedule for patients with disseminated breast cancer. Patients were treated with adriamycin $40mg/m^2$, and vindesine $3mg/m^2$ or vincristine $1.4mg/m2$ on days 1 and 8 of a 28 day cycle together with either flurbiprofen 100mg three times per day or placebo for at least two weeks of each cycle. Between January 1979 and January 1982, 187 patients were randomised, 176 of whom are at present assessable for toxicity and 135 assessable for response.

The results clearly showed that flurbiprofen failed to improve the response of disseminated breast cancer to chemotherapy with vinca/adriamycin. Survival and duration of response for assessable patients who received flurbiprofen was the same as that for those who received placebo. Similarly, toxicity was similar for patients who received flurbiprofen or placebo with no indication that flurbiprofen protects the host against the toxic effects of this type of chemotherapy.

DISCUSSION

In spite of clear cut experimental evidence indicating that administration of prostaglandin analogues or anti-inflammatory drugs can affect the growth and development of tumours in animals, the results of these clinical trials have failed to show any benefit for patients with breast cancer.

It is disappointing that good control of bone metastases can be achieved by administration of various anti-inflammatory drugs to rats, but we have failed to influence development of bone metastases in patients with primary breast cancer given adequate dosages of benorylate for $1\frac{1}{2}$ years. It seems probable that inhibition of rapidly developing osteolytic tumours transplanted directly into rat bones, bear little resemblance to the development of bone metastases in man.

With regard to the interaction of anti-inflammatory drugs and cytotoxic chemotherapy, it was similarly disappointing that administration of flurbiprofen failed to improve the response rate of disseminated breast cancer, or reduce the toxicity of the adriamycin/vinca alkaloid combination. This may relate to inappropriate dosage of flurbiprofen in patients with disseminated cancer compared to animals with discrete transplanted tumours. Alternatively, the experimental observations included an alkylating agent in the chemotherapy combination which unfortunately is not included in our first line disseminated breast cancer schedule.

Finally, the small studies which we have done to evaluate the effect of administation of P.G.s on tumour growth in patients with disseminated breast cancer have failed to show any antitumour effects. The limited availability of these agents for clinical testing has not allowed a proper Phase II evaluation, and it is possible that there is a significant anti-tumour activity which has been missed in the preliminary studies. Further clinical trials with prostaglandin-like agents and agents which can raise endogenous prostaglandin levels are now indicated.

REFERENCES
1. Santoro GM, Philpott GW and Jaffe BM: Inhibition of tumour growth in vivo and in vitro by prostaglandin E. Nature (263): 777-779, 1976.
2. Santoro GM, Philpott GW and Jaffe BM: Prostaglandin A_1 induces differentiation in Friend erythroleukemia cells. Prostaglandins (17): 719-727, 1979.

3. Adolphe M, Giroud JP, Timsit J and Lechat P: Etude comparative des effets des prostaglandines E1, E2, A2, Flapha, Flapha sur la division des cellules HeLa en culture. C R Acad Sci [D] (Paris) (277): 537-540, 1973.

4. Eisenbarth GS, Willman DK and Lebovitz HE: Prostaglandin A_1 inhibition of chrondrosarcoma growth. Biochem Biophys Res Commun (60): 1302-1308, 1974.

5. Favalli C, Garaci E, Santoro MG, Santucci L and Jaffe BM: The effect of PGA_1 on the immune response in B-16 melanoma-bearing mice. Prostaglandins (19): 587-594, 1980.

6. Honn KV, Dunn JR, Morgan LR, Bienkowski M and Marnett LJ: Inhibition of DNA synthesis i Harding-Passey melanoma cells by prostaglandins A_1 and A_2: Comparison with chemotherapeutic agents. Biochem Biophys Res Commun (87): 795-801, 1979.

7. Galasko CSB and Bennett A: Relationship of bone destruction in skeletal metastases to osteoclast activation and prostaglandins. Nature (263): 508-510, 1976.

8. Powles TJ, Clark SA, Easty DM, Easty GC and Neville AM: Inhibition by aspirin and indomethacin of osteolytic tumour deposits and hypercalcaeia in rats with Walker tumour and its possible application to human breast cancer. Br J Cancer (28): 316-321, 1973.

9. Bennett A, Houghton J, Leaper DJ and Stamford IF: Cancer growth, response to treatment and survival time in mice: Beneficial effect of the prostaglandin synthesis inhibitor flurbiprofen. Prostaglandins (17): 179-181, 1979.

10. Powles TJ, Alexander P and Millar JL: Enhancement of anti-cancer activity of cytotoxic chemotherapy with protection tissues by inhibition of P.G. synthesis. Biochem Pharmacol (27): 1389-1392, 1978.

11. Powles TJ, Muindi J and Coombes RC: Mechanisms for development of bone metastases and effects of anti-inflammatory drugs. In: Powles TJ, Bockman R, Honn KV and Ranwell PW (eds) Prostaglandins and Cancer. Alan R. Liss, New York, 1982, pp 541-553.

THE THERAPEUTIC POTENTIAL OF LYMPHOKINES IN HUMAN CANCER

D.C.DUMONDE

1. LYMPHOKINES AS REGULATORY MOLECULES IN THE PHYSIOLOGY OF THE IMMUNE SYSTEM: RATIONALE FOR THEIR THERAPEUTIC INVESTIGATION IN CANCER

1.1 Nature and biological activities of lymphokines

Lymphokines are non-antibody proteins, generated by lymphocyte activation, that act as intercellular mediators of the immunological response. Lymphokines were first delineated in 1969 as substances which effect a restricted range of cellular immune responses such as delayed-type hypersensitivity, allograft rejection and macrophage activation. They were soon shown to be different from immunoglobulins and to be produced under the governing influence of thymus-derived lymphocytes. In the last few years this rather restricted view of lymphokine function has been enlarged by the realization that lymphokines play a fundamental role in the intrinsic regulation of the immune system and in its inter-actions with neuroendocrine mechanisms which are thought to act homeo-statically in the extrinsic regulation of the immunological response (for refs see (1)).

Lymphokines are glycosylated polypeptides or proteins and they exert a multiplicity of biological effects upon most isolated or cultured mesenchymal cell types such as lymphocytes, macrophages, granulocytes, vascular endothelial cells, fibroblasts, chondrocytes and osteoclasts (2). According to the cellular composition of the biological system being studied, lymphokines can be shown to exert cell proliferation or arrest of the cell cycle; stimulation or inhibition of cell motility; phenotypic change or maintenance of differentiation. When injected regionally or systemically into animals, lymphokines can stimulate or suppress the immunological response; they can exert local inflammation including lymphoid tissue hyperplasia; and they can stimulate myelopoiesis. Under certain circumstances lymphokines can be selectively cytotoxic for

283

cultured tumour cells; they can stimulate the microbicidal and tumouricidal activities of cultured macrophages; and, following systemic
injection, can induce host resistance to intracellular infection and to
the growth of transplantable syngeneic tumours. For these reasons lymphokines are viewed as effecting and coordinating the 'inflammatory',
'surveillance' and 'immunoregulatory' functions of T-lymphocytes by acting
as 'cell cooperators' and 'cell traffic regulators' in the intrinsic
physiology of the immune apparatus: to this extent they act as if they
are local hormones of the immune system. Thus recent evidence reveals
that under immunostimulation, lymphokines appear free in the blood plasma;
that lymphoid and myeloid cells possess receptors for certain lymphokines;
and that a variety of cell types respond to lymphokines by alterations
in intracellular levels of cyclic nucleotides. Where a lymphokine seems
to act as an intercellular mediator of white cell activation or maturation
the term 'interleukin' is also used.

     In addition to acting as local hormones of the lymphoid apparatus
there is recent evidence that lymphokines act on the neuroendocrine system
to 'signal' to it the level of immunological reactivity, with the resulting
activation of endocrine mechanisms that act homeostatically in the
extrinsic regulation of the immunological response (3). There is now
substantial evidence to view lymphokines as providing the basis for a
molecular pharmacology of the immune system itself and of its interactions
with other body systems involved in the host response to infection, immunosuppression, trauma, ageing and stress. It is but a short step to consider
that the tumour-bearing host might well be 'at risk' of defective adaptation
in respect of some of these responses; and accordingly that lymphokines
might be of some value in the therapeutic approach to human cancer (see 4).

1.2 Rationale for giving lymphokines to tumour-bearing patients

     Five additional lines of investigation complete this rationale:
(a) in progressive neoplasia the characteristic depression of cellular
immune status is of bad prognosis and may be due to serum factors inhibiting
lymphokine activity or lymphocyte function; (b) lymphokines inhibit tumour
cell growth, metabolism and migration and can stimulate macrophages and
other white cells to tumouricidal capacity; (c) lymphokine injection into
mice augments tumour regression induced by chemotherapy; (d) bacterial
preparations enhancing host resistance may also stimulate lymphokine

production in vivo; and (e) local injection of human lymphoid cell-line lymphokine (LCL-LK) into human metastatic tumour nodules induces their clinical regression. With ethical permission, informed consent and individual compassionate care, some 40 patients with advanced cancer received local and/or systemic injections of human lymphokine derived from the lymphoblastoid cell-line RPMI-1788. The next section summarizes the results of this study carried out between 1976 and 1982 (see 1,4).

2. RESPONSE OF TUMOUR-BEARING PATIENTS TO THE INJECTION OF LYMPHOID
   CELL LINE LYMPHOKINE (LCL-LK)

2.1 Summary of principal findings

My colleagues and I carried out an initial study of the short-term and long-term administration of human lymphoid cell-line lymphokines (LCL-LK) to some 40 patients with advanced cancer resistant to other therapy. LCL-LK was prepared from the RPMI 1788 cell line and given intradermally (I/D), intralesionally (I/L) or intravenously (I/V) to cancer patients; such courses ranged from one week to two years. I/D injection resulted in a sustained inflammatory response very similar to that of the classical tuberculin reaction. I/L injection resulted in local tumour regression with tumour cell necrosis and leucocytic infiltration. I/V injection resulted in transient pyrexia, polymorph leucocytosis, lymphopenia, endocrine changes (raised ACTH, GH, cortisol) and biochemical changes (fall in serum Zn and Fe; elevation of acute phase proteins). Long-term I/V LCL-LK, up to two years, was well tolerated without attributable toxicity and some evidence of patient benefit was obtained. The systemic effects of LCL-LK seemed to involve mechanisms different from interferon; but they confirmed experimental evidence that lymphokines activate extrinsic (neuroendocrine) immunoregulatory circuits. The local effects of LCL-LK supported the view that lymphokines are mediators of delayed hypersensitivity in Man. The study showed how information about lymphokine action in Man is obtainable and how this can be related to lymphokine activities in vitro. The study also provided biological response data and clinical experience upon which to base future protocols for the therapeutic evaluation of lymphokines (see 4).

2.2 <u>Immunopharmacological and clinical implications of the study</u>

Immunopharmacological characterization of responses to intradermal and intralesional LCL-LK would seem to be a useful component to future work; it is likely that the mediator interleukin-1 (IL-1) is involved in both phenomena and that it may facilitate the generation of inflammatory, helper and cytotoxic lymphoid cells at the tumour site itself. The pyrexial, haematological and biochemical responses support the view that lymphokines mediate systemic reactions of delayed hypersensitivity, possibly also via the action of IL-1. The endocrine effects provide evidence for an immune-neuroendocrine link in Man and raise the question whether IL-1 or some other polypeptide lymphokine acts as the intermediary: preliminary evidence suggests that these effects are separable from the pyrexia, indicating that there may be at least two central response pathways in the hypothalamus to systemically injected lymphokine.

In clinical terms the LCL-LK preparations are non-toxic, convenient to dispense, and produce predictable acute-phase responses. Although the above study was not designed to examine clinical efficacy, its results give encouragement to the continued study of this class of biological product. The high degree of patient compliance and the lack of long-term toxicity both provide reinforcement for continued study. A formal phase I/II investigation of LCL-LK in cancer will involve the design strategy implicit in all 'biological response modifiers'; and indeed, the local and systemic reactions to LCL-LK provide a striking example of the concept of biological response modification itself. It seems plausible to suggest that recurrent stimulation of an acute-phase response by intravenous injection of LCL-LK may favourably diminish the side effects of irradiation or chemotherapy. On this basis the 'lymphokine strategy' is aimed at improving the ability of a tumour-bearing host to tolerate existing treatment modalities rather than being aimed at killing the tumour by virtue of the cytotoxic action of lymphokines themselves.

3. FUTURE PERSPECTIVES

There is now enormous industrial and academic interest in the diagnostic and therapeutic potential of lymphokines, lymphokine agonists and lymphokine antagonists. To say (as in 1981) that 'lymphokines are on the move' (5) is (in 1983-4) a masterly understatement. With the introduction of recombinant technology into the lymphokine field, and the

increased success of hybridoma technology, we shall witness an explosion
of clinical interest in lymphokines in the remainder of the 1980's. One
of the exciting possibilities is that lymphokines or their derivatives may
be found to exert biological effects on both the differentiation and/or
metastatic capabilities of tumour cells themselves, as well as on host
defence systems that are compromised by both the tumour and the oncologist:
a concept which has evident implications for haematological malignancies
as well as for 'solid' tumours.

It is our working hypothesis that one or more 'lymphokine strategies'
will be found which will improve the host's ability to tolerate his cancer,
to tolerate existing treatment modalities, and to recover more quickly
from their depressant effect on immunological and other host defence
mechanisms. In the near future, more highly purified or recombinant
lymphokines will become available for clinical evaluation. In the meantime
our approach is simply to study and compare host response to a limited
range of eukaryotic lymphokine preparations of broad spectrum whose
prominent activities can be manipulated (eg presence or absence of interferon, interleukin-1 or interleukin-2) and also specified by means of
acceptable methods of measurement. In this way we plan to contribute to
the further understanding of lymphokines as regulatory molecules in the
biology and management of the host: tumour relationship.

4. REFERENCES

1. Dumonde DC, Hamblin AS: Lymphokines. *In*: Holborow EJ and Reeves WJ
   (eds) Immunology in Medicine, 2nd Ed. Academic Press, New York, 1983,
   pp 122-150.
2. Cohen S, Pick E, Oppenheim JJ (eds): Biology of the Lymphokines,
   Academic Press, New York, 1979.
3. Khan A, Hill NO: Human Lymphokines: the biological immune response
   modifiers. Academic Press, New York, 1982.
4. Fabris N, Gavaci E, Hadden J, Mitchison NA: Immunoregulation, Plenum
   Press, New York, 1983.
5. Paetkau V: Lymphokines on the move. Nature 294: 689-690.

THE INTERLEUKINS

R.J. BOOTH, R.L. PRESTIDGE AND J.D. WATSON

INTRODUCTION

   All blood cells are believed to arise from a common pool of
hemopoietic stem cells.   From early in fetal life and throughout
adult life, these cells differentiate, function for a short period
and are replaced.   Although the regulatory mechanisms that channel
stem cells into a particular pathway of development are unknown,
there are a variety of humoral mediators which stimulate the
growth and differentiation of blood cell types in culture and it
is a reasonable assumption that some of these may belong to
families of hormones which are responsible for the development of
cells *in vivo*. The term "Interleukin" was proposed at the Second
International Lymphokine Workshop in 1979 to describe such a class
of lymphokines involved in communication "between leukocytes".
What follows is a brief summary of the properties of the interleukins and a discussion of their potential application to cancer
therapy.

INTERLEUKIN 1 (IL-1)

   IL-1 is a glycoprotein of molecular weight 12-16,000 produced
by activated macrophages which displays a range of amplifying
effects on immunological and inflammatory reactions.   Many agents
that induce IL-1 production are potent adjuvants and it is
conceivable that IL-1 may play an important role in mediating
their nonspecific immunoenhancing effects *in vivo* (1).   Activated
lymphocytes can also stimulate macrophages to produce IL-1 either
directly by Ia-restricted cell contact or indirectly by secreting
macrophage-activating lymphokines such as IL-3 (2).   Recently,
murine keratinocytes (2) have been shown to produce a factor which

shares many of the characteristics of IL-1.

IL-1 is not directly mitogenic for T lymphocytes but acts on a subset of helper T cells, activated by antigens or mitogens, to induce the production of the T cell growth factor IL-2 (3). In this respect IL-1 provides a differentiative signal to activated IL-2-producer T cells. IL-1 can also exert effects on cells of the B lymphocyte lineage by promoting both proliferation and the production of antibody-forming cells (4). As well as T and B lymphocytes, IL-1 appears to affect a much wider range of target cells that participate in inflammatory reactions. It stimulates prostaglandin production by cells of the hypothalamic fever centre, production of acute phase proteins by hepatocytes, and fibroblast growth and collagenase and prostaglandin production by rheumatoid synovial cells (2).

INTERLEUKIN 2 (IL-2).

IL-2 is a lymphokine produced by a class of helper T lympho-cytes following activation by antigen (or mitogen) and IL-1. Both murine and human IL-2 display considerable size and charge hetero-geneity, much of which can be attributed to variable carbohydrate content. Human IL-2 is normally isolated as a single chain protein of molecular weight near 16,000, while murine IL-2 appears to exist as a dimer of two 16-18,000 chains (5).

The major role of IL-2 is that of a growth factor for activated T cells. Following activation with antigens or mitogens T cells respond by expressing surface receptors for IL-2. Subsequent proliferation is then controlled only by the lymphokine. IL-2 has been used to maintain in culture long-term proliferating antigen-specific clones derived from helper, suppressor or cytotoxic T lymphocytes (3). It appears, therefore, that most classes of T cells are able to express IL-2 receptors and respond to its signal. Early reports suggested that IL-2 could also act on purified B lymphocytes but it is likely that the effects were due to the influence of IL-2 on residual helper T cells. Recent studies have indicated that IL-2 can augment *in vitro* natural killer (NK) cell activity but this effect appears to be due, at least in part, to the induction of interferon-γ (6).

INTERLEUKIN 3 (IL-3).

The term IL-3 was recently introduced to describe a factor in conditioned medium from concanavalin A-stimulated murine lymphocytes that induced the expression of an enzymeα-steroid dehydrogenase in cultures of nu/nu splenic lymphocytes (7). Various cloned T cell lines also produce IL-3 but the most convenient source is the myelomonocytic line WEHI-3 which constitutively produces high titres. Thus, unlike IL-1 and IL-2 which are exclusively products of macrophages and T lymphocytes respectively, IL-3 is produced by cells of both these lineages. A variety of colony stimulating factors (CSF) have been associated with IL-3-containing supernatants and recently it was established using a purified homogeneous preparation, that IL-3 was responsible for many of these activities (8). Thus, a single factor with a molecular weight of 28,000 appears to affect the growth of cells from a range of hemopoietic lineages. IL-3 may act on multi-potential stem cells found in the bone marrow to generate lineage-specific cells which may include most of the specialised cell types of the blood. Alternatively, the factor may stimulate the growth of progenitors already committed to the particular lineages (9).

POTENTIAL THERAPEUTIC APPLICATIONS OF INTERLEUKINS.

The role of IL-1 as a stimulator of inflammatory and immuno-logical reactions (1) suggests a possible application as an adjuvant-like adjunct to other therapeutic regimens. The useful-ness of IL-3 as a therapeutic agent is less obvious, although its effects on the cells of various hemopoietic lineages point to potential future applications in the treatment of hemopoietic malignancies. However, it is IL-2 that offers the most immediate promise due to its potent T cell growth-promoting properties and ability to activate NK cells. Three approaches are at present being explored.

(1) *In vitro* activation of tumour-specific, IL-2-producer and helper T lymphocytes followed by reinjection into the tumour-bearing host. Such "adoptive immunotherapy" has been used to eliminate large subcutaneous Moloney sarcomas from rats (10) and,

in combination with cyclophosphamide, to treat mice bearing
disseminated Friend virus-induced leukemia (11).

(2) IL-2-mediated expansion of antigen-activated cytotoxic T
cells *in vitro* followed by reinjection into the tumour-bearing
host. Mills *et al* (12) demonstrated that spleen cells taken from
mice bearing the syngeneic mastocytoma P815, and incubated *in
vitro* for 5 days with IL-2 and irradiated P815 stimulator cells,
developed cytotoxic lymphocytes which were effective at killing
P815 cells *in vivo*. Under certain conditions, a significant
fraction of mice treated with cytotoxic lymphocytes survived the
P815 tumour indefinitely. As a prelude to using such methods in
the treatment of human tumours, Vose and Bonnard (13) have
developed a method for stimulating human lymphocytes with tumour
cells *in vitro*, purifying antigen-specific activated blast cells
and generating tumour-specific cytotoxic T lymphocytes.
Conceivably, IL-2 could be used to expand such clones rapidly to
produce large numbers of tumour-specific cells for use in treatment.

(3) Direct administration of IL-2 to patients to augment tumour-
specific cytotoxic and helper T lymphocytes and NK cell activities.
Cheever *et al* (14) have demonstrated that the effectiveness of
"adoptive immunotherapy" using long-term cultured tumour-specific
T lymphocytes can be greatly enhanced by exogenously-administered
IL-2 presumably by promoting *in vivo* survival and growth of the
adoptively-transferred cells. Recently, Hefeneider *et al* (15)
have tested the *in vivo* effect of highly-purified IL-2 on cellular
immune responses. By employing an immunisation protocol known
to generate cytotoxic activity against allogeneic tumour cells in
mice, they showed that administration of IL-2, either with or 2
days after tumour administration, resulted in an augmented
cytotoxic T cell response. Furthermore, purified IL-2 given to
naive recipients not challenged with antigen substantially
potentiated NK cell activity. Clearly, the prospects for the use
of IL-2 in the treatment of human tumours depend on the
availability of large quantities of highly-purified material. The
recent successful cloning of the human IL-2 gene in *E.coli* (16)
therefore offers great promise for the future of immunotherapy.

REFERENCES

1. Staruch MJ, Wood DD. The adjuvanticity of interleukin 1 *in vivo*. J Immunol(130):2191-2194,1983.
2. Oppenheim JJ, GeryI: Interleukin 1 is more than an interleukin. Immunol Today(3)113-119,1982.
3. Gillis S, Watson J: Interleukin-2-dependent culture of cytolytic T cell lines. Immunol Rev(54):81-109,1981.
4. Booth RJ, Prestidge RL, Watson JD: Constitutive production by the WEHI-3 cell line of B cell growth and differentiation factor that co-purifies with IL-1. J Immunol(131): 1289-1293,1983
5. Caplan B, Gibbs C, Paetkau V: Properties of sodium dodecyl sulfate-denatured IL-2. J Immunol(126):1351-1354,1981.
6. Kawase I, Brooks CG, Kuribayashi K, Olabuenaga S, Newman W, Gillis S, Henney CS: Interleukin-2 induces γ-interferon production: participation of macrophages and NK-like cells. J Immunol(131):288-292,1983.
7. Ihle JN, Rebar L, Keller J, Lee JC, Hapel AJ: Interleukin 3: Possible roles in the regulation of lymphocyte differentiation and growth. Immunol Rev(63):5-32,1982.
8. Ihle, JN, Keller J, Henderson LE, Copeland TD, Fitch F, Prystowsky MB, Goldwasser E, Schrader JW, Palaszynski E, Dy M, Lebel B: Biologic properties of homogeneous interleukin 3. I. Demonstration of WEHI-3 growth factor activity, MCGF, PSF, CSF and HCSF. J Immunol(131):282-287,1983.
9. Watson JD, Prestidge RL: Interleukin 3 and colony-stimulating factors. Immunol Today(4):278-280,1983.
10. Fernandez-Cruz E, Woda BA, Feldman JD: Elimination of syngeneic sarcomas in rats by a subset of T lymphocytes. J Exp Med(152):823-841,1980.
11. Greenberg PD, Cheever MA, Fefer A: Eradication of disseminated murine leukemia by chemoimmunotherapy with cyclophosphamide and adoptively-transferred immune syngeneic Lyt1⁺2⁻ lymphocytes. J Exp Med(154):952-963,1981.
12. Mills GB, Carlson G, Paetkau V: Generation of cytotoxic lymphocytes to syngeneic tumors by using co-stimulator (IL-2): *In vivo* activity. J Immunol(125):1904-1909,1980.
13. Vose BM, Bonnard GD: Human tumour antigens defined by cytotoxicity and proliferative responses of cultured lymphoid cells. Nature (London)(296):359-361,1982.
14. Cheever MA, Greenberg PD, Fefer A, Gillis S: Augmentation of the anti-tumor therapeutic efficacy of long-term cultured T lymphocytes by *in vivo* administration of purified interleukin 2. J Exp Med(155):968-980,1982.
15. Hefeneider SH, Conlon PJ, Henney CS, Gillis S: *In vivo* interleukin 2 administration augments the generation of alloreactive cytolytic T lymphocytes and resident natural killer cells. J Immunol(130):222-227,1983.
16. Taniguchi T, Matsui H, Fujita T, Takaoka C, Kashima N, Yoshimoto R, Hamuro J: Structure and expression of a cloned cDNA for human IL-2. Nature (London)(302):305-310,1983.

THE ROLE OF POLYAMINES IN CELL DIFFERENTIATION

P.K. BONDY, J.L. RYAN, Z.N. CANELLAKIS

1. INTRODUCTION

The polyamines, putrescine (Put), spermidine (Spd) and spermine (Spm) are aliphatic flexible molecules derived from decarboxylation of ornithine by the enzyme ornithine decarboxylase (ODC). Put, the primary product, is converted to Spd and Spm by sequential addition of aminopropyl groups derived from S-adenosylmethionine which has been decarboxylated by the enzyme SAM-decarboxylase. The polyamines are present in all living cells, where they are essential for growth (1).

The exact physiological role(s) of the polyamines are not clear, but they provide endogenous cations because of the positive charges on their amino groups at physiological pH; they modulate the configuration and transcription of DNA; they participate in the post-translational modification of proteins; and they produce derivatives which have important physiological activity. These latter include γ-aminobutyric acid (GABA) and the monoacetylated derivatives of the polyamines themselves (2,3). In addition, the N,N'-diacetyl derivative of Put can induce differentiation of many types of cells in culture (4). The importance of polyamines for cellular differentiation is, however, still under study.

In intact multicellular organisms the definition of differentiation may seem intuitively obvious; but in cells in culture it is necessary to define the term with some rigour. For the purposes of this discussion, we consider differentiation to consist of several components: A. The cells enter resting (G_o) or terminal growth phase; B. Protein synthesis terminates, sometimes after a burst of synthesis of specific products such as hemoglobin or keratin; C. The cells assume an adult morphology.

295

2. PROCEDURE

Murine erythroleukemia cells (MELC) obtained from Dr. Charlotte Friend's laboratory were induced to differentiate by exposure to N,N'-diacetylputrescine (tetramethylenebisacetamide, TMBA), its hexa-methylene analogue (HMBA) or dimethylsulfoxide (DMSO) (5). Different-iation was evaluated by appearance of hemoglobin, as manifested by benzidine positive staining. Mouse splenic lymphocytes were stimulat-ed to undergo mitosis and initiate synthesis of immunoglobulins by exposure to purified bacterial lipopolysaccharide (LPS)(6). The concentration of polyamines and their derivatives was measured by high performance liquid chromatography (HPLC) as previously described (7). Polyamine biosynthesis was inhibited by α-difluoromethylornithine (DFMO), which is an irreversible inhibitor of ODC, and by methylglyoxal bis-(guanylhydrazone) (MGBG), which inhibits SAM-decarboxylase (8).

3. RESULTS

MELC undergo changes when exposed to inducing agents, which lead to "commitment" to differentiation (5). Within the first 24 hours, they have entered terminal cell division. During the next few days they begin to form hemoglobin, which can be taken as an indication of differentiation. The levels of polyamines are altered by induction. When TMBA is used, the intracellular Put level is increased, because part of the TMBA is hydrolyzed to Put in the cell; and when HMBA is used, hexamethylenediamine appears within the cell, but Put remains at normal pre-induction levels. The levels of total cell-associated Spd and Spm are reduced after induction with both agents and with DMSO; but Spd is increased by MGBG because Spm can be converted to Spd but MGBG prevents conversion of Spd to Spm. The most impressive alteration occurs in the membrane and nuclear fractions, and affects both Spd and Spm (9).

Another form of metabolic control occurs when lymphocytes are exposed to LPS (6). In this case, a cell in G_o is induced to convert to an active state in which it divides rapidly and secretes immunoglobulins. Inducers of differentiation such as HMBA inhibit

the conversion of resting lymphocytes to active secreting plasma cells
(Table 1) (6), although HMBA alone has does not activate lymphocytes.

Table 1

EFFECTS OF ACETYLATED POLYAMINES
on IMMUNOGLOBULIN SECRETION

CONDITIONS	Exper 1	Exper 2
	Number of Plaque-forming Colonies	
LPS	201+40	43+15
LPS + HMBA	45+10	10+ 6

Mean +S.D.

Table 3

ANTAGONISTS AND POLYAMINE
CONCENTRATIONS
nmol/5x10⁷ cells

Additions	Put	Spd	Spm
Control	2	42	72
DFMO	0	0	25
MGBG	127	57	35
DFMO/MGBG	1	1	50

DFMO = 8 mM; MGBG = .008 mM.
Measured at 72 hrs' incubation.

Table 2

POLYAMINE ANTAGONISTS
and MELC DIFFERENTIATION

Conditions	Benzid (% +)	Viable (%)
Control	0	98
DFMO	0	87
MGBG	0	90
HMBA	60	95
HMBA/DFMO	0	90
HMBA/MGBG	8	65
HMBA/DFMO/MGBG	52	54
DMSO	50	72
DMSO/DFMO	33	75

DFMO: 8 mM; MGBG: .007 mM;
HMBA: 4 mM; DMSO: 1.5%;
Induction: HMBA: 72 hr; DMSO: 144 hr
Blocking agents added 24 hr
before inducers.

The addition of HMBA or TMBA (not shown) causes conversion of a high
percentage of the MELC cells to benzidine positive within 72 hours, and
the conversion of Put to GABA is enhanced (data not shown). Inhibitors
of polyamine biosynthesis prevent differentiation in this system when
added separately, although differentiation proceeds when these
inhibitors are added in combination (Table 2) (9).

Intracellular polyamine levels at the end of the incubation are
shown in Table 3. As expected, DFMO completely inhibits Put and Spd
production while MGBG results in accumulation of Put.

DISCUSSION

These observations indicate that the polyamines participate in the
process of cell differentiation in vitro, but their exact function is
not known. On the other hand, in some situations, when the blocking
agents are administered they appear to stimulate rather than depress
differentiation. Some of the effects of the blocking agent DFMO
reported in the literature are shown in Table 4.

Table 4

EFFECTS OF POLYAMINE MANIPULATIONS ON CELL MATURATION

IMMATURE	DFMO	HMBA	"MATURE"	Ref.
MELC	←	→	Erythrocyte	(4,9)
Marrow stem				
in vitro	←		Mature WBC,	(10)
in vivo	→		RBC, etc.	(11)
3T3 fibroblast	←		Adipocyte	(12)
E. gracilis plastid	←*		Photoauto-troph	(13)
Neuroblastoma	→**	→	Neurite formation	(14,15)
Chick blastocyst	←		Gastrulla	(16)
Lymphocytes in vivo	→		Helper T cells	(17)
PHS stim in vitro		←	Activated B Cells	(6)
Embryonal carcinoma	→		Fibroblast morphology	(18)

* blocker: α-methylornithine; ** blocker: α-fluoromethylornithine

We feel that certain conclusions can be drawn about the role of polyamines in differentiation. The concentration of Put seems not to be critical, since differentiation is suppressed by MGBG even when Put is present in high concentrations (Tables 2 and 3) It is also clear from our work and that of others that cell growth is suppressed relatively easily by inhibitors of polyamine synthesis, whereas prevention of differentiation requires profound reduction of the levels of Spd and Spm. On the other hand, when DFMO and MGBG are both present, and polyamine synthesis is maximally suppressed, almost all of the surviving cells differentiate (Table 2). Even under these circumstances, when Put and Spd have been maximally suppressed, the level of Spm remains unaltered. Since Spm can be converted metabolically to both Spd and Put, there is never a time in this type of experiment when all traces of the polyamines are removed.

Although the evidence at hand at present is not conclusive, it strongly suggests that the major polyamines participate in the early phases of "commitment" to differentiation in vitro. By the time differentiation has actually occurred, the initial alterations of the polyamine distribution have disappeared, so they may be of little importance in the late phases of the process.

REFERENCES
1. Williams-Ashman HG, Canellakis ZN: Polyamines in mammalian biology and medicine. Perspect Biol Med (22):421-453, 1979.
2. Canellakis ZN, Milstone LM, Marsh LL, Young PR, Bondy PK: GABA from putrescine is bound in macromolecular form in keratinocytes. Life Sci (33):599-603, 1983.
3. Canellakis ZN, Lande LA, Bondy, PK: Factors modulating the activity of ornithine decarboxylase in rat HTC cells. Medical Biology (59):300-307, 1981.
4. Canellakis ZN, Bondy PK: Diacetylputrescine induces differentiation and is metabolized in Friend erythroleukemia cells. In: Bachrach U, Kaye A, Chayen R (ed) Advances in Polyamine Research. Raven Press, New York, 1983, vol 4 pp 769-778.
5. Marks PA, Rifkind RA: Erythroleukemic differentiation. Ann Rev Biochem (47):419-448, 1978.
6. Ryan JL, Bondy PK, Gobran L, Canellakis ZN: Acetylated diamines inhibit endotoxin-induced lymphocyte activation. Submitted.
7. Bondy PK, Canellakis ZN: High performance liquid chromatography in the separation and measurement of di-and polyamines and their derivatives. With methods for the specific preparation of isomers of their monoacetyl derivatives. J Chromatogr. (244):371-379, 1980.
8. Pegg AE, McCann PP: Polyamine metabolism and function. Am J Physiol (243)(Cell Physiol 12):C212-C221, 1982.
9. Canellakis ZN, Chari R, Bondy PK: Aspects of Polyamine Metabolism in Differentiating Friend Erythroleukemia Cells.
10. Verma DS, Sukara PS: An essential role for polyamine biosynthesis during human hematopoietic differentiation. Cancer Res (42):3046-3049, 1982
11. Niskanen E, Kallio A, McCann PP, Baker DG: The role of polyamine biosynthesis in hematopoietic precursor cell proliferation in mice. Blood (61):740-745, 1983
12. Bethell DR, Pegg AE,: Polyamines are needed for the differentiation of 3T3-L1 fibroblasts into adipose cells. Biochem Biophys Res Commun (102):272-278, 1981.
13. Schuber F, Aleksijevic A, Blee E: Comparative role of polyamines in division and plastid differentiation of Euglena gracilis. Biochim Biophys Acta (675):178-187, 1981.
14. Chen KY, Nau D, Liu AY-C: Effects of inhibitors of ornithine decarboxylase on the differentiation of mouse neuroblastoma cells. Cancer Res (43):2812-2818, 1983.
15. Palfrey C, Kimhi Y, Littauer UZ, Reuben RC, Marks PA: Induction of differentiation in mouse neuroblastoma cells by hexamethylene bisacetamide. Biochem Biophys Res Commun (76):937-942, 1977.
16. Löwkvist B, Heby O, Emanuelsson H: Essential role of the polyamines in early chick embryo development. J Embryol Exp Morph (60):83-92, 1980.
17. Sharkis SJ, Luk GD, Collector MI, McCann PP, Baylin ST, Sensenbrenner LL: Regulation of hematopoiesis II: The role of polyamine inhibition on helper or suppressor influences of the thymus. Blood (61):604-607, 1983.
18. Schindler J, Kelly M, McCann PP: Inhibition of ornithine decarboxylase induces embryonal carcinoma cell differentiation. Biochem Biophys Res Commun (114):410-417, 1983.

POLYAMINES, IMMUNE RESPONSE AND TUMOUR GROWTH CONTROL

W. A. BOGGUST,   S. O'CONNELL   AND   A. DRUMM,

INTRODUCTION AND SUMMARY

Polyamines may control primary tumour growth and metastasis by the
proliferative and cytotoxic effect of their oxidation products on both
neoplastic and infiltrating cells. Spleen cells of mice responding to
antigenic stimulation with SRBC and to tumour have elevated polyamine
oxidase activity, like tumour macrophages, and their numbers are increased
by polyamine administration. Accordingly, increased primary tumour mass,
associated with increased infiltration and reduced metastasis may be regulated by a polyamine-polyamine-oxidase-induced increase in the numbers of
cytotoxic cells reacting to the tumour.

EXPERIMENTAL

He-La cells were seeded at 10^4 cells/ml with put.2HCl, spermd.3HCl,
sper.4HCl, oxidised put.(1), acrolein, monoacet.put., diacet.put. in standard
medium (2) with 2% calf serum and in put- and sper-oxidase-free medium (calf
serum 70 mins at $65^{\circ}C$) with 0.5% mouse serum. Proliferation rates (cell
count increase in 4 days at $37^{\circ}C$ (2)) are shown in tables 1 and 4.

Three month LACA and WHT/Ht female mice were inoculated i.p. with 500
x 10^6 washed SRBC. Spleen cell suspensions were prepared daily in Ringer's
sol. at $4^{\circ}C$. Amine oxidase was assayed by incubating cells with 10 μg put.
2HCl and sper.4HCl in 2 ml Ringer's sol. for 20 hrs at $37^{\circ}C$ followed by
dansylation of residual P.A. (3). P.A. oxidase was assayed in spleen
cells of syngeneic WHT/Ht mice after 14 days growth of carcinoma (1,4)
(tables 2 and 3).

WHT/Ht mice inoculated with SRBC were injected daily i.p. with 0.2 ml
0.25% CMC-saline containing put.2HCl (183 μg/g) or sper.4HCl (0.25 μg/g) or
solvent only. Spleen antibody-forming cells, assayed daily by the plaque
technique (5) are expressed (table 6) as relative mean numbers of plaques
per 10^6 cells calculated as % of count for normal spleens.

301

Table 1. Proliferation rate of HE-LA cells expressed as % of control in standard medium with added polyamines and related compounds.

Putrescine (μg/ml)

.01	.02	.04	.05	.06	.10
111±8.7	125±15.5	145±15.1	155±16.2	125±17.6	119±4.0

Spermidine

.005	.010	.015	.020	.025	.100
101±1.7	131±10.6	128±19.2	138±14.8	105±8.1	82±10.7

Spermine

.002	.004	.005	.006	.010	.020
106±1.9	109±9.1	138±7.8	119±10.6	103±6.8	101±5.0

Oxidised putrescine

.001	.002	.003	.004	.005	.010
105±6.9	111±7.0	134±10.9	123±17.7	100±7.4	94±3.2

Acrolein

.001	.002	.003	.004	.01	.50
105±3.1	150±15.6	146±15.6	138±3.7	94±20.3	81±8.8

N-acetylputrescine

.02	.04	.06	.08	.10	.15
106±0.6	122±1.4	134±8.1	138±9.0	124±3.6	99±1.8

N.N'diacetylputrescine*

.06	.10	.12	.15	.20	.50
112±3.7	132±8.4	141±9.6	136±2.3	113±6.4	93±3.6

means ± SD, n = 5 or 6, *20% serum

Table 2. Amine oxidase activity in spleens of LACA mice as μg putrescine degraded by 30 M cells following inoculation with 500×10^6 SRBC. (means ± SD, n = 5 or 6)

Days after inoculation

0	3	5	7	8	10
.60±.12	1.07±.34	1.54±.48	2.72±.42	3.23±.37	1.76±.48

Table 3. Amine oxidase activity in spleens of normal and tumour-bearing WHT/Ht mice as μg substrate degraded by 25 M cells (means ± SD)

	Normal	Tumour
Putrescine	1.18±.51 (n = 5)	6.89±2.01 (n = 18)
Spermine	1.00±.48 (n = 6)	5.23±1.25 (n = 16)

Cell suspensions of tumours in WHT/Ht mice receiving daily i.p. injections of P.A., Razoxane or CMC-saline (1,4), prepared with trypsin, pancreatin and collagenase (4.0, 1.2 and 2.0 mg/ml) were counted in 2 size ranges: large and intermediate, mainly neoplastic cells (20-45μ) and small (10-15μ) including lymphocytes; preliminary findings are shown in table 7. Glass adherent tumour macrophages (6) were frozen and thawed; eluates were assayed for P.A. oxidase (table 5).

Table 4. Proliferation rate of HE-LA cells expressed as % of control in medium without serum polyamine oxidases with added polyamines and related compounds (means ± SD, n = 5 or 6).

Putrescine (μg/ml)					
.02	.03	.04	.05	.06	.10
105±3.4	124±8.9	137±7.6	143±9.5	127±6.0	117±6.9
Spermidine					
.005	.010	.015	.020	.025	.050
102±3.8	112±7.0	120±23.9	125±10.3	117±13.2	94±5.7
Spermine					
.002	.004	.005	.006	.010	.020
96±4.5	86±9.2	83±4.2	78.5±4.0	70±6.1	69±6.6
Oxidised putrescine					
.0006	.0010	.0020	.0030	.0040	.0050
107±3.7	120±5.9	132±16.4	151±14.4	123±16.0	92±6.3
Acrolein					
.005	.010	.025	.050	.100	.250
107±2.0	126±3.5	121±2.8	113±2.9	88±4.4	59±3.0

Table 5. Amine oxidase activity of macrophages in tumours of WHT/Ht mice as μg putrescine degraded (means ± SD, n = 7 or 8).

Macrophages	1 x 10^6	2 x 10^6
	2.38±0.85	4.01±0.49

Table 6. Relative mean numbers of plaques per 10^6 spleen cells formed after inoculation with SRBC in normal WHT/Ht mice and mice receiving daily injections of putrescine and spermine.

Days after inoculation	0	3	4	5	6	7	8	9	12
Controls	100	–	105	135	122	177	327	152	157
SD ±	9.1		3.0	12.1	11.6	40.9	17.4	15.2	18.1
Putrescine	–	–	116	185	174	258	369	162	189
SD ±			2.8	13.2	25.6	31.4	38.5	35.9	12.1
Spermine	–	104	136	191	166	375	544	188	187
		7.6	4.8	26.0	24.1	22.7	22.6	17.6	28.3

n = 5, SD, standard deviation as % of values found.

Table 7. Composition of tumours of mice receiving putrescine and
Razoxane compared with control tumours.

Ratio : small cells/large and intermediate cells		
CMC-saline (controls)	Putrescine	I.C.R.F.-159
0.87±0.07	1.98±1.07	0.45±0.23

RESULTS AND DISCUSSION

Added polyamines increase He-La proliferation at specific optimum concentrations, put.> spermd.> sper. Put. and sper. may be replaced by their
enzyme oxidation products including acrolein (1,7). At higher concentrations,
inhibition and cytotoxicity occur. Mono- and diacetyl-put. increase proliferation after hydrolysis to put. by serum enzymes.

Put. and spermd. but not sper. also regulate proliferation in systems
without extrinsic P.A. oxidase and their oxidation products do the same.
P.A. oxidation may stimulate cell division and P.A. oxidases are intimately
concerned, occurring intrinsically in proliferating malignant cells, as
inferred from changes in P.A. levels in homogenates and cultures treated
with P.A.-oxidase inhibitors (2,8), or extrinsically in serum or macrophages
and infiltrating cells in tumours. Accordingly changes in growth rate are
attributed to oxidation of polyamines adjacent to proliferating cells.

The cytotoxicity of polyamines is attributed to their oxidation products
including acrolein (7). Our findings of increased cell proliferation by
oxidised put. and acrolein at critical low concentrations and inhibition
at higher levels correspond to the behaviour of their precursor P.A. in the
presence of P.A. oxidase.

After daily injection of P.A. in mice inoculated with SRBC the peak
numbers of antibody-producing spleen cells reached at day 8 are much increased. The largest relative increases, on day 7, amounted to 137% and
192% of control values for put. and sper. respectively. Spleen cell put.-
oxidase also rises, reaching a maximum increased 5-fold relative to controls
on day 8 and then declining. Spleens of mice with 14-day tumour show a 6-
fold increase in put. oxidase and a 5-fold increase in sper. oxidase relative
to normal. Tumour macrophages have high P.A. oxidase activity.

Accordingly, antigen stimulating production of spleen cells forming
antibodies to SRBC, presumably B-lymphocytes, simultaneously induces increased spleen cell P.A.-oxidase activity coinciding with development of
the immune response. P.A. increase the response by promoting an increase
in spleen antibody-forming cells, possibly by P.A.-oxidase-induced pro-

liferation. T-lymphocytes also may be modified by P.A. with significant consequences for growth and survival of malignant cells in the primary tumour, in the circulation and at sites of potential metastatic growth.

Tumour P.A.-oxidase is augmented by infiltrating lymphoid cells and tumour macrophages previously implicated in control of tumour growth and sometimes present in large numbers (6). As cell proliferation reflects the P.A./P.A.-oxidase status of the environment and added P.A. increase primary tumour growth in mice and reduce metastasis, growth in tumours with spontaneously raised P.A. levels (1) may be regulated by these cellular factors thus accounting for the immunological stimulation of primary tumours by spleen cells (9) and the inhibition of metastasis.

Since both tumour mass and spleen antibody-forming cell numbers are increased by P.A. the former may reflect increased infiltration by circulating lymphoid cells including T-lymphocytes cytotoxic to malignant cells. Our preliminary findings show increased infiltration in tumours of mice receiving P.A. and decreased infiltration with the immunosuppressive drug Razoxane, thus supporting the hypothesis for a causal relationship between increased tumour growth rate and reduced metastasis.

REFERENCES

1. Boggust WA, O'Connell S: Proc 9th Internat Symp Biol Charact of Human Tumours, Bologna 1981 (pub. October 1983).
2. Boggust WA: Changes in polyamine concentrations in relation to the proliferation of He-La cells IRCS Med Sci (8): 600-601, 1980.
3. Seiler N: Use of the Dansyl reaction in biochemical analysis. Methods in Biochem Anal (18): 259-337, 1970.
4. Boggust WA, O'Connell S, Carroll R, Wilson P: Inhibition of metastatic tumour development in WHT/Ht mice by putrescine, spermidine and spermine administration. IRCS Med Sci (8): 597-598, 1980.
5. Hunt SV: Cunningham plaque assay for antibody-secreting cells. In: Hall DO, Hawkins SE (eds) Laboratory Manual of Cell Biology. EUP London, 1975, pp.259-263.
6. Evans R: Macrophages in syngeneic animal tumours. Transplant (14): 468, 1972.
7. Kimes BW, Morris DR: Preparation and stability of oxidised polyamines. Biochim Biophys Acta (228): 223, 1971.
8. Boggust WA, O'Connell S: Changes in cells induced by drugs inhibiting experimental tumours etc. In: Davies W, Harrap KR, Stathopoulos G (eds) Human Cancer, Charact and Treatment. Excerpta Medica, Amsterdam, 1980, pp.374-386.
9. Prehn RT: The immune reaction as a stimulator of tumor growth. Science (176): 170-171, 1972.

ACKNOWLEDGEMENT

Acknowledgement is made to Saint Luke's Cancer Research Fund and the Irish Tobacco Manufacturers' Advisory Committee.

POTENTIAL USE OF RETINOIDS IN CANCER PREVENTION AND TREATMENT

G.J.S. RUSTIN

INTRODUCTION

A role for vitamin A in oncology has been suspected since the 1920's
when it was reported that rats fed a diet deficient in vitamin A developed
carcinoma of the stomach (1). Despite there being good reasons for using
vitamin A in oncology there remains confusion as to its method of action
and its administration is not without hazards. Excessive intake of vitamin A
can cause numerous side effects, including severe hepatocellular damage.
Chemical modification of vitamin A alcohol retinol, results in numerous
compounds called retinoids. As most synthetic retinoids are not stored in
the liver they do not appear to damage that organ and this has opened the
way to more extensive use of retinoids in oncology.

GROWTH INHIBITION

In vitro.   The growth of many different cell types can be inhibited
in culture when retinoids are added. There is however considerable variability,
for example of 6 human melanoma lines Lotan (2) found only 2 showed growth
inhibition whilst 1 actually showed stimulation after addition of retinoic
acid. Most in vitro studies have used 10^{-5} molar concentrations of retinoids
whilst it is dangerous to maintain a concentration above 10^{-6} molar in human
serum. As the growth inhibitory effects are usually reversible on removal
of the retinoid only the few tumours which have satisfactory growth inhibition
at concentrations of retinoids less than 10^{-7} molar, are candidates for
retinoid therapy.

In vivo.   Most tumours used in the N.C.I. screening programme are
resistant to retinoids unless the dose is sufficient to cause severe hyper-
vitaminosis A. There are exceptions, transplantable rat chondrosarcoma
being the most convincing with several different retinoids causing inhibition
of tumour growth at non-toxic doses (3). The growth inhibitory effects may
be partly mediated through immunological mechanisms as demonstrated by retinyl

307

palonitate inhibiting growth of S91 murine melanoma when transplanted into allogeneic mice but not when transplanted into synergeneic mice (4).

<u>Clinical Studies</u>. The earliest clinical studies were performed after vitamin A had been shown to have a therapeutic effect on epithelial skin tumours induced by DMBA in mice. Bollag and Ott (5) in 1971 showed that topical vitamin A acid induced a complete response in 5 of 16 patients with basal cell carcinomas. Since then oral retinoids have been shown to be effective in the treatment of actinic keratoses, multiple superficial and isolated basal cell carcinomas, squamous cell carcinomas and keratoacanthomas (6). Recently responses have been seen in cutaneous deposits of mycosis fungoides after oral cis retinoic acid therapy (7). Amongst 35 evaluable patients with solid tumours the author (8) found no tumour responses after a minimum of 1 month of oral etretinate. However, of 11 patients with advanced malignant melanoma 2 patients had stabilisation of disease, 1 with subcutaneous and lymph node disease for 29 weeks and 1 with brain metastases for 36 months. Meyskens (9) saw partial responses in 2 of 18 patients given cis retinoic acid for advanced malignant melanoma and in 6 of 24 patients with advanced squamous cell carcinomas. Further studies are required to determine whether combining retinoids which are not myelosuppressive with cytotoxic drugs will have any therapeutic benefit.

The retinol and retinoic acid cellular binding proteins may have a role in treatment of established tumours. In most human tumours examined 1 or both receptors are present at a higher concentration than in normal surrounding tissue. I am at present trying to discover whether this difference can be utilized in drug targeting.

DIFFERENTIATION

The anti-carcinogenic role of retinoids may be modulated through their known capacity to induce differentiation of cells such that they mature and are then incapable of proliferation. Their capacity to induce differentiation has been well demonstrated in mouse embryonal carcinoma cells in cell culture. After exposure of the F9 nullipotent cell line to concentrations of retinoic acid as low as 10^{-9}M multiple phenotypic changes indicative of differentiation into endoderm were seen (10). Mice bearing malignant murine embryonal carcinomas have been treated with oral retinoids with evidence of differentiation and intra-tumour injections of retinoic acid dissolved in DMSO have produced growth inhibition. I therefore treated 8 patients with metastatic malignant teratoma who had failed cytotoxic chemotherapy with the synthetic retinoic etretinate and was unable to detect any evidence of differentiation. This is compatible with a recent study in which retinoic acid failed to induce differentiation in 7 human teratocarcinoma cell lines (12).

Breitman and colleagues (13) have demonstrated that 8/8 human pro-myelocytic leukaemia (PML) cells in primary culture could be induced to differentiate by low doses of retinoic acid. Although he was unable to see differentiation in the cells of 18 patients with non-PML myeloid leukaemia after addition of retinoic acid Douer and Koeffler (14) found that 1 μM retinoic acid caused > 50 % inhibition of clonal growth of cells from 5 of 7 patients with myeloid leukaemia other than PML. Recently several groups have been looking at synergism between retinoic acid when combined with dexamethasone, serum differentiating factors or agents that increase intra-cellular cAMP.

ANTICARCINOGENESIS

The potential for retinoids as anticarcinogens is demonstrated in animal studies where they can prevent the development of many carcinogen induced tumours. Considerable variability exists between retinoids both in their anticarcinogenic capacity and in their toxicity. A therapeutic index has been developed by Bollag (15) which is calculated from the degree of regress-ion of chemically induced papillomas in mice following retinoid therapy and the grade of toxicity manifested as weight loss, desquamation of the skin, hair loss and bone fractures. Retinoids can prevent the development of many carcinogen induced cancers including cancer of the skin, respiratory tract, prostate, urinary tract and mammary gland. Retinyl acetate has been shown to reduce the incidence of MNU induced mammary cancers in rats and to have a synergistic effect when combined with 2-bromo-alpha-ergocryptine, tamoxifen or oopherectomy (16). Hydroxyphenyl retinamide appears to have the best therapeutic effect against nitrosamine induced bladder cancers in mice (17). This compound should enter clinical trials in man in 1984 after completion of animal toxicology. Etretinate has been used in 2 trials in patients with recurrent superficial bladder tumours. In a Finnish study (18) 11/15 patients on etretinate for 1 year had no tumours, or < 50% the number of pre trial tumours compared to 4/15 om placebo (p<0.01). A Swiss study (19) confirms this improvement but larger numbers wil be required to see if the invasive carcinomas can be prevented.

Epidemiological studies support the anticarcinogenic role of vitamin A.

17/20 dietry studies and a recent prospective study show significant inverse relation between high dietry intake of foods rich in vitamin A and development of cancer (20,21). As these observations are also compatible with beta carotene being the preventative agent as this compound is non toxic an intervention study of 30 mg beta carotene every 2 days has now begun in American physicians. Until animal studies have confirmed the value of beta carotene, intervention studies in high-risk groups with retinoids appear the best way forward.

REFERENCES

1. Fujimaki Y. Formation of carcinoma in albino rats fed on deficient diets. J. Cancer Res. 10: 469-477, 1926.
2. Lotan R. Effects of vitamin A and its analogue (retinoids) on normal and neoplastic cells. Bio Chimica and Bio Physica Acta. 605: 33-91, 1980.
3. Trown PW, Burk MJ, Hansen R. Inhibition of growth and regression of transplantable rat condrosarcoma by three retinoids. Cancer Treat. Rep. 60: 647-653, 1976.
4. Felin EL, Loyd B, Cohen MH. Inhibition of the growth and development of transplantable murine melanoma by vitamin A. Science. 189: 886-888, 1975.
5. Bollag W, Ott F. Therapy of actinic-keratoses and basal cell carcinomas with local application of vitamin A acid. Cancer Chemotherapy Rep. 55: 59-60, 1971.
6. Grupper CH, Berretti B. Cutaneous neoplasia and etretinate. Proc. 13th Int. Cong. Chemotherapy Vienna 1983; part 201: 24-27.
7. Kessler JF, Meyskens FL, Levine N, Lynch, Jones SE. Treatment of cutaneous T-cell lymphoma (Mycosis Fungoides) with 13 cis-retinoic acid. Lancet 1: 1345-1347, 1983.
8. Rustin GJS, Bagshawe KD. Trial of an aromatic retinoid in patients with solid tumours. Br. J. Cancer. 45: 304-308, 1982.
9. Meyskens FL, Gilmartin E, Alberts DS, Levine NS, Brooks R, Salmon SE, Surwit EA. Activity of Isotretinoin against squamous cell cancers and preneoplastic lesions. Cancer Treat. Rep. 66: 1315-1319, 1982.
10. Strickland S, Mahdavi V. The induction of differentiation in terato-carcinoma cells by retinoic acid. Cell. 15: 393-403, 1978.
11. Speers WC. Conversion of malignant murine embryonal carcinomas to benign teratomas by chemical induction of differentiation in vivo. Cancer Res. 42: 1843-1849, 1982.
12. Matthaei KI, Andrews PW, Bronson DL. Retinoic acid fails to induce differentiation in human teratocarcinoma cell lines that express high levels of cellular receptor proteins. Exp. Cell Res. 143: 91-102, 1983.
13. Breitman TR, Keene BR, Hemmi H. Retinoic acid induced differentiation of fresh human leukaemia cells and the human myelomonocytic leukaemia cell lines, HL-60, U-937 and THP-1. Cancer Surveys 2: 263-291, 1983.
14. Douer D, Koeffler HP. Retinoic acid, inhibition of colonal growth of human myeloid cells. J. Clin. Invest. 69: 277-283, 1982.
15. Bollag W. Vitamin A and retinoids: from nutrition to pharmacology in dermatology and oncology. Lancet. 860-863, 1983.
16. Moon RC, McCormick DL, Mehta RG. Inhibition of carcinogenesis by retinoids. Cancer Res. (suppl) 43: 2469-2475, 1983.

311

17. Hicks RN, Turton JA, Tomlinson CN, Gwynne J, Nandra K. The effect of two retinoids on the response of an inbred mouse strain to the bladder carcinogen M-butyl-N-(4-hydroxibutyl) nitrosamine (BBN). Proc. Nutrit. Soc. 42: 11A, 1983.
18. Alrtnan O, Tarkkanen J, Grohn P, Heinonen E, Pyrhonen S, Saila K. Tigason (etretinate) in prevention of recurrence of superficial bladder tumours. Lur. Urol. 9: 6-9, 1983.
19. Studer UE, Biedermann C, Chollet D, Karrer P, Kraft R, Toggenburg H, Vonbank F. The place of retinoids in the treatment of recurrent superficial bladder carcinomas. Proc. 13th Int. Cong. Chemotherapy Vienna. 201: 22-23, 1983.
20. Peto R, Doll R, Buckley JD, Sporn MB. Can dietry beta carotene materially reduce human cancer rates? Nature. 290: 201-208, 1981.
21. Shekelle RB, Lepper M, Shuguey L, Maliza C, Raynor WJ, Rossof AH. Dietry vitamin A risk of cancer in Western Electric Study. Lancet ii. 1185-1190, 1981.

CHAPTER IV

DESIGN AND DEVELOPMENT OF NEW DRUGS

INOSINE 5'-PHOSPHATE DEHYDROGENASE AS A TARGET FOR CANCER
CHEMOTHERAPY. RESULTS WITH 3-DEAZAGUANINE, TIAZOFURIN AND
2-β-D-RIBOFURANOSYLSELENAZOLE-4-CARBOXAMIDE (PD-111232)

T.J. BORITZKI, D.W. FRY, J. BESSERER, P.D. COOK and R.C. JACKSON

1. THE RATE-CONTROLLING ROLE OF IMP DEHYDROGENASE

IMP dehydrogenase is the first and rate-limiting enzyme of
the guanine nucleotide branch of the purine biosynthetic pathway.
Table 1 summarizes maximal activities of enzymes of purine ribonucleotide interconversion in cytosol preparations from rat liver
and the rapidly growing transplantable hepatoma 3683.

Table 1. Enzymes of purine metabolism in rat liver and hepatoma

Enzyme	Rat liver Hepatoma 3683 (nmol/hr/mg protein)		Hepatoma activity as % liver activity
IMP dehydrogenase	2	26	1300
GMP synthetase	10	55	550
GMP kinase	6800	8160	120
GDP kinase	12000	24000	200
SAMP synthetase	36	112	310
SAMP lyase	290	508	175
AMP kinase	99000	9900	10
AMP deaminase	6000	25800	430

Source: references 1 - 6.

IMP dehydrogenase had the lowest activity of the purine ribonucleotide biosynthetic enzymes in normal liver (and in other normal
tissues). Although it showed the greatest proportional increase
of all these enzymes in hepatomas, it remained rate-limiting for
the pathway (1, 2). Elevations in activity of IMP dehydrogenase
have also been described in kidney tumours, colon carcinoma,
sarcoma and leukaemia (7 - 10). These results suggested that IMP
dehydrogenase should be a sensitive target for cancer chemotherapy.

2. 3-DEAZAGUANINE

This purine base analogue, synthesized by Cook et al.(11) has antitumour activity in several systems, particularly mouse and rat mammary carcinomas (12). As the ribonucleotide it is an effective inhibitor of IMP dehydrogenase (13). It is also incorporated into nucleic acid (14). Recently, 3-deaza-GMP was shown to be a potent inhibitor of an enzyme of the purine de novo biosynthetic pathway, AICAR transformylase, with $K_i = 0.1$ µM (15). 3-Deazaguanine also inhibits protein synthesis in L1210 cells(16). Studies in our laboratory showed that 100 µM guanine, guanosine, hypoxanthine or adenine gave protection of HCT-8 human colon carcinoma cells from 60 µM 3-deazaguanine, with considerable partial protection even if the rescue agent was delayed for 4 hr after 3-deazaguanine. It is possible that adenine and hypoxanthine protected by depletion of cellular PRPP. Table 2 shows the effects of 3-deazaguanine or 3-deazaguanine plus adenosine on ribonucleotide pools in human lymphoblastoid cells following a 2 hr treatment.

Table 2. Formation of 3-deazaguanine nucleotides and effects on cellular ribonucleoside triphosphates in WI-L2 cells

Culture	Cellular nucleotides (nmole/10^9 cells)						
	3DGMP	3DGDP	3DGTP	CTP	UTP	ATP	GTP
Control	–	–	–	147	428	1890	520
3DG (67µM)	65	229	378	126	401	1615	262
3DG (67µM)+ Ado(100µM)	–	66	108	124	270	2440	359

These pools were measured by HPLC, using detection at 305 nm for the 3-deazaguanine nucleotides. 3-Deazaguanine reduced GTP to 50% of control within 2 hr. Adenosine decreased formation of 3-deazaguanine nucleotides and antagonized the effect on GTP. 3-Deazaguanine (100µM) was found to cause a 2.8-fold increase in IMP pools of HCT-8 cells, peaking at 2 hr after addition of drug. This elevation is much less than that found with tiazofurin, and may reflect the inhibition of AICAR transformylase by 3-deazaGMP.

3. TIAZOFURIN

Tiazofurin, synthesized by Robins et al.(17) has potent antitumour activity against Lewis lung carcinoma and other murine

systems, with minimal host toxicity. Tiazofurin has been shown
to be converted within cells to an analogue of NAD which acts as
a potent inhibitor of IMP dehydrogenase (18,19). This appears to
be the primary site of action of tiazofurin, since its effects
are reversed by guanine or guanosine, but not by adenine or hypoxanthine. A problem in the phase 1 clinical trials has been hyper-
uricaemia, perhaps a result of the marked accumulation of IMP in
treated cells (Table 3). This condition may be alleviated by
administration of allopurinol. Tissue culture studies with WI-L2
cells showed that allopurinol (100µM) neither enhanced nor antagonized the inhibitory effect of tiazofurin at 3.5, 7 or 15 µM.

4. 2-β-D-RIBOFURANOSYLSELENAZOLE-4-CARBOXAMIDE (PD-111232)

This compound, the selenium analogue of tiazofurin, was synthesized by Srivastava and Robins (20). It is about 10-fold more
potent than tiazofurin, in vitro and in vivo (21). Its effects
on cells in culture are reversed by guanine or guanosine, but not
by hypoxanthine or adenine. The effects of PD-111232 on ribonucleotide pools, in comparison with other IMP dehydrogenase inhibitors, are shown in Table 3. These data refer to a 2 hr treatment
time, with inhibitor at 10 µM in each case.

Table 3. Effects of IMP dehydrogenase inhibitors on WI-L2
cell ribonucleotide pools

Culture	IMP	GMP	UDP	UTP	CTP	ADP	ATP	GDP	GTP
			(nmole/10^9 cells)						
Control	17	77	170	514	185	700	2240	204	630
			(percent of control)						
Tiazofurin	1560	23	125	148	154	95	123	49	48
PD-111232	2080	19	124	158	146	80	100	34	32
Mycophenolic acid	2110	21	113	189	183	72	118	37	36
Bredinin	1580	82	113	126	112	97	93	63	47
Bredinin aglycone	1230	108	111	98	90	95	87	68	55
Ribavirin	ND	ND	ND	131	126	97	116	55	61

PD-111232 had the most pronounced anti-guanylate effect of the
inhibitors tested. The cellular dGTP pool was also depressed (21).
Like tiazofurin, PD-111232 inhibits the synthesis of both RNA and
DNA, and treated cells increase in size, indicating unbalanced
growth. The inhibition of partially purified IMP dehydrogenase

from L1210 cells was compared using the NAD analogues of tiazofurin (TAD) and PD-111232 (SeAD). The K_i values were 57 nM for
TAD and 33 nM for SeAD. This difference may partially explain
the difference in potency between tiazofurin and PD-111232, but
other factors are probably also involved.

5. KINETICS OF INHIBITION OF THE GUANYLATE PATHWAY

A possible explanation for the great sensitivity of cells to
IMP dehydrogenase inhibition may be found in the kinetic properties of the pathway, as studied by computer modelling (22).
Biosynthesis of ATP from IMP (v3 in Fig.1) requires GTP, which is
a substrate for SAMP synthetase. Conversely, synthesis of GTP
(v2 in Fig.1) requires ATP at 3 sites (GMP synthetase, GMP kinase,
GDP kinase). Fig.1 (top) shows v3 as a function of (GTP). The
steady-state values of v2 may also be plotted as a function of
GTP, since the concentration of ATP, upon which v2 depends, is,
in turn, dependent on the GTP level. Fig.1 (top) shows a family
of such curves (A-E) corresponding to different IMP dehydrogenase
activities. These curves are sigmoid, because of the high-order
ATP-dependence of v2. Because IMP dehydrogenase is inhibited by
GMP, the curves show inhibition at high GTP levels (which are
accompanied by high GMP). In the steady state, since roughly
equal amounts of GTP and ATP are used for nucleic acid synthesis,
v2=v3. These points are shown in Fig.1 (top). For a given activity of IMP dehydrogenase there may be 1, 2 or 3 steady points
(where there are 3, the middle one will be unstable). Fig.1
(centre) shows the steady state values (v2=v3=v4) as a function
of IMP dehydrogenase activity. Consider a system on the upper
limb of this curve, with a level of IMP dehydrogenase slightly
greater than that at point B; v4 is comparatively high. Slight
inhibition of IMP dehydrogenase will bring the system to the
upper of the 2 points marked B; v4 is still high. If IMP dehydrogenase is now inhibited further, the only steady state the system
can assume is on the lower limb of the curve, to the left of the
lower point B. This corresponds to a very low rate of nucleic
acid synthesis (v4). Thus a minor degree of inhibition of IMP
dehydrogenase has resulted in extensive shutdown of nucleic acid
synthesis. At present we have no experimental evidence for

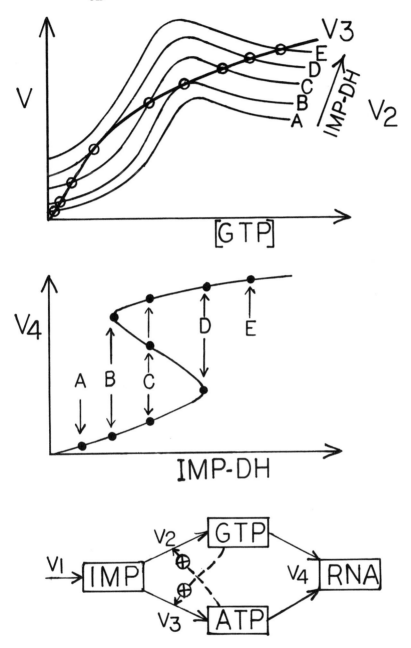

FIGURE 1.   Multistability in the purine ribonucleotide
            biosynthetic pathway.

multistability of the purine pathway, but our kinetic simulation has shown that, based upon the known kinetic properties of the enzymes, this behaviour is possible, and may explain the sensitivity of tumour cells to inhibition of IMP dehydrogenase.

REFERENCES

1. Jackson RC, Weber G, Morris HP: IMP dehydrogenase, an enzyme linked with proliferation and malignancy.Nature(256):331-333,1975.
2. Jackson RC, Morris HP, Weber G: Properties of IMP dehydrogenase in normal and malignant rat tissues.Biochem J(166):1-10,1977.
3. Jackson RC, Morris HP, Weber G: Enzymes of the purine ribonucleotide cycle in rat hepatomas. Cancer Res(37)3057-3065,1977.
4. Weber G, Lui MS, Faderan MA, Natsumeda Y: Molecular targets of anti-IMP dehydrogenase chemotherapy. Adv Enz Reg(22)in press,1984
5. Criss WE, Litwack G, Morris HP, Weinhouse S: AMP kinase isozymes in rat liver and hepatomas. Cancer Res(30):370-375,1970.
6. Boritzki TJ, Jackson RC, Morris HP, Weber G: GMP synthetase and GMP kinase in rat hepatomas. Biochim Biophys Acta(658)102,1981.
7. Jackson RC, Goulding FJ, Weber G: Enzymes of purine metabolism in renal cell carcinoma. J Natl Cancer Inst(62):749-754,1979.
8. Weber G, Hager JC, Lui MS, Prajda N: Biochemical patterns of colon carcinoma xenografts. Cancer Res(41):854-859,1981.
9. Weber G, Burt ME, Jackson RC, Prajda N: Purine and pyrimidine enzymic pattern in sarcoma. Cancer Res(43):1019-1023,1983.
10. Becher HJ, Lohr GW: IMP dehydrogenase activity in normal and leukaemia blood cells. Klin Wochenschr(57):1109-1115,1979.
11. Cook PD, Rousseau RJ, Mian AM, meyer RB, Robins RK: Synthesis of 3-deazaguanine. J Am Chem Soc(98):1492-1498,1976.
12. Khwaja TA: 3-Deazaguanine, a candidate drug for the chemotherapy of breast cancer. Cancer Treat Rep(66):1853-1858,1982.
13. Streeter DG, Koyama HHP: Inhibition of purine ribonucleotide biosynthesis by 3-deazaguanine. Biochem Pharmacol(25):2413,1976.
14. Schwartz P, Hammond D, Khwaja TA: Biochemical pharmacology of 3-deazaguanine. Proc Am Assoc Cancer Res(18):153,1977.
15. Smejkal RM, Page T, Nyhan WL, Jacobsen TJ, Mangum JH, Robins RK: Novel nucleoside inhibitors of guanosine metabolism as antitumor agents. Adv Enz Reg(22):in press,1984.
16. Rivest RS, Irwin D, Mandel HG: 3-Deazaguanine: inhibition of initiation of translation. Cancer Res(42):4039-4044,1982.
17. Robins RK, Srivastava PC, Narayanan VL, Plowman J, Paull KD: 2-β-D-ribofuranosylthiazole-4-carboxamide, a novel potential antitumor agent. J Med Chem(25):107-108,1982.
18. Cooney DA, Jayaram HN, Gebeyehu G, Betts CR: The conversion of tiazofurin to an analogue of NAD. Biochem Pharmacol(31):2133,1982.
19. Kuttan R, Robins RK, Saunders PP:Inhibition of IMP dehydrogenase by metabolites of tiazofurin. BBRC(107):862-868,1982.
20. Srivastava PC, Robins RK: Synthesis and antitumor activity of selenazole-4-carboxamide C-nucleoside. J Med Chem(26):445,1983.
21. Fry DW, Boritzki TJ, Besserer J, Jackson RC, Cook PD, Robins RK: Studies of the biochemical mechanism of action of the novel tiazofurin analog PD111232. Abstracts,13th Int Chemotherapy Congress, Vienna, 1983.
22. Jackson RC:Kinetic simulation. Int J Bio-Med Comp(11):197,1980.

ANTITUMOUR ACTIVITY AND PHARMACOLOGY OF CCRG 81010 (NSC 353451, M&B 39565, 8-carbamoyl-3-(1-chloroethyl)imidazo[5,1-d]-1,1,3,5-tetrazin-4(3H)-one)

J.A. HICKMAN AND M.F.G. STEVENS,

CCRG 81010 is one of the most potently active experimental antitumour agents which has been tested against murine tumours in vivo and it accomplishes the cure of animals bearing most of the ascitic or solid tumours (1-3). The rationale for its synthesis and screening arose from long term interests in the chemistry and pharmacology of molecules which contain triazene (N-N-N) linkages (4,5) and in the pharmacology of the nitrosoureas (6). Figure 1 shows the structure of CCRG 81010 together with that of the clinically useful antitumour triazene DTIC and a generalised formula for the chloroethylnitrosoureas. Structural similarities are apparent and indeed these similarities have been shown to extend to the broad spectrum of antitumour activity demonstrated by CCRG 81010 and to its mechanism of action, both of which will be outlined here.

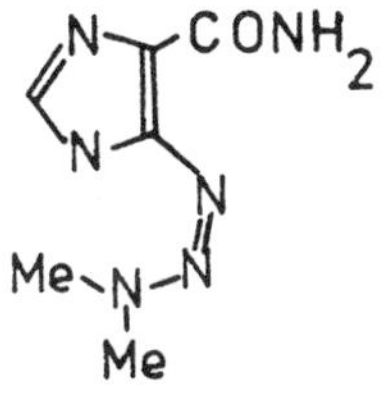

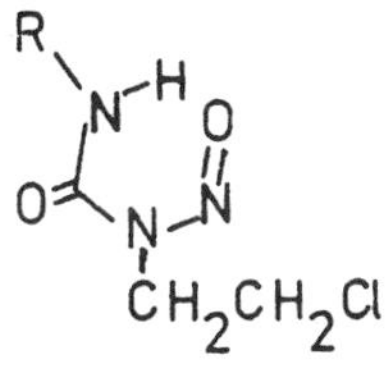

FIGURE 1. The structure of (1) DTIC, (2) CCRG 81010 and (3) RCNU, for example CCNU would be R=cyclohexyl

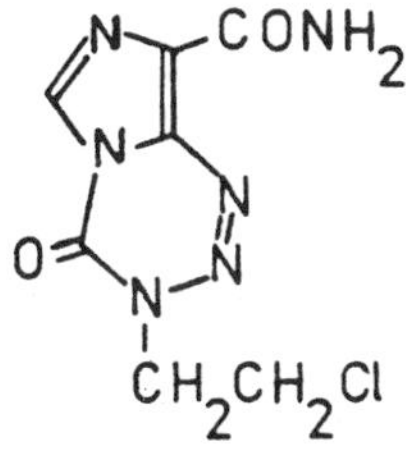

Chemical studies of certain imidazotetrazinones, of which CCRG 81010 is a member, had shown that it was possible, under relatively non-polar conditions, for this type of molecule to cleave and release diazoazoles and isocyanate moeities (2). Results of our studies on the mechanism of action of nitrosoureas had rather surprisingly suggested that the murine TLX5 lymphoma, but not the L1210 leukaemia, were sensitive to carbamoylating species released on nitrosourea breakdown (6) and CCRG 81010 at that stage was screened as a potential releaser of chloroethyl isocyanate. In fact no such cleavage takes place under physiological conditions (of polarity and pH) and, anyway, we

found CCRG 81010 to cure the L1210 leukaemia in vivo, a result not compatible
with the action of a carbamoylating agent. The mechanism of chemical cleavage
of CCRG 81010 under physiological conditions is shown in figure 2 (2) and from
this the clear similarities between CCRG 81010, the triazenes and nitrosoureas
are apparent: CCRG 81010 cleaves to generate the chloroethyltriazene MCTIC,
nucleophilic attack upon which leads to chloroethylation as is the case with
the nitrosoureas (7)

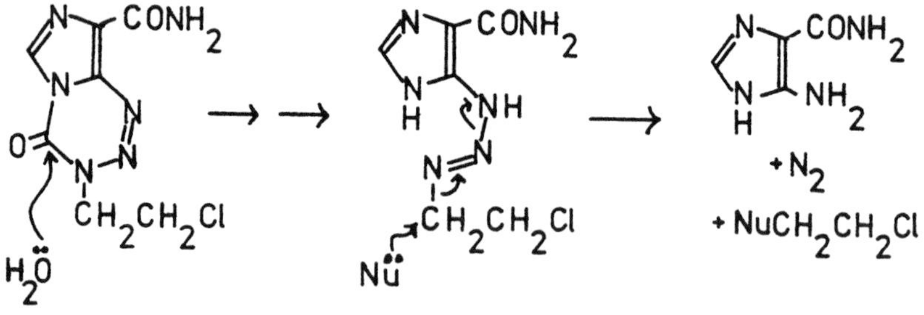

CCRG 81010   MCTIC

FIGURE 2. Decomposition of CCRG 81010 to MTIC and subsequent chloroethylation
of nucleophile

The results of the screening of CCRG 81010 against murine tumours in vivo
are shown in a standard summary form in table 1 where comparison is made with
the activity of a number of clinically useful agents. Clearly CCRG 81010
ranks with the best of these in the murine systems. In addition to curative
activity against the P388 and L1210 leukaemias and the colon 26 carcinoma
(disease free animals alive 60 days injection of 10^5 cells i.p. or s.c.) it
also cures the TLX5 lymphoma, the solid M5076 reticulum cell sarcoma, Lewis
Lung carcinoma, PC6A plasmacytoma and colon 38. Against the solid tumours the
therapeutic index is equivalent or better than that achieved with the
nitrosoureas and cyclophosphamide.

The experimental activity of CCRG 81010 is clearly superior to that of
the triazene DTIC (table 1) and (not shown) to the product of its
decomposition MCTIC (figure 2) - a highly unstable compound which had shown

TABLE 1. ACTIVITY* OF CCRG 81010 AND OTHER DRUGS IN THE NCI MUSE TUMOUR PANEL

Drug	L1210	P388	B16	LL	Colon 26	C38	CD8F$_1$
CCRG 81010	++	++	++	++	++	++	+
Nitrogen mustard	++	++	++	-	++	+	+
BCNU	++	++	++	++	++	+	++
DTIC	++	+	+	++	-	+	+
cis-Platinum	++	++	++	++	++	+	++
Cyclophosphamide	++	++	++	++	++	++	++
Methotrexate	++	++	-	+	-	-	+
Adriamycin	++	++	++	++	++	-	++

* NCI activity criteria (A. Goldin, J.M. Venditti, J.S. MacDonald,
F.M. Muggia, J.E. Henney and V.T. DeVita, Europ. J. Cancer, 1981,
17, 129-142.

- = inactive

activity against the L1210 leukaemia in an i.p. tumour/i.p. drug test (8). In
fact, CCRG 81010 is a remarkably stable molecule, with a chemical half life of
about 1h in human plasma. More importantly, it is acid stable, unlike the
triazenes (9) and so may be administered orally where, in an L1210 test, it
exhibited activity equivalent to that when it was given i.p. (3).

Cross resistance in the murine systems is perhaps as would be predicted
from the proposed pathway of decomposition (figure 2) given its similarities
to the nitrosoureas. Both the L1210 and TLX5 lymphomas made resistant to BCNU
showed complete cross resistance to CCRG 81010 and it was not cross resistant
with β-chloroethylamine type alkylating agents such as cyclophosphamide, using
the L1210 resistant line.

Cross resistant patterns of this type and its broad spectrum of activity
(table 1) indeed supported the idea that breakdown in vivo of CCRG 81010
occurred to give the chloroethyltriazene MCTIC, which in turn will react in a
similar manner as the nitrosoureas, as it contains an inherent
chloroethyldiazo species. However as stated as above, we found no chemical
evidence for the release of carbamoylating agent under physiological

conditions and biological studies which compare CCRG 81010 with BCNU clearly show them to be quite different in this respect. For example BCNU potently inhibits the activity of glutathione reductase, an enzyme supremely sensitive to carbamoylating agents, whereas CCRG 81010 had no effect (10).

Similarities to the nitrosoureas were seen in studies of DNA damage in L1210 cells treated for 2 hours with CNU, MCTIC or CCRG 81010. DNA-DNA cross-links were observed, under conditions of alkaline elution of the cellular DNA, which were equivalent in number for all three drugs at equitoxic concentrations. The rate of formation differed: a peak of crosslinking was reached in 6h with CNU whereas both MCTIC and CCRG appeared to alkylate more slowly with the peak of DNA-DNA crosslinks appearing at 9h (11).

The most enlightening and conclusive evidence for the mechanism of action of this potent new drug comes from studies of DNA damage induced in two human cell lines in vitro (12). These studies also provide for optimism regarding the potential clinical usefulness of CCRG 81010 (at present in phase 1 trial). CCRG 81010 was found to be 7 times more cytotoxic to the transformed VA13 cell line than than the 'normal' IMR 90 line, and in the VA13 line DNA-DNA crosslinks were observed which were proportional in number to cytotoxicity. In the IMR 90 line no DNA-DNA crosslinks were observed, even at high concentrations (2 log cell kill) although DNA-protein crosslinks were equivalent to those seen in VA13 cells, showing equivalence of drug-chromatin interaction. The sensitive VA13 line has been designated as Mer$^-$, and lacks the ability to repair methylation (and presumably other alkylations) at 0^6 of guanine. IMR90 cells are repair competent. It thus appears that 0^6 of guanine is the target for CCRG 81010. Presumably chloroethylation at this locus then "converts" to a crosslink by slow loss of chloride ion. The size of the differential toxicity between the two lines is higher than than seen for BCNU or CCNU, an encouraging result which may relate to the lack of carbamoylation inherent in CCRG 81010 and/or to what we at present believe might be structural features of the molecule which optimise reaction at 0^6 of guanine. The latter hypothesis is at present under investigation.

Acknowledgements. We thank the Cancer Research Campaign, SERC, May and Baker Ltd., Rhone Poulenc and the National Cancer Institute for resources, scientific or financial and for manpower. Especial acknowledgements should be made to our two ex-graduate students who were there at the beginning in 1981, Dr Robert Stone and Dr Neil Gibson.

References

1. Hickman, J.A., Gibson, N.W., Stone, R., Stevens, M.F.G., Lavelle, F. and Fizames, C. M & B 39565. A novel heterocycle with potent antitumour activity in mice. Proc. 13th Int. Cancer Congr. (UICC) p559, 1982.

2. Stevens, M.F.G., Hickman, J.A., Stone, R., Gibson, N.W., Baig, G.U., Lunt, E. and Newton, C.G. Antitumour imidazotetrazinones. 1. Synthesis and chemistry of 8-carbamoyl-3-(2-chloroethyl)imidazo [5,1-d]-1,2,3,5-tetrazin-4(3H)-one. J. Med. Chem. in press.

3. Hickman, J.A., Langdon, S.P., Gibson, N.W., Chubb, D., Stevens, M.F.G., Lavelle, F., Fizames, C. and Atassi, G. Experimental antitumour activity of M&B 39565, a potent and novel antitumour heterocycle. In preparation for Cancer Research.

4. Baig, G.U. and Stevens, M.F.G. Triazines and related products, Part 22. Synthesis and reactions of Imidazo[5,1-c][1,2,4]triazines. J. Chem. Soc. Perkin I, 1424-1432, 1982.

5. Gescher, A., Hickman, J.A., Simmonds, R.J., Stevens, M.F.G. and Vaughan, K. Studies of the mode of action of antitumour triazenes and triazines - II. Investigation of the selective toxicity of 1-aryl-3,3-dimethyltriazenes. Biochem. Pharmac. (30) 89-93 (1981).

6. Gibson, N.W. and Hickman, J.A. The role of isocyanates in the toxicity of antitumour nitrosoureas. Biochem. Pharmac. (31) 2795-2800, 1982.

7. Weinkam, R.J. and Lin, H.S. Reactions of 1,3-bis(2-chloroethyl)-3-cyclohexyl-1-nitrosourea in aqueous solution. J. Med. Chem. (22) 1193-1198, 1979.

8. Shealy, Y.F., O'Dell, C.A. and Krauth, C.A. 5-[(3-(2-chloroethyl)-1-triazenyl]imidazo-4-carboxamide and a possible mechanism of action of 5[3,3-bis(2-chloroethyl)-1-triazenyl]imidazo-4-carboxamide. J. Pharm. Sci. (64) 177-180, 1975.

9. Vaughan, K. and Stevens, M.F.G. Monoalkyltriazenes. Chem. Soc. Rev. 377-397, 1978.

10. Horgan, C.M.T., Stevens, M.F.G. and Tisdale, M.J. Preliminary investigations of the mode of action of CCRG 81010 (M & B 39565) Br. J. Cancer (48), 132, 1983.

11. Gibson, N.W., Erickson, L.C. and Hickman, J.A. Effects of the antitumour agent 8-carbamoyl-3-(2-chloroethyl)imidazo[5,1-d]-1,2,3,5-tetrazin-4(3H)-one on the DNA of mouse cells. Cancer Research, in press.

12. Gibson, N.W., Hickman, J.A. and Erickson, L.C. DNA cross-linking and cytotoxicity in normal and transformed human cells treated in vitro with 8-carbamoyl-3-(2-chloroethyl)imidazo[5,1-d]-1,2,3,5-tetrazin-4(3H)-one. Cancer Res. in press.

NEW PYRIMIDINE NUCLEOSIDES WITH POTENT ANTIVIRAL ACTIVITY

B. LEYLAND-JONES

Several years ago, the Organic Chemistry Laboratory of the Memorial
Sloan-Kettering Cancer Center embarked upon a program for the synthesis
of 2'-substituted arabinosyl-pyrimidine nucleosides as potential anticancer
and/or antiviral agents. Cytosine arabinoside, a potent antitumor drug,
also inhibits the multiplication of several DNA viruses in cell culture.
Therapeutic trials of cytosine arabinoside in herpes infections in animal
models were not encouraging because its therapeutic to toxic ratio approached
unity. Although arabinofuranosyluracil and some of its 5-alkylated derivatives
had been shown to exhibit anti-herpes virus activities, the more attractive
of these was arabinosylthymine which was active against HSV types I and II,
as well as against equinine herpes virus. It was therefore obvious that the
nature of the substituent at C-5 of the pyrimidine nucleoside was an important
factor in the determination of biological activity. Since activity was noted
for both the arabino- as well as for 2'-deoxyribo-pyrimidine nucleosides, the
C-2' substituent must also play a role. Fox and Watanabe therefore undertook
the synthesis of a series of 5-substituted-1-(2'deoxy-2'-fluoro- β-D-ara-
binofuranosyl) pyrimidines as potential antiviral agents.

Based upon Fox and Watanabe's past work, it was clear that the direct introduction of a halogeno function in the 2'-"up"(arabino) position would be
difficult if not impossible, because of the neighboring group participation
by the 2-carbonyl function of the pyrimidine moiety in any displacement
reactions. They therefore developed a 9-step synthesis of a suitably
protected 2'-deoxy-2'-fluoro-arabinofuranosylbromide, a key sugar intermediate, from readily available di-isopropylidene-α- d-allofuranose (1).
This synthesis was amenable to large-scale preparations. The syntheses
of various 5-substituted derivatives of 2'-fluoro-ara-C was achieved by
condensation of the key 2'-fluoro-arabinofuranosylbromide mentioned above
with appropriately substituted trimethylsilylated cytosines to afford

327

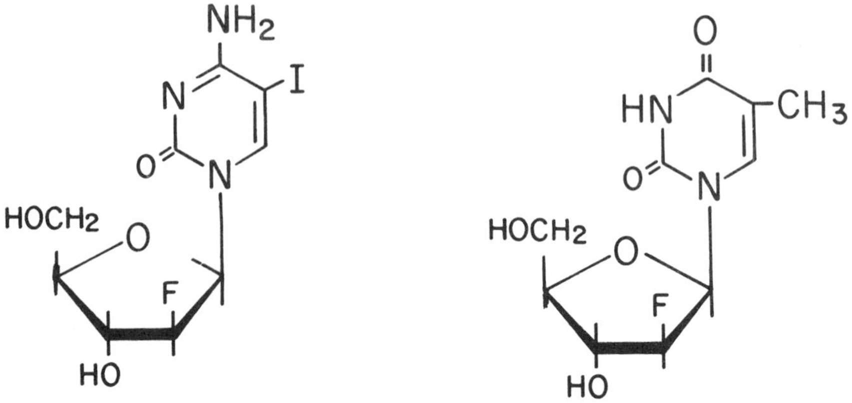

FIGURE 1

blocked nucleosides which were then deprotected with methanolic ammonia to nucleosides.

The most potent compound developed from the series was 2'-fluoro-5-iodo-ara C or FIAC (Fig. 1) (1). From tissue culture (in vitro) results, FIAC exhibited strong suppression of replication of herpes simplex I and II, herpes zoster and CMV (2). FIAC suppressed by 90% the replication of various strains of herpes simplex virus types I and II at concentrations of 0.0025 to 0.0125 μm. Cytotoxicity was minimal as determined by trypan blue dye exclusion with normal Vero, Wi-38, and NC-37 cell proliferation; the 50% inhibitory dose was 4 to 10 μm in a 4-day assay. When compared with other antiviral drugs, FIAC was active at much lower concentrations than arabinosylcytosine, iodo-deoxyuridine, and arabinosyladenine. It was slightly more active against herpes simplex virus type I than acyclovir and slightly more toxic to normal cells (2). FIAC's activity was further documented in in vivo models in mice and guinea pigs (1, 2). The mechanism of action of FIAC is similar to that of acyclovir utilizing the functional differences between pyrimidine nucleoside kinase enzymes of viral infected cells and those of normal cells. Following administration FIAC is selectively activated in vivo through phosphorylation by viral kinase enzymes to the active nucleotide FIAC-monophosphate (1,2).

Chou et al (3) have studied the metabolic disposition and fate of i.v. [2-^{14} C] FIAC in vivo in rats and mice. Their studies disclose that the major circulating nucleoside in mice is FIAU, the deaminated metabolite of FIAC. In rats, less than 10% of the administered FIAC is deaminated. FIAU is itself a potent antiherpes agent, although more cytotoxic than FIAC (1).

Our initial studies in immunosuppressed patients with severe herpes virus infections demonstrated that FIAC could be given at 400 mg/sq m/day for 7 days with minimal toxicity (4). Moreover, we observed prompt stabilization and improvement in cutanous VZV infections in all patients who received > 120 mg/sq m/day. Based upon these encouraging results, we initiated a double-blind randomized comparison of FIAC against Ara-A in 34 immunosuppressed patients with VZV infections. FIAC was administered intravenously 400 mg/sq m x 5 days on a 10 minute infusion b.i.d. schedule. Ara-A was infused 400 mg/sq m over 12 hours daily x 5 days.

The median time to the appearance of last new lesion (2 days) and the median time to first crusting of lesions (3 days) were shorter (P < .001) in patients who received FIAC relative to those who received Ara-A (5 and 7 days respectively). FIAC also reduced pain within 72 hours in a signif- icantly greater proportion of patients when compared to Ara-A (P=0.004). FIAC caused few toxic reactions (mild nausea and transient elevation in serum glutamyl oxaloacetic transaminase activity). FIAC proved therefore to be therapeutically superior to Ara-A for the treatment of varicella zoster infections in immunosuppressed patients.

More recent studies have been designed to define the metabolic fate of FIAC in man, and to define a suitable Phase II oral schedule. Single doses of [2-^{14}C]-FIAC, either 50 or 100 mg/sq m, were injected i.v. on day 1 in three patients with varicella zoster infections; 24 hours later the same dose was given p.o. Plasma and urine were taken during 24 hours after each dose and analyzed by high-pressure liquid chromatography (5). Recovery of radioactivity in urine in each 24-hr was, after i.v. injection 60-83% of dose; after p.o. 37-59%. Urine radioactivity in % of dose after i.v. injection consisted of 11-13% of unchanged drug, 30-56% of 2'-fluoro-5-iodo-1-β-D-arabinosyluracil (FIAU) 7-8% of 2'-fluoro-1-β-D-arabinosyl- uracil, 0.2-0.5% of 2'-fluoro-5-iodo-1-β-D-arabinosylcytosine, and misc., 7-10%. These substances were present in urine after p.o. doses though conspicuously less FIAU was found. They were also in plasma shortly after giving [2-^{14}C] FIAC. Deamination to FIAU was rapid: by 10 min. after i.v. injection 45-86% of plasma radioactivity consisted of FIAU while FIAC accounted for only 5-10%. By 8 hr FIAU was ca. 50% of plasma radioactivity and FIAC was <2%. Since FIAU is nearly as potent against herpes as is FIAC, it is significant that, as late as 12 hr. after i.v. and p.o. doses, plasma concentrations of FIAU exceeded those inhibiting HSV-1 replication in vitro by 90%. These studies suggest that FIAC should also show significant antiviral activity in man by both intravenous and oral routes at lower doses than those reported in the current clinical trials.

FMAU, 2'-fluoro-5-methyl-ara-uracil, (Fig 1) is of clinical interest both as an antileukemic and as an antiviral drug. FMAU is highly active in vitro and in vivo against P815 and L1210 cell lines resistant to cytosine arabinoside (Ara-C). In mice inoculated intracerebrally with Herpes Simplex Virus Type II, FMAU is one hundred-fold more potent than adenine arabinoside (Ara -A) cyclovir (AVC), or 2'-fluoro-5-iodo-1-β-D-arabinoside (FIAC). We conducted a Phase I trial of FMAU in patients with advanced cancer. The dose levels studied were 2,4,8,16,32,64, and 128 mg/sq m/day IV for 5 days. Dose-limiting toxicity occurred at 32 mg/sq m and consisted of transient, mild encephalopathy. Severe encephalopathy with extrapyramidal dysfunction occurred at 64 and 128 mg/sq m and contributed to two deaths. No toxicity was observed below 32 mg/sq m. Because of its potent antileukemic and antiviral activity, future trials of low doses of FMAU in patients with Ara-C resistant leukemia and in immunosuppressed patients with viral infections are under consideration.

1. Fox JJ, Lopez C, Watanabe KA: 2-Fluoro-arabinosyl pyrimidine nucleosides: chemistry, antiviral, and potential anticancer activities. In: Vega S (ed) Medicinal chemistry advances, 1981, pp 27-40.

2. Lopez C, Watanabe KA, Fox JJ: 2-Fluoro-5-iodo-araacytosine, a potent and selective anti-herpes virus agent. Antimicrob Agents Chemotherap. (17): 803-806, 1980.

3. Chou TC, Feinberg A, Grant AJ, Vidal P, Reichman W, Watanabe KA, Fox JJ, and Philips FS: Pharmacologic disposition and metabolic fate of 2'-fluoro-5-iodo-1- β -D-arabinofuranosylcytosine in mice and rats. Cancer Res (41): 3336-3342, 1981.

4. Young CW, Schneider R, Leyland-Jones B, Armstrong D, Tan CTC, Lopez C, Watanabe KA, Fox JJ, Philips FS: Phase I evalution of 2'fluoro-5-iodo-1-β-D-arabinofuranosylcytosine in immunosuppressed patients with herpes virus infection. Cancer Res (43): 5006-5009, 1983.

5. Leyland-Jones B, Feinberg A, Vidal P, Fanucchi M, Williams L, Young C, Fox J, Philips F: Human metabolism of 2'fluoro-5-iodo-1-β -D-arabino-sylcytosine (FIAC). Proceedings of the Amer. Assoc. for Cancer Res. (24): 136, 1983.

LIPOPHILIC INHIBITORS OF DIHYDROFOLATE REDUCTASE

CHARLES A. NICHOL, CARL W. SIGEL, and DAVID S. DUCH

1. INTRODUCTION

The evaluation of lipophilic inhibitors of dihydrofolate reductase (DHFR) as anticancer agents is a continuing effort because of the development of clinical resistance to methotrexate (MTX) and its limited spectrum of activity. The temperature-sensitive entry of MTX into cells is carrier-dependent and, in some tumors, MTX uptake is so slow that the cells are unresponsive to this drug. The very rapid temperature-insensitive passage of lipophilic DHFR inhibitors across cell membranes accounts for their activity against MTX-resistant cells and for their better entry into various tissues including brain. Among the many heterocyclic DHFR inhibitors which were synthesized as potential antibacterial and antiparasitic agents, some were too potent as inhibitors of mammalian DHFR and were tested as anticancer agents (1,2). Extensive studies of diaminopyrimidines, such as metoprine (DDMP), and diaminotriazines, such as triazinate (Baker's antifol), indicated some useful features but limited efficacy at tolerated doses and unsuitable pharmacokinetics led to the search for other compounds (2). Subsequently, several diaminopyridopyrimidines and diaminoquinazolines were found to be as potent as MTX as inhibitors of DHFR and cell growth and, like MTX, their toxic effects can be prevented by calcium leucovorin (2-4). Since these lipophilic DHFR inhibitors cannot form polyglutamates, comparison of their properties with those of MTX is of particular interest in view of the likelihood that the formation of MTX-polyglutamates may contribute to the cytotoxicity and hepatotoxicity of MTX (5,6). Currently, BW301U, 2,4-diamino-6-(2,5-dimethoxybenzyl)-5-methylpyrido[2,3-d]pyrimidine, has been selected for clinical evaluation. Before reviewing the properties of BW301U, it is in keeping with the theme of this conference on "Selective Drug

Development" to discuss aspects of our studies indicating that it is feasible and practical to explore biochemical reactions which might underline adverse effects.

2. METHOTREXATE: A PUTATIVE INHIBITOR OF NEUROTRANSMITTER SYNTHESIS

The unconjugated pterin, tetrahydrobiopterin (BH$_4$), is the cofactor for tyrosine and tryptophan hydroxylases and interference with the biosynthesis of this cofactor could impair synthesis of the neuro-transmitters, dopamine and serotonin. Several reports have indicated that the reduction of 7,8-dihydrobiopterin by DHFR is the final step in the biosynthesis of BH$_4$. Evidence that 7,8-dihydrobiopterin is converted to BH$_4$ by DHFR (7) and that DHFR is present in brain (8,9) led to the suggestion that some of the adverse CNS effects of MTX could be due to interference with neurotransmitter synthesis (9). Such a prospect deserved closer examination since lipophilic DHFR inhibitors might have a greater effect than MTX because of their entry into the CNS. Upon examination of neuroblastoma N115 cells growing in medium supplemented with thymidine and hypoxanthine, we found that a normal rate of BH$_4$ biosynthesis continued in the presence of sufficient MTX to completely inhibit DHFR (10). Also, there was no decrease in the BH$_4$ content of tissues (adrenal, pineal, pituitary or brain) from rats which received MTX (10 mg/kg i.p. for 4 days) along with leucovorin. Metoprine also had no effect on the BH$_4$ content of brain (10). The biosynthesis of BH$_4$ from GTP in cell-free preparations of bovine adrenal medulla proceeds by a DHFR-independent pathway (11). The conflicting reports on BH$_4$ biosynthesis can be resolved by recognition of two pathways: (i) a DHFR-dependent pterin salvage pathway and (ii) the de novo biosynthesis of BH$_4$ from GTP which is not impaired by DHFR inhibitors (11,12). Consequently, interference with the biosyn-thesis of dopamine and serotonin by DHFR inhibitors appears to be unlikely. Since very high concentrations of MTX can inhibit dihydro-pteridine reductase in vitro (13), it would be prudent to examine new DHFR inhibitors for any action on this enzyme.

3. INHIBITION OF HISTAMINE DISPOSITION BY LIPOPHILIC DHFR INHIBITORS

Heterocyclic compounds of diverse structure can interfere with the disposition of histamine by inhibiting histamine-N-methyltransferase

(HMT) (14,15). Some DHFR inhibitors were found to have higher affinity for HMT than the substrate, histamine (Km, 9.5×10^{-6} M) and several also inhibited diamine oxidase (histaminase) (15,16). MTX has essentially no effect on histamine metabolism, whereas the Ki's of metoprine and triazinate for HMT are 1×10^{-7} M and 6×10^{-7} M, respectively. Among quinazoline compounds, methasquin inhibited both HMT and diamine oxidase, and one of the most potent inhibitors of HMT was a trimethoxybenzylaminoquinazoline (TMQ, JB-11) (16). Methylation is the main means of disposition of histamine in brain and a single dose of either metoprine or TMQ (10 mg/kg i.p.) elevated histamine levels in rat brain (15,16). DHFR inhibitors which also inhibit HMT clearly lack desired selectivity. Since HMT inhibition was not corre-lated with DHFR inhibition, it was feasible to select compounds with the least effect on histamine metabolism. Subsequently, a large number of potent DHFR inhibitors were examined as inhibitors of HMT and diamine oxidase *in vitro*, and for their effects on histamine levels *in vivo* (16). This exclusion process led to the selection of a series of diaminopyridopyrimidines among which BW301U was eventually selected for clinical evaluation. Although some of the adverse effects of triazinate and metoprine might be related to effects on histamine metabolism, no direct measurement of changes in histamine levels in cells or body fluids were made during Phase I/II clinical studies. Consequently, the extent to which elevation of histamine levels in patients may be related to any limiting adverse reactions remains to be determined and it seems reasonable to monitor this in future studies.

4. BIOLOGICAL PROPERTIES OF THE DIAMINOPYRIDOPYRIMIDINE, BW301U

This compound is as potent as MTX as an inhibitor of DHFR *in vitro* and as an inhibitor of the growth of cells in culture (17). Its toxicity *in vivo* is prevented by calcium leucovorin (folinic acid) but BW301U differs from MTX in that both leucovorin and thymidine are required to prevent its cytotoxicity in Sarcoma 180 cell cultures (3). In contrast to MTX, entry of BW301U into cells is rapid and is temperature-inde-pendent, indicating passage across cell membranes by diffusion. Also, there is no competition between BW301U and leucovorin for uptake into cells indicating that cell entry would not be altered by transport changes associated with resistance to MTX. Indeed, BW301U is highly active against a Walker 256 carcinosarcoma which is refractory to MTX (3). It is anticipated that BW301U will behave like metoprine which is active against a MTX-refractory murine tumor (M5076) and the occurrence of collateral sensitivity to metoprine in MTX-resistant cells deserves further study (18). There is a good rationale for combinations of MTX with lipophilic DHFR inhibitors to minimize the emergence of resistant cells or to suppress the growth of heterogenous cell populations now recognized in solid tumors (19-21).

The very slow clearance of metoprine ($T\frac{1}{2}$ of 8 to 14 days) in patients presented real problems in dose scheduling (22). The pharmacokinetic profile of BW301U in rats and dogs is quite different from that of metoprine and is similar to that of MTX (23). In the initial Phase I/II studies of BW301U in cancer patients with normal hepatic and renal functions, the plasma half-life ranged from 2.3 to 9 hours following i.v. infusion (24). Our laboratory studies have focused on the selection of an agent with favorable properties regarding pharmacokinetic profile, increased tissue penetration and minimal side-effects which hopefully provide some basis for selectivity and efficacy.

REFERENCES

1. Hitchings GH (ed): Inhibition of folate metabolism in chemotherapy. Vol. 64, Handbook of Experimental Pharmacology, Springer-Verlag, New York, 1983.
2. McCormack JJ: Dihydrofolate reductase inhibitors as potential drugs. Medicinal Reviews (1): 303-331, 1981.
3. Duch DS, Edelstein MP, Bowers SW, Nichol CA: Biochemical and chemotherapeutic studies on 2,4-diamino-6-(2,5-dimethoxybenzyl)-5-methylpyrido[2,3-d]pyrimidine (BW301U), a novel lipid-soluble inhibitor of dihydrofolate reductase. Cancer Res. (42): 3987-3994, 1982.
4. Bertino, JR: Toward improved selectivity in cancer chemotherapy. Cancer Res. (39): 293-304, 1979.
5. Galivan J: Evidence for the cytotoxic activity of polyglutamate derivatives of methotrexate. Mol. Pharmacol. (17): 105-110, 1980.
6. Ashton RE, Millward-Sadler GH, White JE: Complications in methotrexate treatment of psoriasis with particular reference to liver fibrosis. J. Investig. Dermatol. (79): 229-232, 1982.
7. Kaufman S: Metabolism of the phenylalanine hydroxylation cofactor. J. Biol. Chem. (242): 3934-3943, 1967.
8. Duch DS, Bigner DD, Bowers SW, Nichol CA: Dihydrofolate reductase in primary brain tumors, cell cultures of central nervous system origin and normal brain during fetal and neonatal growth. Cancer Res. (39): 487-491, 1979.

9. Abelson HT: Methotrexate and central nervous system toxicity. Cancer Treat. Rep. (62): 1999-2001, 1978.
10. Duch DS, Lee CL, Edelstein MP, Nichol CA: Biosynthesis of tetra-hydrobiopterin in the presence of dihydrofolate reductase inhibitors. Mol. Pharmacol. (24): 103-108, 1983.
11. Nichol CA, Lee CL, Edelstein MP, Chao JY, Duch DS: Biosynthesis of tetrahydrobiopterin by de novo and salvage pathways in adrenal medulla extracts, mammalian cell cultures and rat brain in vivo. Proc. Natl. Acad. Sci. U.S.A. (80): 1546-1550, 1983.
12. Nichol CA, Viveros OH, Duch DS, Abou-Donia MM, Smith GK: Metabolism of pteridine cofactors in neurochemistry. In: Blair JA (ed) Chemistry and biology of pteridines. Walter de Gruyter & Co., New York, 1983, p 131-151.
13. Craine JE, Hall ES, Kaufman S: The isolation and characterization of dihydropteridine reductase from sheep liver. J. Biol. Chem. (247): 6082-6091, 1972.
14. Cohn VH: Inhibition of histamine methylation by antimalarial drugs. Biochem. Pharmacol. (14): 1686-1688, 1965.
15. Duch DS, Bowers SW, Nichol CA: Elevation of brain histamine levels by diaminopyrimidine inhibitors of histamine N-methyl transferase. Biochem. Pharmacol. (27): 1507-1509, 1978.
16. Duch DS, Edelstein MP, Nichol CA: Inhibition of histamine metabo-lizing enzymes and elevation of histamine levels in tissues by lipid-soluble anticancer folate antagonists. Mol. Pharmacol. (18): 100-104, 1980.
17. Grivsky EM, Lee S, Sigel CW, Duch DS, Nichol CA: Synthesis and antitumor activity of 2,4-diamino-6-(2,5-dimethoxybenzyl)-5-methylpyrido[2,3-d]pyrimidine. J. Med. Chem. (23): 327-329, 1980.
18. Sirotnak FM, Moccio DM, Goutas LJ, Kelleher LE, Montgomery JA: Biochemical correlates of responsiveness and collateral sensitivity of some methotrexate-resistant murine tumors to the lipophilic antifolate, metoprine. Cancer Res. (42): 924-928, 1982.
19. Sedwick WD, Kutler M, Frazer T, Brown OE, Laszlo J: New dose-time relationships of folate antagonists to sustain inhibition of human lymphoblasts and leukemic cells in vitro. Cancer Res. (39): 3612-3618, 1979.
20. Hamrell M, Laszlo J, Brown OE, Sedwick WD: Toxicity of methotrexate and metoprine in a dihydrofolate reductase gene-amplified mouse cell line. Mol. Pharmacol. (20): 637-643, 1981.
21. Goldie JH, Goldman AJ, Gudanskas GA: Rationale for the use of alternating non-cross-resistant chemotherapy. Cancer Treat. Rep. (66): 439-449, 1982.
22. Cavallito JC, Nichol CA, Brenckman WD, DeAngelis RL, Stickney DR, Simmons WS, Sigel CW: Lipid-soluble inhibitors of dihydrofolate reductase. I. kinetics, tissue distribution, and extent of metabolism of pyrimethamine, metoprine and etoprine in the rat, dog, and man. Drug Metab. Dispos. (6): 329-337, 1978.
23. Duch DS, Sigel CW, Bowers SW, Edelstein MP, Cavallito JC, Foss RG, Nichol CA: Lipid-soluble inhibitors of dihydrofolate reductase: selection and evaluation of the 2,4-diaminopyridopyrimidine BW301U and related compounds as anticancer agents. In: Nelson JD, Grassi C (eds) Current Chemotherapy and Infectious Diseases. American Society for Microbiology, Washington, D.C., 1980, p 1597-1599.
24. Blum MR, Sigel CW, Williams TE: unpublished data.

REVIEW OF PHASE I-II CLINICAL TRIALS WITH VINZOLIDINE (VZL), A NEW ORALLY ACTIVE SEMISYNTHETIC VINBLASTINE DERIVATIVE

R.L. NELSON

INTRODUCTION

Vinzolidine is a semisynthetic oxazolidinedione derivative of vinblastine (Figure 1). It was chosen for clinical development because of marked oncolytic activity against a wide spectrum of transplanted murine tumors when administered either orally or parenterally. In adult rhesus monkeys the absolute oral bioavailability of VZL was found to be about 20% in a PO/IV crossover study, compared to 9% for vinblastine; terminal half lives in this study were 22.8 hr and 9.6 hr for VZL and vinblastine respectively.

The single dose LD_{50} for VZL in rats was 104 mg/m^2 (PO) and 28 mg/m^2 (IV), the ratio corresponding well with the rhesus monkey bioavailability study. When administered orally on a weekly or twice weekly basis to rodents and dogs, VZL caused moderate reversible myelosuppression which proved to be the dose limiting toxicity, with no evidence of neuropathy. The lowest toxic dose (TDL) was 6 mg/m^2 orally twice weekly in the Beagle dog.

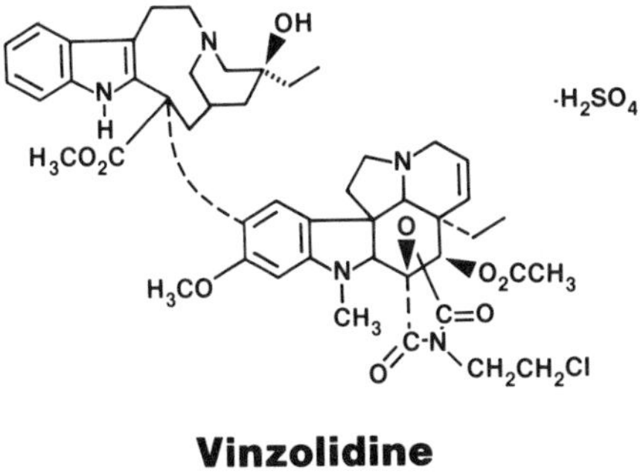

Vinzolidine

Figure 1. Chemical structure of vinzolidine (M.W. = 982.6)

PHASE I STUDIES

VZL has been given to 61 patients in 3 phase I studies, each of which investigated a different dosage schedule. The initial phase I clinical trial employed a once weekly dosage regimen based on previous experience with other vinca alkaloids using this schedule, the elimination half life of about 24 hr in the monkey, and the absence of cumulative toxicity in rodents and dogs with twice weekly dosing. The initial dose given was 0.6 mg/m^2 orally, with escalations permitted every 2nd - 3rd dose. As the study progressed evidence of cumulative marrow depression was observed, as well as a very prolonged terminal serum half life of 101 hr (49-164 hr) which led to abandoning this schedule. Oral doses of 15-25 mg/m^2 were tolerated by most patients, who eventually developed mild to moderate stable leukopenia and slowly progressive peripheral neuropathy which proved to be completely reversible when dosing was stopped.

In a second phase I study VZL was given as a single oral dose every 2 wks, and was found to be very well tolerated at doses of 30-35 mg/m^2. Toxicity consisted of readily reversible granulocytopenia (nadir day 7-11, recovery day 12-15), mild reversible peripheral neuropathy, mild nausea/vomiting, moderate diarrhea, moderate lassitude, transient eosinophilia, and occasional mild alopecia. In a third phase I study VZL was administered orally on a 5 day schedule in which the day 1 dose was 6 times the day 2-5 dose, with a cycle time of 3 wks. This regimen, based on pharmacokinetic considerations, represented an attempt to simulate a constant infusion schedule and maintain body stores of drug at steady state levels for 5-7 days. Side effects were identical to those seen on the 2 wk schedule. The tolerated dose was 45 mg/m^2 total dose per 3 wk cycle.

It is noteworthy that in all three phase I studies wide variation was noted among patients in that specific dose which, in a given patient, resulted in clinically tolerable moderate leukopenia. This variability was not observed within a given patient upon repeated dosing at the same dose. When administered orally on a chronic basis, the between patient variability appears to be much greater than the within patient variability for VZL dose.

PHASE II STUDIES

Phase II studies are in progress at 6 centers, with 8 investigators employing 3 dose regimens. As of September 7, 1983 a total of 227 patients had been treated with VZL on 16 study protocols. Target diseases included leukemia, Hodgkin's and non-Hodgkin's lymphoma, multiple myeloma, lung, breast, colorectal, and pancreas carcinomas, AIDS-associated Kaposi's sarcoma, and certain cancers individually selected by the human tumor stem cell assay.

An analysis of therapeutic response by disease category for all patients is presented in Table 1. To be considered evaluable for response all patients had to have either measurable or evaluable disease. Phase I patients must have received at least 2 cycles of treatment at a dose of VZL causing any degree of myelosuppression. Phase II patients must have received 2 or

Table 1. Analysis of response to treatment by tumor type

		Evaluation Status			Major Response Status	
	Total	Too Early	Inevaluable	Evaluated	Responders	Failures
Diagnosis						
Leukemia	6	0	1	5	0	5
Hodgkin's	18	2	0	16	8 (50%)	8
Non-Hodgkin's	43	10	3	30	7 (23%)	23
Mycosis Fungoides	5	0	0	5	1 (20%)	4
Multiple Myeloma	5	2	0	3	0	3
Non-Small Cell Lung	47	7	13	27	4 (15%)	23
Colon	23	9	6	8	0	8
Breast	20	4	6	10	1 (10%)	9
Prostate	6	0	6	0	0	0
Kidney	9	3	6	0	0	0
Kaposi Sarcoma	12	3	3	6	1 (17%)	5
Other Sarcoma	6	0	2	4	0	4
Ovary	6	3	2	1	1 (100%)	0
Miscellaneous	21	4	7	10	0	10
Totals	227	47	55	125	23	102

Analysis Date: September 7, 1983

more cycles of treatment as specified in the treatment protocol, regardless of whether or not any toxicity was observed. Only objective complete and partial remissions of 4 wk or greater duration were considered responders; minor responses and stable disease patients were included in the failure category.

Although no complete remissions have been achieved, very encouraging activity of VZL has been documented by four investigators in patients with heavily pretreated Hodgkin's disease (8/16 responders; median duration 9+ wks). VZL also appears to have clinically meaningful activity in all types of non-Hodgkin's lymphomas, with an overall response rate of 20-25% in heavily pretreated patients. Three complete remissions have been seen (lymphocytic lymphoma = 14 wks; histiocytic lymphoma = 51+ wks; mycosis fungoides = 28 wks). There is some suggestion of activity in patients with previously untreated non-small cell lung cancer. Isolated responses have been reported in patients with breast and ovarian carcinoma, and Kaposi's sarcoma.

Table 2. Summary of patient study status and reasons for exit from study

---

Of 227 Patients Treated on Study to Date:
  66 Remain on Study
    47 are too early for efficacy evaluation
    13 are responders who remain on study because of continued benefit
    6 are in a stable or minor response status and remain on study
  161 Are Off Study
    29 Died While on Study
        22 from cancer progression
        5 from drug-related toxicity
        2 from complications not related to study drug or cancer
    132 Exited from Study Alive
        110 because of cancer progression
        8 because of patient request
        7 because of intolerable drug-related toxicity
        2 at the discretion of the investigator
        1 because lost to follow-up
        4 because of other reason not related to study drug toxicity

---

Analysis Date: September 7, 1983

With expansion of the VZL trials into phase II, the large variability in the tolerated dose among patients noted in the three phase I studies was accentuated. Five VZL-related deaths from granulocytopenic sepsis have occurred (see Table 2). This has prompted cessation of new patient accrual on all VZL studies until further clinical pharmacology investigations with intra-venously administered VZL have resolved the reasons for the large interpatient variability in sensitivity to a given dose. Possible mechanisms for this variability include variations in oral absorption, metabolism, disposition kinetics, intrinsic marrow sensitivity, or a combination of two or more of these factors.

CONCLUSIONS

VZL has demonstrated marked clinically meaningful antitumor activity when given orally to patients with heavily pretreated lymphomas of all types. There is a suggestion of useful activity in patients with previously untreated non-small cell lung cancer. However VZL has unpredictable marrow toxicity when administered orally and has been related to five deaths from granulocytopenic sepsis. The major dose limiting toxicity of VZL is schedule-dependent myelosuppression consisting of readily reversible granulocytopenia. The between patient variability is much greater than the within patient variability in sensitivity to a given dose when VZL is given orally with repeated administration every 2-3 wks. There is no evidence of cumulative bone marrow toxicity with an every 2 week or every 3 week schedule. Other side effects, including peripheral neuropathy, nausea/vomiting, diarrhea, lassitude, and alopecia are generally mild and clinically manageable. Early pharmacokinetic studies show an exceptionally long elimination half life with variability among patients which may be related to variability in sensitivity to a given dose. Studies employing radiolabeled VZL administered intravenously are planned which may reveal the mechanism for the interpatient variability in toxicity seen with oral administration of this drug.

NEW DEVELOPMENTS IN ANTHRACYCLINES

A. DI MARCO, A.M. CASAZZA, T. FACCHINETTI

The cytotoxic effect of Anthracyclines (Anthr) may be related to different parameters: a) affinity to DNA as expressed by the values of K_{app}, b) cellular uptake, which can be related to partition coefficient lipids/ water, c) interactions with cell membrane. On the basis of wide experimental evidence, it is generally accepted that DNA, present as nucleoproteins in chromatin, is the last target of Anthr in the cell (1). However, in spite of the same inhibitory effect on DNA and RNA polymerases, the ability to inhibit cellular proliferation changes dramatically as observed for doxorubicin (DX) and some of its analogues, indicating that the increase in potency could be related to the increased ability in crossing the cell membrane. It has been demonstrated that Anthr uptake into the cell occurs by passive diffusion, while it has been suggested that the efflux in nucleated cells is carrier mediated (2). It is pertinent to note that,while it is possible to interfere with the expression of acquired resistance to daunorubicin (DNR) by structural analogs through an interference with the extrusion mechanism, (3) only some compounds are able to interfere with the expression of the resistance to DX. This may indicate that the pump, which is supposed to operate in the efflux of Anthr from the cell , does not operate in the same way for DNR and DX or their analogs.

The cell membrane is necessarily involved in the uptake of these drugs and can be irreversibly damaged by pure contact reaction, as indicated in rat hepatocytes using DX-polyglutaraldehyde complex, which does not penetrate the cell, but still possesses cytotoxic activity comparable to that of the free drug (4). This can be related to a perturbation of the membrane

345

structure, direct or mediated through the stimulation of superoxide radicals formation by the drug, as documented for liver microsomes, mitochondria, nuclei (5).

Alteration of the membrane phospholipids (PHL) leads to an impairment of enzymatic activity of PHL dependent enzymes present at membrane level, such as PHL dependent adenyl-cyclase. Anthr cell membrane interactions could also involve the glycocalix membrane component, which is known to modulate cell permeability to the drug and cell ion transport.

It is commonly accepted that DNR and DX effects are more consistant in cells that are in S phase. Further studies suggested an effect of the drug on earlier cellular events. In fact an increase in the fast phase of the 45 Ca^{2+} influx and a reduced rate of the slow phase of the efflux of Ca^{2+} with a consequent increase in total exchangeable calcium pool was observed in HeLa cells in the presence of DX (6). Also a later increase in intracellular Na^{+} was observed in HeLa cells (6).

It is known that chromatin must be modified in order to be duplicated or transcribed, and it has been proposed that the specific repression of gene expression is determined by hystones, by the sequence of DNA, and by the ionic environment. A possible link between Anthr effects on cell membrane and nucleic acids could be found in the Anthr induced ions transport changes. Recently it has been reported that reinitiation of DNA synthesis induced by serum in chick embryo fibroblasts is preceeded by an earlier peak in ions fluxes (Na^{+}, Rb^{+}) and phosphorylation of chromosomal proteins (7) which in turn are supposed to promote the dissociation of histones from DNA.

This should increase the probability of Anthr to intercalate the available regions of DNA. In fact the K_{app} of Anthr for chromatin is considerably reduced compared to that for isolated DNA (8).

Alteration of the ion transport system in differentiated cells, such as myocardial cells, can damage their specialized structures in a highly selective manner. A kinetic analysis of Ca^{2+} flux in cultures of spontaneously beating myoblasts showed that DX is able to suppress the early phase of exchangeable Ca^{2+} pool (9), which is an expression of the ion transport through the glycocalix, and increases the rate constant and the Ca^{2+} efflux during the two phases of slow exchange, which represent the intracellular calcium pool The same effect was confirmed in different experimental systems by Villani et al. (10). This is in agreement with the observation that DX, at very low concentration, specifically inhibits the Na^+/Ca^{2+} exchange system of heart .sarcolemma; while the $Ca^{2+} - Mg^{2+}$ dependent ATPase is not affected (11). These observations explain the reduced ability of Ca^{2+} to travel between heart sarcoplasma and medium. Alterations in cellular Ca^{2+} content and kinetics can involve systems regulating ion flux and metabolic effects. It has been demonstrated that DX exerts an inhibitory effect on the phosphorylation of cytosolic proteins in the heart, which can be competitively reversed by phosphorylserine (PHS), cardiolipin and calmodulin (CMD) (12). DX by itself has little or no effect on the basal phosphorylation seen in the absence of Ca^{2+}, PHS, or CMD: similarly the cAMP or cGMP dependent phosphokinase is not inhibited (12). To what extent the inhibition of the two phosphorylation systems may be important for a selective toxicity for different cells and tissues and particularly for the cardiomyopathy is presently unclear.

The *in vitro* effects of Anthr on ions transport mechanisms are strongly affected by the stereochemistry of the carbohydrate moiety: modifications at the 4'position result in a increased cytotoxicity and potency concomitant with an increase in lipids solubility and a decrease in effects on ions transport and in cardiotoxicity (13).Further experimental studies suggest a correlation between ability to alter Ca^{2+} exchange and cardiotoxicity of Anthr in animals: epirubicin (11, 13) and esorubicin (13), which are less cardiotoxic than DX,have less effect on Na^{+}/Ca^{2+} exchange in dog heart sarcolemma, while inhibition of DNA and RNA synthesis in mice hearts is similar to that observed for DX. These studies show that an effect of DNR and DX on ionic exchanges is present in HeLa cells as well as in embryonic myocardial cells. However, while in the tumor cells, cell death is a relatively late event, compared to the early damage to the mechanism of ions transport, in the higly differentiated systems the lesion of the regulating mechanism immediately results in the loss of contractile functions. To what extent this is connected with chronic cardiotoxicity is not clear; it can be assumed that the initial lesion at the level of the cellular membrane results in alternations of mitochondrial and myofibral structures and functions leading to irreversible damage.

References

1. Di Marco A, Arcamone F, Zunino F.: Daunomycin, adriamycin and structural analogs: biological activity and mechanism of action. In: Corcoran J W

and Hahn FE (ed) Antibiotics vol 3. Springer Verlag Inc. 1975.

2. Danø K : Acquired cellular resistance to Anthracycline in experimental systems: a review. In: Hansen H H (ed) Anthracyclines and Cancer Therapy. Excerpta Medica, Amsterdam, 1983, pp 26-38.

3. Danø K: Personal communication.

4. Rogers K and Tökes Z: Synthesis of Adriamycin-coupled polyglutaraldehyde microspheres and evaluation of their cytostatic activity. Proc. Natl. Acad. Sci. USA 79 (6): 2026-2030, 1982.

5. Myers C E: The role of free radical damage in the genesis of Doxorubicin cardiac toxicity. In: Muggia F M, Young C W, Carter S K (ed) Anthracycline antibiotics in Cancer Therapy. M. Nijhoff Publ., 1982, pp 295-297.

6. Dasdia T, Di Marco A, Goffredi M, Minghetti A, and Necco A: Ion level and Calcium Fluxes in HeLa cells after Adriamycin treatment. Pharm. Res. Comm. (11) 1, 19-29, 1979.

7. Pouyssegur J, Chambard J C, Franchi A, Paris S, Van Obberghen-Schilling E: Growth factor activation of an amyloride-sensitive Na^+/H^+ Exchange system in quiescent fibroblast: Coupling to ribosomal protein S6 phosphorylation. Proc. Natl. Acad. Sci. USA (79) 13: 3935-3939, 1982.

8. Zunino F, Di Marco A, Zaccara A, and Gambetta R A: The interaction of DNR and DX with DNA and chromatin. Biochim, Biophys.Acta(607): 206-214, 1980

9. Dasdia T, Di Marco A, Minghetti A, and Necco A: Effect of DX on Calcium exchange of cultured heart cells. Pharm. Res. Comm. (11) 10: 881-889, 1979.

10. Villani F, Favalli L and Piccinini F: Relationship between the effect on Ca^{2+}turnover and early cardiotoxicity of DX and 4' epi-DX in guinea pig heart muscle. Tumori (66): 689-697, 1980.

11. Caroni P, Villani F, Carafoli E: The cardiotoxic antibiotic DX inhibits the Na^+/Ca^{2+} exchange of dog heart sarcolemmal vescicles. Febbs. Let. (130) 2: 184-186, 1981.

12. Katoh N, Wise B C, Wrenn R W, and Kuo J F: Inhibition by Adriamycin of calmoduline sensitive and phospholipid sensitive calcium dependent phosphorylation of endogenous proteins from heart. Bioch. J. (198):199-205 (1981).

13. Casazza AM, Di Marco A, Bonadonna G, Bonfante V, Bertazzoli G, Bellini O, Pratesi G, Solcia L, Ballerini L.: Anthracyclines: Current Status and New Developments. In: Crooke, Reich (ed) Acad. Press N.Y, 1980, pp 403-430.

NITROSOUREAS-STILL A CHALLENGE FOR DEVELOPMENTAL CANCER CHEMOTHERAPY

GERHARD EISENBRAND

1. INTRODUCTION

Although 2-chloroethyl-N-nitrosoureas (CNU's) are highly active antineoplastic agents with a broad antitumour spectrum in experimental systems, in the clinic their usefulness is limited. The most important limiting factor in CNU therapy is their delayed and cumulative myelotoxicity. Much effort has been spent therefore to develop analogues with more favorable properties.

First generation CNU's like BCNU, 1,2-bis(2-chloroethyl)-1-nitrosourea, CCNU, 1-(2-chloroethyl)-1-nitroso-3-cyclohexylurea, and Me-CCNU, 1-(2-chloroethyl)-1-nitroso-3-(4-methyl)cyclohexylurea have been introduced into the clinic in rather rapid sequence and have shown activity in several human neoplasms. Chlorozotocin (CZT), 2-[3-(2-chloroethyl)-3-nitrosoureido]-D- desoxyglucopyranose, was the first water-soluble analogue to be tested clinically (Johnston et al, 1975). This second generation CNU showed reduced myelotoxicity in animal experiments and in the clinic (Talley et al, 1981) but also was therapeutically considerably less active than other CNU's in several experimental systems.(Summarized by Spreafico et al, 1981).

Lipophilicity is considered to be essential for high antineoplastic activity, especially towards intracerebral tumours. To comply with this requirement, a promising CNU should therefore be both, well water soluble and lipophilic. An example for a third-generation analogue is HECNU, 1-(2-chloroethyl)-1-nitroso-3-(2-hydroxyethyl)urea. HECNU is about 30 times more water soluble than BCNU, but prefers the lipophilic phase, when distributed between octanol and water (log P = 0.3).

2. MECHANISM OF ACTION

CNU's are monofunctional and bifunctional alkylating agents. They decompose into 2-chloroethyldiazotate or an equivalent bifunctional electrophile and into an isocyanate. Alkylation and crosslink formation between DNA bases is considered an important factor in CNU activity and the biomolecular events connected with crosslink formation have been investigated in detail (Ludlum & Tong, 1981; Tong et al, 1982). Carbamoylation of biomolecules by the isocyanate has also received much attention. Inhibition of DNA repair, reduction of rodent-liver glutathione levels, inhibition of gluthathione reductase in erythrocytes and further effects due to protein carbamoylation (summarized by Reed, 1981) have been described. The biological significance of carbamoylation however remains uncertain.

3. ANTINEOPLASTIC ACTIVITY OF SELECTED CNU'S

In structure-activity studies, we have synthesized and investigated a wide spectrum of CNU-analogues (Eisenbrand et al, 1981). Some were rather promising and two, HECNU and acetamido-CNU, 1-(2-chloroethyl)-1-nitroso-3-(methylene carboxamido)urea have been investigated in more detail, in comparison to clinically applied first- and second generation CNU's. They have been tested in a very wide spectrum of experimental rodent tumours, including many transplantation tumours (Spreafico et al, 1981), human xenografts in nude mice (Fiebig, 1982), and autochthonous tumours, such as DMBA-induced acute leukemia (Berger, 1979) or DMBA-induced mammary carcinoma (Fiebig et al, 1980) and others. In most of these experimental tumour systems, the new analogues were more effective antineoplastic agents than clinically used CNU's. HECNU was especially highly active against intracerebrally (i.c.) implanted tumours, such as anaplastic mouse mammary carcinoma (Radacic et al, in prep.), murine ependymoblastoma

(Spreafico et al, 1981), astrocytoma HT 60 of the rat (Fiebig & Schmähl, 1979) or i.c. implanted rodent leukemias. (Spreafico et al, 1981; Zeller et al, 1978).

4. DNA-DNA INTERSTRAND CROSSLINKING IN RODENT BONE MARROW

Since the main dose-limiting target of CNU's is considered to be the bone marrow, formation and subsequent removal of DNA-DNA interstrand crosslinks in the bone marrow of rats after a single i.p. injection (100 µmol/kg) of BCNU, HECNU, acetamido-CNU and CZT were studied (Bedford & Eisenbrand, in press.). All four agents produced crosslinks, however to a considerably varying extent. HECNU and acetamido-CNU were much more effective in inducing interstrand crosslinks than BCNU and CZT. For HECNU and acetamido-CNU crosslinking was found to peak at 24 hours after injection, followed by a decrease at 36 and 48 hrs. No peak in crosslinking was seen for BCNU and CZT. The kinetics of crosslink disappearance were identical for BCNU, a strongly, and CZT, a weakly carbamoylating analogue. The much greater potential of crosslink formation of HECNU and acetamido-CNU correlates with the higher antineoplastic effectiveness of these two analogues in a wide series of rodent tumour systems.

5. LONG TERM TOXICITY AND CARCINOGENICITY

In long term toxicity studies BCNU, CZT, HECNU, acetamido-CNU and several further CNU's were intravenously applied to rats every 6 weeks at dose levels of 9.5 - 150 mg/m², respectively. Treatment was discontinued either when severe lethal toxicity became apparent or after the maximum number of ten applications had been applied. Animals were observed for lifetime. The results revealed extreme differences in long term toxicity. BCNU by far was the most toxic compound, causing very short median survival times (MST) in all dosages, except the lowest. CZT was very toxic at 75 mg/m², but could be fully applied at lower dosages. In contrast to BCNU and CZT, HECNU and acetamido-CNU were much better tolerated, as exemplified by higher total doses, and by much longer MST. (Habs, 1980;

Eisenbrand et al, 1981).

BCNU also was exeptional in its carcinogenic potency, inducing high incidence of malignant tumours in lung and neuro-
genous tissues, within very short induction times. The other
agents also showed neoplastic effects, with a prevalence for
lung and nervous tissue, but tumour incidences were much lower
(Habs, 1980; Eisenbrand, et al, 1981). The results are parallel
to results of previous studies in rats with BCNU, HECNU, CZT
and some further CNU's, given once weekly by i.p. injection
(Eisenbrand, 1979; Habs et al, 1979). In these studies BCNU
and CZT were found to be potent, locally acting carcinogens,
inducing malignant tumours in the i.p. cavity, whereas HECNU
did not induce local tumours.

6. CLINICAL PHASE I AND ONGOING PHASE II STUDIES

54 patients are evaluable in phase I and 22 until now in
phase II. Dose limiting toxicity of HECNU consists of delayed
thrombo- and leucocytopenia with a nadir after 24 and 35 days,
respectively, occuring in low frequencies at the MTD of 120 mg/m²
(thrombocytopenia < 50.000 = 4 %; leukocytopenia < 2.000 =
11 %). Besides nausea and vomiting (24 % and 25 % at 120 mg/m²),
no other toxicities were observed. Partial remissions (PR)
were observed in 3/10 patients with stomach cancer, 1/3 melanomas, 1/8 epidermoid cancers of the lung and 1/1 parotid
cancer. A steep dose-response relationship for toxicity and
a flat dose-response curve for antitumour activity (one PR
already at 60 mg/m²) indicate a large therapeutic index. The
recommended dose for broad phase II trials is 120 mg/m², i.v.,
q. 6 weeks in untreated patients (Fiebig et al, 1983).

7. FUTURE DEVELOPMENTS

The above results show that even within a group of thorough-
ly investigated antineoplastic agents, new and promising analogues might be detected, provided relevant test methods are
applied. Our future developmental work will be directed towards more selective drug targeting. Methods for attaching
CNU groups to amino acids and oligopeptides have been developed.

Such derivatives are used to link CNU groups to appropriate carrier molecules, especially to steroids or to specific proteins. By this approach it is hoped that a greater selectivity of antitumour therapy with CNU's will be reached.

ACKNOWLEDGEMENTS

Work summarized here was supported in part by the German Ministry for Research and Technology (BMFT). Parts have also been carried out within the activities of the EORTC screening and pharmacology group.

REFERENCES

1. Bedford, P., Eisenbrand, G., DNA damage and repair in the bone marrow of rats treated with four chloroethylnitrosoureas, Cancer Research, in press
2. Berger, M., Chemotherapie der Rattenleukämie L 5222 und von autochthonen Leukämien, die durch DMBA induziert wurden, Dissert., Univers. Heidelberg, 1979
3. Eisenbrand, G.; Habs, M.; Zeller, W.J.; Fiebig, H.; Berger, M.; Zelesny, O., Schmähl, D., New nitrosoureas - Therapeutic and long term toxic effects of selected compounds in comparison to established drugs, in: Serrou, B.; Schein, P.S.; Imbach, J.L., (Eds.) Nitrosoureas in Cancer Treatment, INSERM Sympos. N. 19, 175-191 (1981)
4. Eisenbrand, G., Carcinogenic action of BCNU analogues after repeated application to SD-rats, Proc. Am. Ass. Cancer Res. 20, 46 (1979)
5. Fiebig, H.H.; Eisenbrand, G.; Zeller, W.J.; Zentgraf, R., Anticancer activity of new nitrosoureas against Walker carcinosarcoma 256 and DMBA-induced mammary cancer of the rat, Oncology, 37, 177-183 (1980)
6. Fiebig, H.H.; Schmähl, D.; Development of models for brain tumours in rats and their responsiveness to chemotherapy with nitrosoureas, Proc. Am. Ass. Cancer Res., 20, 276 (1979)
7. Fiebig, H., Wachstum und Chemotherapie menschlicher Tumoren in der thymusaplastischen Nacktmaus, Habil. Schrift Med. Fak. Univ. Freiburg (1982)
8. Fiebig, H.H.; Schuchhardt, C.; Henss, H.; Eisenbrand, G.; Löhr, G.W.; Phase I study of the water-soluble nitrosourea 1-(2-hydroxyethyl)-3-(2-chloroethyl)-3-nitrosourea (HECNU), Proc. Am. Ass. Cancer Res., 24, 139 (1983)
9. Habs, M., Experimentelle Untersuchungen zur Cancerogenen Wirkung zytostatischer Arzneimittel, Habilitationsschrift Univ. Heidelberg (1980)
10. Habs, M.; Eisenbrand, G.; Schmähl, D., Carcinogenic activity in Sprague-Dawley rats of 2-[3-(2-chloroethyl)-3-nitrosoureido]D-Glucopyranose (Chlorozotocin), Cancer Letters, 8, 133-137 (1979)

11. Johnston, T.P., Mc Caleb, G.S. and Montgomery, I.A., Synthesis of chlorozotocin, the 2-chloroethyl analog of the anticancer antibiotic streptozotocin, J. Med. Chem., 18, 104-106 (1975)

12. Ludlum, D.P.; Tong, W.P., Modification of DNA and RNA bases by the nitrosoureas, in: Serrou, B.; Schein, P.S.; Imbach, J.L., (Eds.) Nitrosoureas in Cancer Treatment, INSERM Sympos. No. 19, 21-31 (1981)

13. Reed, D.J., Metabolism of Nitrosoureas, in: Prestayko, A.W.; Baker, L.H.; Crooke, S.T.; Carter, S.K.; Schein, P.S. (Eds.) Nitrosoureas, current status and new developments, 51-67, Acad. Press., New York (1981)

14. Spreafico,I.; Filippeschi, S.; Falautano, P.; Eisenbrand, G.; Fiebig, H.H.; Habs, M.; Zeller, W.J.; Schmähl, D.; van Putten, L.M.; Smink, T., The Development of novel nitrosoureas, in: Prestayko, A.W.; Crooke, S.T.; Baker, L.H.; Carter, S.K.; Schein, P.S., (Eds.), Nitrosoureas, current status and new developments, Academ. Press., New York, 175-191, (1981)

15. Talley, R.W., Samson, M.K., Browlee, R.W., Samhouri, A.M., Fraile, R.J., Baker, L.H., Phase II evaluation of chlorozotocin (NSC-178258) in advanced human cancer, Europ. J. Cancer, 17, 337-343 (1981)

16. Tong, W.P.; Kirk, M.C.; Ludlum, D.B., Formation of crosslink 1-[N^3-deoxycytidyl]-2-[N^1-deoxyguanosinyl]-ethane in DNA treated with N,N'-bis (2-chloroethyl)-N-nitrosourea, Cancer Res. 42, 3102-3105, (1982)

17. Zeller, W.J., Eisenbrand, G., Fiebig, H.H., Chemotherapeutic activity of new 2-chloroethylnitrosoureas in rat leukemia L 5222. Comparison of bifunctional and water-soluble derivatives with BCNU, J. Natn. Cancer Inst. 60, 345-348, (1978)

FURTHER OBJECTIVES IN THE DEVELOPMENT OF PLATINUM DRUGS

M.J. CLEARE

Cisplatin, either as a single agent or, more usually, in combination therapy, is active against several human tumours, particularly those of genito-urinary origin. While it has undoubtedly broadened the spectrum of tumours which are amenable to chemotherapy, its contribution is still quite limited. While cisplatin has improved responses for cervix, bladder, prostate and head and neck cancer, it has, to date, only made a major impact on long term survival for ovarian and, particularly, testicular tumours(1). Also, its efficacy is somewhat compromised by the occurrence of major toxic side effects such as nephrotoxicity, myelosuppression, nausea and vomiting and ototoxicity. Although hydration techniques have reduced nephrotoxicity, which is the major dose limiting factor, higher doses can sometimes result in the appearance of peripheral neuropathy

symptoms after several treatments. This has stimulated efforts to identify alternative complexes which retain the useful anti-tumour properties of cisplatin while having reduced toxicity. Studies have concentrated on complexes of the type $\underline{cis}$-$[PtX_2A_2]$ (where A_2 = two monodentate or one bidentate amine ligand and X_2 = two monodentate or one bidentate anionic ligand). The chemistry of such species has been discussed in detail elsewhere(2) but it is sufficient here to emphasise that the strength of the Pt-N (amine) bond is a dominating feature which means that the X groups are relatively reactive compared to the A groups which are inert to substitution. Early studies(3,4) clearly established two simple criteria for activity, namely the requirements for a neutral complex with adjacent ($\underline{cis}$) reactive X groups and these criteria have held for all compounds tested to date.

Hundreds of compounds with a wide variety of A and X groups have been tested and many active species reported against animal tumours(5). The following broad conclusions can be drawn to date and objectives for future

357

work inferred.

A GROUPS

Although the A groups have little effect on the reactivity of the complex (unless they are very bulky and cause steric hindrance) they appear to have a major effect on anti-tumour properties as shown by animal tests. Effective A groups identified to date include n- and iso-alkylamines, alicyclic and heterocyclic amines, diaminoalkanes, diaminocycloalkanes and diamino acids. Current clinical trial data suggest that variations due to amine type are not as significant as indicated by animal tests.

Platinum(IV) complexes of the type cis-$[PtCl_4A_2]$ and cis-$[PtCl_2(OH)_2A_2]$ have been shown to be active against animal tumours, and can have equal activity to their Pt(II) analogues(5). Pt(IV) amine complexes are inert (especially in the absence of light) and can be considered relatively unreactive in the analysis outlined below. One compound, cis-$[PtCl_2(OH)_2(isopropylamine)_2]$ (CHIP - JM9), is currently on clinical trial.

However, one particular area needs to be resolved, namely that of cross resistance with cisplatin. Recent studies have concentrated on bidentate amine ligands, particularly those containing saturated or aromatic hydro-carbon rings. For example, the 1,2-diaminocyclohexane nucleus (1,2-dac) has proved to be a prolific structure for active complexes in combination with a variety of leaving groups(6). Similarly effective are ligands based on substituted 1,3-diaminopropane systems(7), particularly those involving cycloalkanes in the 2-carbon position (e.g. 1,1-diaminomethyl-cyclohexane - 1,1-damcha). These bidentate amine complexes are active against a line of the L1210 tumour which was around 50-fold resistant to cisplatin(5,8). Complexes without bidentate amines were inactive against the resistant tumour. The lack of cross resistance was independent of leaving group (X) and applied to Pt(II) and Pt(IV) species. It is inferred that this could be related to the chelating diamine structure. This interesting addition to preclinical screening has yet to be demonstrated in the clinic. Trials on [Pt(TMA)(1,2-dac)] (JM82) and [Pt(SO_4)(H_2O)(1,1-damcha)] (TNO-6) may provide some clues. It is undoubtedly an important requirement for second or third generation drugs that they show activity against tumours which have become resistant to cisplatin.

X GROUPS

These determine the reactivity of the complex and animal tests indicated that three classes of active species could be identified on a kinetic basis(2,5). (1) Reactive species which hydrolyse readily in solution, e.g. complexes with NO_3 and SO_4 ligands, highlighting the significance of the initial blood uptake phase for active complexes of this type. (2) Species with intermediate hydrolysis activity, e.g. complexes with chloride and chloroacetate ligands. (3) Complexes with bidentate carboxylate ligands, e.g. oxalates and malonates which are inert in vitro to such an extent that an in vivo activation mechanism has been postulated(2). Examples of all three classes are on clinical trial and a structure-toxicity relationship can be defined with toxic side effects clearly reduced for the less reactive species(5). Of particular interest are complexes with bidentate carboxylate ligands, particularly malonates. Animal tests have shown that these ligands, in combination with many amines have good activity, although they are more effective against solid tumours than leukemia(5). The more reactive chloro species are more effective against murine leukemia L1210(5). Several analogues with a variety of X groups gave much lower nephrotoxicity indicators in animals compared to cisplatin with malonates particularly promising. All analogues tested showed significant myelosuppression generally comparable to cisplatin.

Clinical trials in progress seem to confirm the strong relationship between toxicity and reactivity. The relatively unreactive malonate species CBDCA (JM8) has been subjected to major Phase 1, 2 and 3 studies at the Royal Marsden Hospital and has shown greatly reduced nephro- and audio-toxicities with reduced nausea and vomiting. Myelosuppression is dose limiting with the therapeutic dose around $400mg/m^2$. Activity is at least comparable to cisplatin for ovarian (Table 1) and has given the best reported single agent response for small cell carcinoma of the bronchus (61% for new patients).

Reactive compounds such as $[Pt(SO_4)(H_2O)(1,1\text{-damcha})]$ (TNO-6) and $[Pt(SO_4)(H_2O)(1,2\text{-dac})]$ appear to have toxicity and stability problems. Another less reactive species is JM9 (CHIP), a Pt(IV) analogue on trial at the Roswell Park Memorial Hospital, Buffalo, and the Christie Hospital, Manchester. Phase 1 results indicate low renal toxicity with myelosuppression dose limiting at $270mg/m^2$(5).

Table 1. Clinical trials on 2nd generation Pt drugs

CBDCA (JM8)	—	Phase 3 Trial, randomised study with cisplatin for advanced ovarian carcinoma.

Location: Royal Marsden Hospital

Treatment: Cisplatin 5 x 100mg/m² + 5 x 20mg/m² monthly doses
            JM8   10 x 400mg/m² monthly doses

Clinical Result: Cisplatin 37 patients 6CR (17%) 15PR (40%)
                  JM8   34 patients 7CR (21%) 8PR (24%)

Toxicity:

	Cisplatin	JM8
Nephrotoxicity	71%	15%
Myelosuppression	31%	36%
Ototoxicity	87%	13%
Peripheral Neuropathy	48%	15%

Data of A.H. Calvert, E. Wiltshaw, J.W. Baker, I.E. Smith (to be published)

The major disadvantage of the less reactive compounds is low potency
and the consequent high dose required. The general relationship between
reactivity, toxicity (particularly nephrotoxicity) and potency is
summarised below.

Leaving Group	Class 1, e.g. H_2O/SO_4	Class 2, e.g. Cl	Class 3, e.g. malonate/oxalate (Pt(IV) species)	
Toxicity	High	⟶		Low
Potency	High	⟶		Low
Dose Level	Low	⟶		High

Optimum Compound Window

An important goal in optimising the overall therapeutic effectiveness
of Pt drugs would be to increase potency to a level where toxicity is still
acceptable. This would probably involve a compound closer to malonate than
chloride in reactivity. Bidentate oxygen chelates forming 7-membered
chelate rings should be more reactive than the malonates (6-membered
rings). The best example of this system studied to date is [Pt(TMA)(1,2-
dac)] which is on clinical trial at the Sloan Kettering Institute in New
York. This is only soluble in alkaline solution (1% $NaHCO_3$) in which it
exhibits intermediate reactivity(2), although a high clinical dose of
640mg/m² is observed(5). Again myelotoxicity appears dose limiting
although some renal effects have been reported.

This approach is worthy of further study although lack of solubility
may be a major problem. A less myelotoxic Pt drug would be highly

desirable but there are no indications from studies to date that this is possible.

ORAL DRUGS

The complexes evaluated clinically to date have all been administered by injection or infusion schedules where the latter, in particular, require highly developed hospital facilities. The patient population amenable to treatment with Pt drugs would be increased substantially by an orally active compound, especially one which had the added benefit of greater control of drug toxicity.

Recent studies by Siddik et al (reported at this meeting in poster form) indicate that the oral route for certain platinum amine complexes offers considerable potential (Table 2). Preliminary results on cisplatin, CBDCA and CHIP indicate oral activity while holding out some possibilities for moderation of toxicity.

Table 2. Anti-tumour activities of Pt complexes given by oral administration

Compound	ADJ/PC6A			Walker 256			L1210
	LD_{50}	ED_{90}	TI	LD_{50}	ED_{90}	TI	% ILS at MTD
Cisplatin	140	24	5.8	114	59	1.9	24
CBDCA	235	99	2.4	566	400	1.4	ND
CHIP	290	69	4.2	449	370	1.2	ND

TI = Therapeutic Index (LD_{50} in mg/kg/ED_{90} in mg/kg). ND = Not determined. ILS and MTD = Increase in Life Span at Maximally Tolerated Dose (50mg/kg). Data of Z.H. Siddik, P.M. Goddard, F.E. Boxall, C.F.J. Barnard, K.R. Harrap.

SYNTHETIC DIRECTIONS

Synthesis effort on new platinum complexes is dedicated increasingly towards functionalised amines in addition to ligands with potential inherent activity, e.g. triazines(9). However, the activity for cisplatin analogues screened to date suggests that highly refined 'targeting' and selectivity for the active site will be required for a successor to the second generation analogues with the low toxicity discussed above. Complexes of platinum with 'biomolecules' such as peptides(10) and saccharides(11) have been prepared and preliminary studies have confirmed the feasibility of attaching platinum to polyamine structures with a range of chain lengths(12). Similarly, enhanced inhibition of DNA synthesis has been demonstrated for platinum complexed anti-tumour immunoglobulins in comparison with $\underline{cis}$-[PtCl$_2$(NH$_3$)$_2$](13).

CONCLUSIONS

The major objectives in the further development of platinum drugs may be summarised as follows. (1) An improved spectrum of activity. The major problem with Pt drugs – as with most other chemotherapeutic agents – remains that of selectivity. Some form of biological targeting is likely to be needed. (2) An active drug which can be administered orally with acceptable toxicity. Feasibility for this approach has been established. (3) A drug which is not cross resistant to cisplatin or one of the other second generation Pt drugs. Animal tests suggest this may be possible. (4) The current second generation drugs have considerably reduced potency compared to cisplatin. Structural modifications might lead to a drug which maintains the reduced toxicity and maximises potency. (5) Ideally a drug with reduced myelotoxicity is required. Evidence from animal and clinical studies to date suggest that this is unlikely to be achieved.

REFERENCES

(1)   J.R. Durant in "Cisplatin: Current Status and New Developments", (Eds. A.W. Prestayko, S.T. Crooke and S.K. Carter), p.317, Academic Press, 1980.
(2)   M.J. Cleare, P.C. Hydes, D.R. Hepburn and B.W. Malerbi, in Ref. (1), p.149.
(3)   M.J. Cleare and J.D. Hoeschele, Bioinorg.Chem., 2, 187 (1973).
(4)   T.A. Connors, M. Jones, W.C.J. Ross, P.D. Braddock, A.R. Khokhar and M. Tobe, Chem-Biol. Interactions, 5, 415 (1972); ibid 11, 145 (1975).
(5)   M.J. Cleare in 'Structure-Activity Relationships of Anti-Tumour Agents', (Developments in Pharmacology; 3), Ed. D.N. Reinhoudt, T.A. Connors, H.M. Pinedo and K.W. van de Poll, Martinus Nijhoff, The Hague, 1983.
(6)   G.R. Gale and S.J. Meischen, U.S. Patent Appl. No. 769,888.
(7)   J. Berg, E.J. Bulten and F. Verbeek, U.K. Patent Appl. No. 2,024,823A.
(8)   J.H. Burchenal, L. Lokys, J. Turkevich, G. Irani and K. Kern, Recent Results Cancer Res., 74, 146 (1980).
(9)   M. Julliard, G. Vernin and J. Metzger, Synthesis, 1982, 1, 49.
(10) W. Beck and M. Girnth, Arch.Pharm.(Weinheim), 1981, 314, 955.
(11) W. Beck and G. Thiel, (BASF) E.P. Appl. No. 0059911A, (Chem.Abstr., 1983, 98, 34900).
(12) C.E. Carraher Jr., W.J. Scott, J.A. Schroeder and D.J. Giron, J.Macromol.Sci.Chem., 1981, A15 (4), 625.
(13) E. Hurwitz, R. Kashi and M. Wilchek, J.N.C.I., 1982, 69, 47.

CHAPTER V

CHROMATIN AS A TARGET IN CANCER CHEMOTHERAPY

THE STRUCTURE OF ACTIVE GENES AND HMG PROTEINS IN NORMAL AND
TRANSFORMED CELLS

G.H. GOODWIN

1. INTRODUCTION

   Regulation of gene activity is thought to be at least partly
controlled by changes in the chromatin structure of genes. A
number of differences between active and inactive genes have
been extensively documented but the relationship between them
and the mechanism by which they effect gene structure is not
known (1). These differences are: (i) active genes are in a
configuration which is more sensitive to attack by DNAse I;
(ii) active genes are marked by DNAse I 'hypersensitive' regions
and (iii) DNA of active genes have less 5-methyl-cytosine.
It is also believed that nucleosomes on active genes have
HMG proteins bound to them. The results presented in this
report are concerned with the structure of active genes in
normal and transformed cells and the HMG proteins in such cells.

2. RESULTS
(i) The structure of the adult β^A-globin gene in early embryonic
    (5 day) and adult (16 day) chick red blood cell lineages
   The β^A-globin gene is expressed in 16 day red blood cells
(RBC) but not 5 day cells (2). However, in both cell lines the
^{A} gene is in a structure that is more sensitive to DNAse I
digestion than the inactive ovalbumin gene. This was demonstrated by the dot-blot hybridization method (3) and the relative
levels of hybridization of the samples (a,b and d) are shown in
the histogram of Fig. 1. Thus DNAse I-sensitivity is not due
to the process of transcription itself. In order to investigate
what factors are responsible for maintaining this open structure
       365

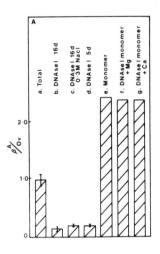

FIGURE 1. Histogram of dot-blot hybridization analyses. Ratios of β^A to ovalbumin sequences quantified by scanning dot-blots of: a - total chicken erythrocyte DNA; b - DNA from DNAse I digested 16-day RBC nuclei; c - DNA from DNAse I digested 16-day RBC nuclei that had been extracted with 0.3M NaCl pH 3; d - DNA from DNAse I-digested 5-day RBC nuclei; e - DNA from 0.1M NaCl-soluble monomer nucleosomes (16-day RBC); f - DNA from DNAse I-digested 0.1M NaCl-soluble monomer nucleosomes (digestion buffer contained Mg^{2+}); g - DNA from DNAse I digested 0.1M NaCl-soluble monomer nucleosomes (digestion buffer contained Ca^{2+}). Ratios were normalised so that the β^A/ov ratio for total chicken erythrocyte DNA was 1.0.

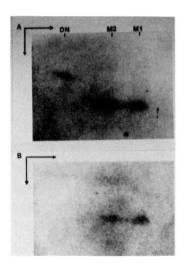

FIGURE 2. Two-dimensional electrophoretic analysis of nucleosomes and dinucleosomes. Salt-soluble RBC nucleosomes were stripped of HMG, H1 and H5 proteins by gel filtration on Sephadex G100 in 0.4M NaCl. The core particles were trimmed to 145 base pairs with micrococcal nuclease and then pure HMG17 added back to bind to on one-third of the nucleosomes. The reconstituted nucleosomes were separated by electrophoresis (left to right) and the DNA then dissociated, denatured and electrophoresed in the second dimension (top to bottom). After transfer of the DNA to DPT paper the blot was probed with (a) the β-globin gene and (b) the ovalbumin gene. M1 is core particle. M2 is core particle associated with HMG protein. DN is the dinucleosome which co-isolates with the monomer nucleosomes.

nuclei were extracted with 0.3M NaCl at pH 3 (4), conditions which remove HMG proteins and histone Hl. Hybridization analysis (Fig. 1, sample c) shows only a very small difference in the level of sensitivity after salt treatment. However, if the nuclei are digested with micrococcal nuclease and the monomer nucleosomes isolated, the DNAse I-sensitive structure is not found when these nucleosomes are subsequently digested with DNAse I (Fig. 1, samples e, f and g). Similar results were obtained using a histone gene probe and with an α-globin probe (data not shown). These results suggest that the major DNAase I-sensitive structure of active genes may not be due to the nucleosomes on such genes being different from inactive nucleosomes but because they are packed into a more open higher order structure. Salt extraction does have a small effect on DNAse I-sensitivity (Fig. 1) and this may be due to the HMG-effect described by Weisbrod (1).

Further data to support the view that nucleosomes bound to active genes are essentially the same as those on inactive genes comes from experiments in which RBC nucleosome core particles were isolated and HMG proteins and lysine-rich histones removed. The nucleosomes were trimmed with micrococcal nuclease and a limited amount of HMG17 was then titrated back onto the core particles so that about one-third of the nucleosomes took up HMG17 and the mixture then separated by polyacrylamide gel electrophoresis. The nucleosomes were blotted and hybridized to β-globin or ovalbumen probes. Fig. 2 shows that the distribution of globin and ovalbumin sequences in the HMG-containing core particles (M2) and the particles devoid of HMG (M1) are essentially the same. However, a dinucleosome (DN) can be seen running behind the monomers which are highly enriched in globin sequences and devoid of ovalbumin sequences. The DNA of this material is 310 base pairs long. These nuclease-resistant dinucleosomes are evidently closely packed chromatosomes. These results suggest that globin-containing nucleosomes are packed together with a shorter linker DNA and may account for the different higher order packing suggested by the above DNAse I experiments.

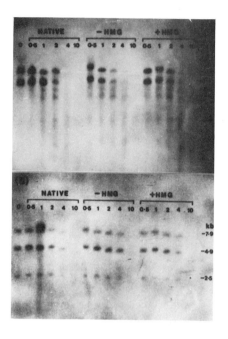

FIGURE 3. DNAse I-sensit-
ivity of the integrated
ASV genes compared to the
serum albumen gene in V1T
cell nuclei in the presence
and absence of HMG proteins.
Native, 0.34M salt-extracted,
and HMG-reconstituted nuclei
were digested with DNAse I
at 0, 0.5, 1, 2, 4 and 10
ug/ml DNAse I and 1 mg/ml
DNA. Southern blots of
Hind III-digested DNA
samples were probed with
(A) ^{32}P-labelled ASV DNA,
and (B) ^{32}P-labelled rat
serum albumen gene DNA.

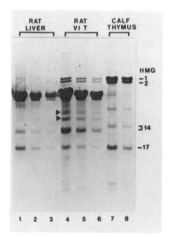

FIGURE 4. Acid-urea poly-
acrylamide gel electro-
phoresis of HMG proteins
from rat liver (lanes 12),
V1T cells (lanes 4-6) and
calf thymus (lanes 7 and
8). The arrow heads show
the doublet of HMG proteins
found in elevated quantities in dividing cells.

(ii) <u>The structure of the avian sarcoma viral provirus (ASV)</u>
   <u>in rat transformed cells (V1T cells)</u>

Nuclei from Rat-1 fibroblasts transformed by the integration of a single copy of the avian sarcoma virus were isolated and digested with increasing amounts of DNAse I and the ASV sequences and (inactive) albumen sequences analysed by Southern blots (Fig. 3). It can be seen that the ASV sequences are more sensitive to digestion by DNAse I than the albumen sequences. Removal or reconstitution of HMG proteins prior to DNAse I digestion of the nuclei had little effect on this sensitivity. The four ASV sub-bands that can be seen on the blots below the main 11.6 and 7.4 Kb bands are due to cutting at 'hypersensitive' sites. DNAse I cutting at these sites is not affected by HMG proteins. Thus the general sensitivity and the hypersensitive sites are not affected by HMG proteins.

(iii) <u>HMG proteins in normal and transformed rat cells</u>

Fig. 4 compares the PCA-soluble proteins from rat liver and V1T cells. It is apparent that V1T cells have a higher ratio of HMG14 to HMG17 than liver cells. V1T cells also have elevated levels of an additional pair of bands running just behind HMG14. Analysis of the untransformed Rat-1 cells and a revertant V1T cell indicate that this doublet is present also, but the HMG14/17 ratio is lower as in liver. Rat thymus contains very little of the slower moving doublet (not shown). Therefore it would appear that compared with non-dividing tissues, proliferating normal and transformed cells in tissue culture contain elevated levels of a pair of additional HMG proteins.

REFERENCES

1. Weisbrod S: Nature (297): 289-295, 1982.
2. Groudine M, Penetz M, Weintraub H: Molecular & Cellular Biology (1) 281-288.
3. Nicolas RH, Wright CA, Cockerill PN, Wyke JA, Goodwin GH: Nucleic Acids Res (11): 753-771, 1983.
4. Villeponteau B, Lasky L, Harary I: Biochemistry (17): 5532-5536, 1978.
5. Larsen A, Weintraub H: Cell (29): 609-622, 1982.

PRETREATMENT OF HUMAN COLON TUMOR CELLS WITH DNA METHYLATING AGENTS INHIBITS
THEIR ABILITY TO PREVENT CHLOROETHYLNITROSOUREA-INDUCED DNA INTERSTRAND
CROSSLINKING

LEONARD C. ERICKSON*, CHANA ZLOTOGORSKI**, AND NEIL W. GIBSON**

INTRODUCTION

Normal human fibroblasts, and a variety of human tumor cell lines, have
been shown to be capable of reactivating Adenovirus which had been damaged by
in vitro exposure to DNA methylating agents (1). Those cells capable of
repairing the damaged viral DNA have been designated Mer$^+$ (Methylation
repair). Other human tumor cell lines are incapable of reactivating damaged
virus, and have been designated Mer$^-$ (1). R. Day and co-workers have shown
that Mer$^+$ cells are also capable of removing methyl groups from the
O^6-position of guanine, whereas Mer$^-$ cells are deficient at the repair of
this lesion (2). In a recent study Yarosh et al. have shown that Mer$^-$ cells
lack the DNA repair enzyme O^6-methylguanine-DNA methyltransferase (3).

The anti-tumor chloroethylnitrosoureas produce DNA interstrand crosslinks
by forming monoadducts on one DNA strand, followed by reaction with the
opposite DNA strand in a delayed second step (4). In several recent reports
we have shown that Mer$^+$ cells are capable of preventing the formation of
chloroethylnitrosourea (CNU) induced DNA interstrand crosslinks (5,6). In
Mer$^-$ cells significant levels of DNA interstrand crosslinks were detected
several hours after exposure of cells to CNU (5,6). We have suggested that in
Mer$^+$ cells O^6-methylguanine-DNA methyltransferase may remove chloroethyl
monoadducts at the O^6-position of guanine before the delayed reaction
produces DNA interstrand crosslinks. The DNA methylating agent MNNG has been
shown to be capable of inhibiting O^6-methylguanine-DNA methyltransferase (7).
In the present study we have examined whether or not the chloroethyl
monoadduct repair can be altered by exposing Mer$^+$ cells to conditions which
might inactivate the O^6-methylguanine-DNA methyltransferase. Furthermore,
we have investigated whether or not this repair system can also prevent DNA

371

crosslinking produced by other clinically useful DNA crosslinking agents such as cis-Pt, melphalan, nitrogen mustard, and a cytoxan derivative.

MATERIALS AND METHODS

Cell Culture. Normal human fibroblasts (IMR-90), SV-40 transformed fibroblasts (VA-13), and human colon carcinoma cells (HT-29) were cultured in Eagle's MEM, containing 10% fetal bovine serum, as previously described (6).

Alkaline Elution. DNA interstrand crosslinking was measured using the proteinase K modification of the alkaline elution method as described by Kohn et al. (8).

Drug Exposure. 1-(2-chloroethyl)-1-nitrosourea (CNU), N-methyl-N'-nitro-N-nitrosoguanidine (MNNG), N-methyl nitrosourea (MNU), methyl methanesulfonate (MMS) were dissolved in 95% ethanol; cis-diamminedichloroplatinum(II) (cis-Pt) was dissolved in MEM: streptozotocin (STZ) was dissolved in 0.01 M sodium citrate; 4-S-(propionic acid)-sulfido-cyclophosphamide (C-2) was dissolved in phosphate buffered saline; nitrogen mustard (HN$_2$) and melphalan (L-Pam) were dissolved in 0.1 N HCl.

RESULTS AND DISCUSSION

The DNA interstrand crosslinking patterns observed in IMR-90 (Panel A) and VA-13 (Panel E) cells exposed to 50 or 100 μM CNU are presented in Fig. 1. Cells were exposed to drug for 1 hour, the medium was changed, and the cells incubated for 6 hours to allow DNA crosslinks to form. Little or no crosslinking was observed in the Mer$^+$ cells (IMR-90), in contrast to the

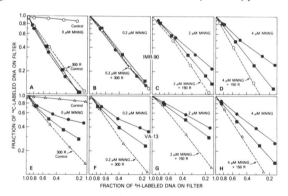

Fig. 1. CNU-induced DNA interstrand crosslinking in IMR-90 and VA-13 cells following pretreatment with various doses of MNNG.

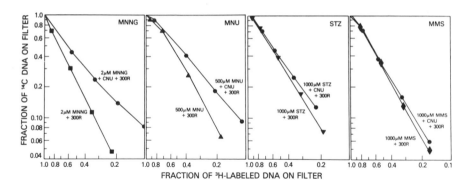

Fig. 2. Effect of pretreatment of HT-29 colon carcinoma cells with various DNA methylating agents prior to exposure of cells to 100 μM CNU.

high levels of crosslinking observed in the Mer⁻ cells (VA-13). However, when cells were pretreated with various doses of MNNG before CNU exposure, the levels of crosslinking observed in the Mer⁺ cells were comparable to the Mer⁻ cells. Thus, when cells were exposed to conditions which should inactivate O^6-methylguanine-DNA methyltransferase (7), Mer⁺ cells temporarily responded as Mer⁻ cells (9). This effect was also observed in another Mer⁺ cell line, HT-29. No interstrand crosslinking has been observed in HT-29 cells exposed to CNU alone. Fig. 2. presents data which demonstrate that MNNG and MNU are capable of inhibiting the DNA repair process by which HT-29 cells avoid the formation of CNU-induced DNA interstrand crosslinks. However, MMS and STZ were much less efficient at inhibiting the chloroethyl monoadduct repair process.

The duration of the DNA monoadduct repair inhibition was studied in HT-29 cells by varying the time of incubation of cells between the MNNG pretreatment, and the CNU exposure. We found that between 3 and 6 hours after the MNNG exposure approximately 50% of the chloroethyl adduct repair capacity had recovered, and after 24 hours of incubation between the MNNG treatment and the CNU exposure all of the repair capacity of the HT-29 cells had been restored (10).

The biological consequences of inhibiting the chloroethyl adduct repair process are presented in Fig. 3. Colony formation assays were utilized to select non-toxic doses of MNNG, MNU, MMS, and STZ, for pretreatment.

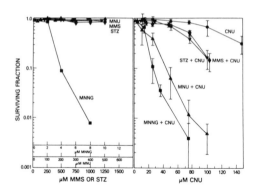

Fig. 3. Colony formation assays with HT-29 cells following a 1 hr exposure to various methylating agents (left panel), or after pretreatment with each agent followed by exposure to varying concentrations of CNU (right panel).

2 μM MNNG, 500 μM MNU, 1000μM MMS and STZ were chosen (left panel). In the right panel the colonying forming ability of HT-29 cells was assessed after pretreatment for 1 hr with each of the methylating agents, followed by a 1 hr exposure to varying concentrations of CNU. It can be seen that the two agents which were most efficient at inhibiting the chloroethyl adduct repair process, and allowed CNU crosslinks to form (MNNG and MNU), greatly increased the cytotoxicity of CNU to the cells. In contrast STZ and MMS, which were inefficient at inhibiting the repair process, only produced a modest increase in the CNU cell killing.

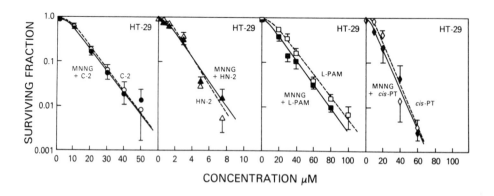

Fig. 4. Colony formation assays with HT-29 cells exposed to C-2, HN$_2$, L-Pam, or cis-Pt with (solid) or without (open) MNNG pretreatment.

Fig. 4 presents colony formation assays of HT-29 cells exposed to varying concentrations of C-2, HN_2, L-Pam, or cis-Pt, with or without pretreatment with 2 μM MNNG. Unlike CNU, the cytotoxicity of these 4 agents was not altered by MNNG pretreatment. In a study to be published elsewhere (N.W.G., C.Z., L.C.E., in preparation) we will show that MNNG pretreatment also does not alter DNA interstrand cross-linking levels produced by these agents. Collectively these data demonstrate that the O^6-guanine repair system is a unique DNA repair system specific for methyl and chloroethyl adducts. Repair proficient cells can be sensitized to killing by the chloroethylnitrosoureas by inhibiting this repair system. Alternative chemotherapy with other alkylating agents may be desirable in repair proficient tumors. (The authors wish to thank Susan Hurst-Calderone for assistance with cell cultures, and Karen Tranchitella for preparation of the manuscript).

REFERENCES

1. Day RS III, Ziolokowski CHJ, Scudiero DA, Meyer SA, Mattern MR: Human tumor cell strains defective in the repair of alkylation damage. Carcinogenesis 1. 21-32, 1980.
2. Day RS III, Ziolokowski CHJ, Scudiero DA, Meyer SA, Lubiniecki AS, Girardi AJ, Galloway SM and Bynum GD: Defective repair of alkylated DNA by human tumor and SV40 transformed human cell strains. Nature 288, 724-727, 1980.
3. Yarosh DB, Foote RS, Mitra S, and Day RS III: Repair of O^6-methylguanine in DNA by demethylation is lacking in Mer⁻ human tumor cell strains. Carcinogenesis 4, 199-205, 1983.
4. Kohn KW: Interstrand cross-linking by BCNU and other 1-(2-chloroethyl)-1-nitrosoureas. Cancer Res. 37, 1450-1454, 1977.
5. Erickson LC, Bradley MO, Ducore JM, Ewig RAG, and Kohn KW: DNA cross-linking and cytotoxicity in normal and transformed human cells treated with antitumor nitrosoureas. Proc. Natl. Acad. Sci. USA 77(1), 467-471, 1980.
6. Erickson LC, Laurent G, Sharkey NA, and Kohn KW: DNA cross-linking and monoadduct repair in nitrosourea treated human tumor cells. Nature 288, 727-729, 1980.
7. Waldstein EA, Cao E, and Setlow RB: Adaptive increase of O^6-methyl-guanine protein in HeLa cells following N-methyl-N'-nitro-N-guanidine treatment. Nucleic Acid Research 10, 4595-4600, 1982.
8. Kohn KW, Ewig RAG, Erickson LC, and Zwelling, LA: Measurement of strand breaks and crosslinks by alkaline elution. In: DNA Repair, A Laboratory Manual of Research Procedures, Vol. 1 (eds. EC Freidberg, and PC Hanawalt), Marcel Dekker, New York, 1981, pp 379-401.
9. Zlotogorski C, and Erickson LC: Pretreatment of normal human fibroblasts and human colon carcinoma cells with MNNG allows chloroethylnitrosourea to produce DNA interstrand cross-links not observed in cells treated with chloroethylnitrosourea alone. Carcinogenesis 4: 759-763, 1983.
10. Zlotogorski C, and Erickson LC: Pretreatment of human colon tumor cells with DNA methylating agents inhibits their ability to repair chloroethyl monoadducts. Carcinogenesis, in press, 1983.

STRUCTURAL REQUIREMENTS FOR DNA INTERCALATION AND THEIR RELEVANCE TO DRUG
DESIGN

M.J. WARING, K.R. FOX & S. HAYLOCK

The intercalation mechanism is known to be very tolerant as regards
the acceptability of aromatic ring systems for insertion between the DNA
base-pairs (1,2). Drugs having two, three, four or more fused six-membered
rings have been characterised as efficient intercalators, and there are
grounds for believing that even the simple side-chains of aromatic amino
acids can intercalate under appropriate conditions (3). In a few studies
the detailed requirements for intercalation in a series of homologous
compounds have been investigated, as for example in the ethidium and
amsacrine (acridinylmethanesulphonanilide) series (4,5). These, too, have
reinforced the view that a wide variety of substituents appended to the
intercalating ring system can be tolerated.

However, when well-characterised intercalative chromophores are to
be linked in pairs to produce bis-intercalating ligands additional constraints
become operative. Such ligands are of current interest as potentially
valuable therapeutic drugs, not least for the treatment of cancer (1,6-8).
One obvious constraint lies in the nature of the flexible chain normally
employed to link the intercalative moieties; it may be inert (as, for
example, a sequence of methylene groups) or it may be deliberately constructed
to contain additional functional groups intended to interact directly with
the DNA. Its mode of attachment to the aromatic rings must be compatible
with their intercalation. Perhaps most obviously its length must be
sufficient to permit bis-intercalation, and that may well require
adherence to the principle of neighbour exclusion (1,2).

One of the first studies on bis-intercalating diacridines revealed
that the minimum length of purely methylene linker chain needed to permit
intercalation of two 9-aminoacridine chromophores was six $-CH_2-$ units (9).
With a slightly shorter chain, having five $-CH_2-$ units, the helix extension
produced by the ligand was not a linear function of the level of binding
but seemed to increase as more drug became bound. We have repeated the

377

experiment using a similar drug having a linker chain containing four
$-CH_2-$ groups and one ether oxygen and found the same peculiar behaviour
(Fig. 1). This result confirms the suggestion that this anomalous response
reflects a slightly-too-short linker rather than any intrinsic peculiarity
of the five-methylene chain. As can be seen, a dimer containing six $-CH_2-$
groups plus two ether oxygens, equivalent in length to a $-(CH_2)_8-$ chain,
behaved in quite normal bis-intercalative fashion yielding a slope (L/Lo
vs D/P) of 2.85 $\pm$ 0.22 which is within the range produced by known bis-
intercalators under these conditions (see Table 1).

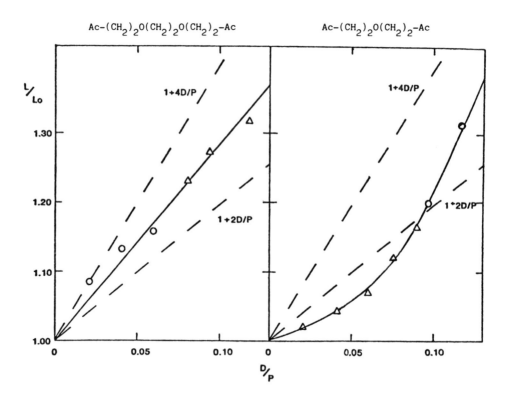

FIGURE 1. Relative length of sonicated rod-like calf thymus DNA fragments
in the presence (L) or absence (Lo) of diacridines. D/P represents the
molar ratio of added drug to DNA nucleotides. The broken lines of slope
4 and 2 correspond to idealised bis-intercalation and simple (monofunctional)
intercalation respectively. The buffer contained 2% (v/v) DMSO. For
experimental details see refs. 9, 10.

It is now clear that the minimum length of linker chain needed to
permit bis-intercalation depends critically upon the nature of the chromo-

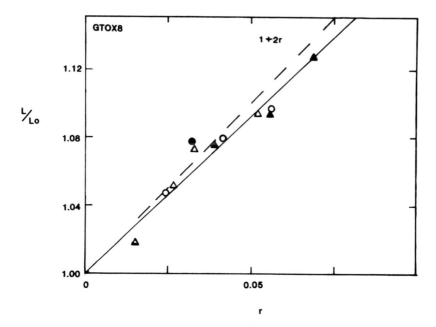

FIGURE 2. Helix-extension plot for nitracrine in buffer containing 2%
(v/v) DMSO, as a function of the actual drug-DNA binding ratio r. The
experimental slope is 1.86 $\pm$ 0.05 and a reference line of slope 2 is
included.

phores, be they identical (homodimers) or not (heterodimers) (6-10). The
rules have been sufficiently clarified to enable the synthesis of successful
tris-intercalators (11,12). Nevertheless there remains much to learn.
Nitracrine is an experimental antitumour drug synthesised by Ledochowski
and his colleagues in Poland (13,14). It is quite a good intercalator,
as judged by its ability to extend the DNA helix (Fig. 2) as well as unwind
it (15,16). Dimeric derivatives of nitracrine have recently been synthesised
by Taylor and Acheson at Oxford and are currently undergoing tests for
biological activity. They are very poorly soluble in water, but by dint
of conducting experiments in 2% (v/v) dimethyl sulphoxide we succeeded in
measuring L/Lo plots for some of them. Controls (Table 1) were performed
to establish norms for bis-intercalators. However, despite our best efforts
the slopes of L/Lo plots for nitracrine dimers fell well below those
anticipated for bis-intercalation and lay even below the value recorded
for the parent compound (Table 1).

Table 1. Gradients of helix-extension plots (L/Lo $\underline{vs}$ D/P) in 0.01 SHE buffer containing 2% (v/v) DMSO. For experimental details see refs. 9, 10.

Drug	Linker	Gradient
C_{10} diacridine	$-(CH_2)_{10}-$	2.68 ± 0.28
C_{12} diacridine	$-(CH_2)_{12}-$	3.22 ± 0.38
Echinomycin	cyclic peptide	3.57 ± 0.02
Nitracrine	none	1.66 ± 0.25
Nitracrine dimers:		
GTOX 4	$-(CH_2)_3NH(CH_2)_3-$	1.18 ± 0.21
GTOX 3	$-(CH_2)_3NCH_3(CH_2)_3-$	1.54 ± 0.13
GTOX 10	$-(CH_2)_4O(CH_2)_4-$	1.08 ± 0.15
GTOX 6	$-(CH_2)_6-$	1.12[*]
GTOX 9	$-(CH_2)_3O(CH_2)_3-$	1.07[*]

[*] precipitation evident, therefore lower limit

These results can be taken to establish no more than the likelihood that some form of intercalative binding to DNA is occurring. It is quite possible that, contrary to experience with previous diacridines (9,10), the linkers of the compounds so far tested were all too short. Another difficulty could be related to butterfly-puckering of the acridinyl ring system due to a preference for adopting the imino form at the 9-amino position. At all events, these dimeric nitracrine derivatives were found to display in exaggerated form many of the untoward properties seen with simpler diacridines, such as low water-solubility and a tendency to provoke precipitation of DNA. These properties may mean that their chromophores are $\underline{too}$ ready to form stacking interactions, and that better drugs would result from synthesising dimers containing weak intercalating ring systems such as occur in the quinoxaline antibiotics (17,18).

This work was supported by grants from the Cancer Research Campaign, the Royal Society, and the Medical Research Council. We thank Tracey Douglas for technical assistance and Drs Graeme Taylor and Morin Acheson for supplying the diacridines.

REFERENCES
1. Waring MJ: DNA modification and cancer. Ann. Rev Biochem (50): 159-192, 1981.
2. Gale EF, Cundliffe E, Reynolds PE, Richmond MH, Waring MJ: The Molecular Basis of Antibiotic Action, 2nd ed., Wiley, London, 1981.

3. Gabbay EJ, Sanford K, Baxter CS, Kapicak L: Specific interaction of peptides with nucleic acids. Evidence for a "selective bookmark" recognition hypothesis. Biochem (12): 4021-4029, 1973.

4. Wakelin LPG, Waring MJ: The unwinding of circular DNA by phenanthridinium drugs: structure-activity relations for the intercalation reaction. Mol Pharmacol (10): 544-561, 1974.

5. Baguley BC, Denny WA, Atwell GJ, Cain BF: Potential antitumour agents. 34. Quantitative relationships between DNA binding and molecular structure for 9-anilinoacridines substituted in the anilino ring. J Med Chem (24): 170-177, 1981.

6. Le Pecq JB, Le Bret M, Barbet J, Roques B: DNA polyintercalating drugs: DNA binding of diacridine derivatives. Proc Natl Acad Sci USA (72): 2915-2919, 1975.

7. Canellakis ES, Fico RM, Sarris AH, Shaw YH: Diacridines - double intercalators as chemotherapeutic agents. Biochem Pharmacol (25): 231-236, 1976.

8. Cain BF, Baguley BC, Denny WA: Potential antitumour agents. 28. DNA polyintercalating agents. J Med Chem (21): 658-668, 1978.

9. Wakelin LPG, Romanos M, Chen TK, Glaubiger D, Canellakis ES, Waring MJ: Structural limitations on the bifunctional intercalation of diacridines into DNA. Biochem (17): 5057-5063, 1978.

10. Wright RGMcR, Wakelin LPG, Fieldes A, Acheson RM, Waring MJ: Effects of ring substituents and linker chains on the bifunctional intercalation of diacridines into DNA. Biochem (19): 5825-5836, 1980.

11. Atwell GJ, Leupin W, Twigden SJ, Denny WA: Triacridine derivative: first DNA tris-intercalating ligand. J Amer Chem Soc (105): 2913-2914, 1983.

12. Hansen JB, Buchardt O: A novel synthesis of tri-, di- and mono-9-acridinyl derivatives of tetra-, tri-, and di-amines. J Chem Soc Chem Commun (1983): 162-164, 1983.

13. Gniazdowski M, Filipski J, Chorazy M: Nitracrine. In: Hahn FE (ed) Antibiotics. V/Part 2. Springer-Verlag, Berlin, 1979, pp 275-297.

14. Denny WA, Baguley BC, Cain BF, Waring MJ: Antitumour acridines. In: Neidle S, Waring MJ (eds) Molecular aspects of anti-cancer drug action. Macmillan, London, 1983, pp 1-34.

15. Filipski J, Marczynski B, Sadzinska L, Chalupko G, Chorazy M: Interactions of some nitro-derivatives of substituted 9-aminoacridine with DNA. Biochim Biophys Acta (478): 33-43, 1977.

16. Wilson WR, Denny WA, Twigden SJ, Baguley BC, Probert JC: Selective toxicity of nitracrine to hypoxic mammalian cells. Brit J Cancer, in press.

17. Waring MJ, Wakelin LPG: Echinomycin: a bifunctional intercalating antibiotic. Nature (252): 653-657, 1974.

18. Waring MJ, Fox KR: Molecular aspects of the interaction between quinoxaline antibiotics and nucleic acids. In: Neidle S, Waring MJ (eds) Molecular aspects of anti-cancer drug action. Macmillan, London, 1983, pp 127-156.

DIALKANESULPHONATES AND CHROMATIN

B.W. FOX, P. BEDFORD AND J. HARTLEY

It was recognised by Finley and co-workers in 1964 (1) that the dialkanesulphonates were a potent group of antitumour agents which, in some but not all cases, also produced a bone marrow depressant action. The mechanism of action of these agents was not understood in the sixties but it was recognised that there was need for bi-functionality, and it was suggested by these workers that the extent of activity with each of these biological systems may be related to the spacing of the two alkylating groups present.

Following Goldacre et al's (2) suggestion that crosslinking reactions may occur with bifunctional alkylating agents, Alexander (3) suggested that optimal activity may be associated with the ability of the intermediate crosslinked material to form a sometimes temporary six membered ring structure. Whereas this hypothesis may still be true for some alkylating reactions in vivo, Finley's results with the cis and trans 1,4 but-2-ene dimesylate did not support this hypothesis since for antitumour activity, the trans form had higher activity than the cis isomer. A similar result was also obtained for mutagenesis in Drosophila (4).

Since this period, a great deal of work has been done on the mode of action of a wide variety of alkylating agents and there are many factors which have now become clear.

1. With nearly all alkylating agents, there is a direct association between antitumour activity and bi- (or poly-) functionality. It is unlikely that any monofunctional agent, where it can be shown that there is no possible conversion of the agent to bifunctionality in vivo, has shown significant antitumour activity.

2. The dialkanesulphonates provide a most valuable system for the investigation of the molecular events occurring, since there is no known enzymic or metabolic sequence assisting the reaction in vivo, and following alkylation, the products are usually non-toxic and unlikely to contribute to any of the biological activities observed. Thus this group of agents represents a clean method of delivering bifunctional alkylating

agents to nucleophilic centres, and whose biological consequences can in all probablity be related directly to the initial chemical reactions occurring.

3. The chemistry of these substances are relatively well known and their preference for nucleophilic sites well recognised. It is possible therefore to undertake true structure-activity studies without implicating metabolic sequences which may be highly tissue and cell dependent. Over the years, it has been recognised that the antitumour activity of these and other alkylating agents are often limited by the efficiency of DNA repair activities within the tumour cell. It has also been shown in some but not all tumour cells that when resistance develops there is an increase in the repair capabilities of these cells to the damage present. We have recently shown (5) that busulphan, for example, induces a very low level of interstrand crosslinks in the DNA of treated cells and that the capacity to remove such lesions is associated with the sensitivity of the cells involved. Thus, we can conclude that tumour cell DNA is attacked by the drug in vivo and that this highly important lesion is in all likelihood, determining the subsequent survival of the tumour cell. We also know that chromosome aberrations are very damaging and possible lethal events and they can often be seen at doses lower than DNA crosslinks can be measured by even the most sensitive biochemical methods available. This implies that lethal DNA-DNA or DNA-protein crosslinks may occur at levels which are not biochemically measurable, and thus any association would not have been recognised in the past.

It is interesting to note that Finley concluded from a comparative study of the effect of a number of dimesylates in bone marrow and their antitumour acivity that the basic cause of damage in the bone marrow and in the tumour cell may not be related. Further evidence for the uniqueness of the interactive events between this type of agent and important nucleophilic sites is provided by the work of Jones and Jones (6) who, during an examination of the effect of meso and +/- dimethylmyleran on the spermatogenic epithelium, observed that the two isomers produced qualitatively different types of damage and that a mixture of the two was markedly synergistic. The most cogent interpretation of these results is that the two isomers produced different lesions at different sites and that their combination would thereby create compounded damage which at the biochemical level would be considerably more difficult to overcome than a single lesion. Recent work in our own Institute suggests that similarly, a difference in site of action of each of these two isomers may also be occurring in the bone marrow. Thus we arrive at the exciting possibility that we may be able to construct new agents by restricting inter-alkylating distances to those which are critical for any particular biological effect. By removing undue flexibility in the molecule, the wide range of possible mechanisms of attack could be reduced to produce a smaller number of unique lesions, so as to achieve antitumour activity without the attendant toxic effects on normal systems.

If we first consider the interaction of such bifunctional agents with DNA, a basic requirement for their chemical ineraction is that the attacking group must be coplanar with the polarity of the electron pair which is being attacked. Furthermore, since the electron rich centres of the DNA bases are known to be in the same plane as the planar ring structure of the bases themselves, this restriction will apply to the attacking molecule itself. Thus, from model calculations on the drug alone we can determine the range of distances permitting this restricted form of attack. The attacking molecule itself will also be subjected to its own internal restrictions of conformation, and when these effects are combined, the possible range of distances permitting biologically effective attack, will be further limited.

Such calculations are now worth pursuing, with the newer techniques availble for measuring crosslinking and repair and with computer technology for determining the least strain configuration of molecules under certain externally imposed restrictions.

We first examined the relative ability of a series of dimethanesulphonate esters of the straight chain diols (7) to produce interstrand crosslinks in DNA, and between DNA and associated protein molecules, by the use of Kohn's (8) alkaline elution technique. The technique was used with and without pronase, so that an estimate of the degree of DNA-DNA as well as DNA-protein crosslinking could be measured. An attempt was made to determine crosslinking at a constant dose level (250μM) on the assumption that all these agents behaved like busulphan (n=4) in that the transport system was by simple diffusion, no active transport systems being involved. It was observed that DNA-DNA interstrand crosslinking occurred with n=1, and n=4-9 with a barely discernable interaction at n=3, and none at all at n=2. The level of crosslinking was maximal at n=6, being several times higher than for busulphan. The optimum level of DNA-protein crosslinking however differed from the DNA-DNA crosslinking, and was maximal at n=8. It was interesting to note that the busulphan (n=4) did not show any DNA-protein binding. The question of the relative importance of the DNA-DNA crosslinking compared to the DNA-protein crosslinking must clearly be evaluated. However, although some relationship may exist between the types of DNA-protein binding produced by neighbouring members of the series around the optimal compound, n=8, it is unlikely that any exists between the n=1 compound, which shows no crosslinking activity either of DNA-DNA or DNA-protein. The main hydrolysis product of the n=1 compound is formaldehyde, which has no antitumour activity at the levels expected to be released from that compound. However, almost the entire level of DNA-protein cross-linking can be related directly to the formaldehyde, although it does not induce any DNA-DNA crosslinks, contrary to the n=1 compound. One could argue from this that the DNA-protein links produced by this drug make no contribution to its antitumour action. However the DNA-DNA crosslinking that the n=1 compound produced appeared to correlate with its antitumour action. This view is supported by the fact that a resistant line developed against the drug was more successful in removing such crosslinks from the cellular DNA compared with the drug-sensitive line. One of us (JH) has recently studied the nature of the protein in the crosslinked material, and has investigated the chromatin structures in the nuclei of cells treated with both formaldehyde and the n=1 compound. We have been able to show that the protein observed in these studies is almost entirely nucleosomal in origin. By gel electrophoretic analyses of the histone extractable from treated cells as well as the histone bound to the DNA, it has been shown (9) that the compositin of the histones on the DNA is the same as whole histone, indicating that the nucleosome is bound intact. This is in agreement with the known properties of formaldehyde which is capable of binding DNA and nucleohistone.

The optimal level of DNA-DNA interstrand crosslinking is shown by 1,6-dimethanesulphonoxy hexane (n=6). However, this agent (like busulphan, n=4) does not produce DNA-protein links. With the n=8 compound however, the production of DNA-protein crosslinks is optimal, and we (9) have shown that a histone-DNA link is involved, but only with histone H3. The possible functional importance of DNA-DNA crosslinking remains to be determined, but from a plot of total crosslinking activity versus cell killing for the whole series of bifunctional methanesulphonates, the relationship is approximately linear except for the n=8 compound which appears to be more cytotoxic than its level of DNA-DNA crosslinking would indicate.

To attempt to limit the degree of flexibility of the two alkylating centres, and to limit the nucleophilic sites that are capable of being attacked, a series of aromatic dimethanesulphonates were made. The interesting series of benzene di(methanesulphonoxyethyl) derivatives were shown to be of equal toxicity in rats but only the ortho-derivative possessed antitumour activity, and this very effectively so. Thus, the evidence suggests that DNA-DNA interstrand crosslinking is very important in determining antitumour action, and that some types of DNA-histone interaction may be biologically important but the binding of the whole nucleosome to DNA does not appear to contribute significantly to cytotoxicity. Further, it appears that by limiting bifunctional alkylation to fewer, more critical sites it may be possible to enhance antitumour effectiveness, whilst decreasing toxicity towards critically important normal systems.

REFERENCES

1. Finley WH, Carlson WW, Frommeyer WB, Woods JW: The bone marrow depressant and antitumour properties in animals of some new alkylating agents. Cancer (17): 1271-1277, 1964.

2. Goldacre RJ, Loveless R, Ross WCJ: Mode of production of chromosome abnormalities by nitrogen mustards: possible role of crosslinking. Nature (163): 667-669, 1949.

3. Alexander P: Reactions of carcinogens with macromolecules. Adv Cancer Res (2): 1-72, 1954.

4. Fahmy OG, Fahmy MJ: Cytogenic analysis of action of carcinogens and tumour inhibitors in Drosophila melanogaster: XI Mutagenic efficiency of mesyloxy esters on sperm in relation to molecular structure. Genetics (46): 1111-1123, 1961.

5. Bedford P, Fox BW: Repair of DNA interstrand crosslinks after busulphan. Cancer Chemother Pharmacol (8): 3-7, 1982.

6. Jones AR, Jones P: Alkylating esters, VIII The action of the isomers of dimethylmyleran on spermatogenesis. Experientia (30): 178-179, 1974.

7. Bedford P, Fox BW: DNA-DNA interstrand crosslinking by dimethane sulphonic acid esters. Biochem Pharmacol (32): 2297-2301, 1983.

8. Kohn KW, Erikson LC, Ewig RAG, Friedman CA: Fractionation of DNA from mammalian cells by alkaline elution. Biochemistry (15): 4629, 1979.

9. Hartley J, Fox BW (in preparation).

DNA REPAIR CHARACTERISTICS OF WALKER RAT CARCINOMA CELLS SENSITIVE AND RESISTANT TO CIS-DIAMMINEDICHLOROPLATINUM(II) (CISPLATIN) AND DIFUNCTIONAL ALKYLATING AGENTS

J.J. ROBERTS, C.J. RAWLINGS and F. FRIEDLOS

1. INTRODUCTION

Studies on cultured cells have indicated the likely relevance of platinum DNA binding to cytotoxicity following their treatment with cis-diamminedichloroplatinum(II) (cisplatin) (1,2). DNA has been shown to be the only macromolecular target that is large enough to undergo more than one hit per molecule at pharmacologically relevant doses (1). Current evidence favours the view that damage to DNA leads to the inhibition of DNA synthesis and this in turn leads to cell death probably as a consequence of associated chromosomal damage. Cisplatin and di-functional alkylating agents can react with DNA to form both inter- and intra-strand crosslinks, crosslinks between DNA and protein and mono-functional adducts. A correlation between interstrand crosslinking and cytotoxicity has been demonstrated in the case of cis and trans diamminedichloroplatinum(II)-treated Hela (3) Chinese hamster (4) and mouse cells (5,6). Again, investigations in mouse leukaemia cells and normal and transformed human cells of varying sensitivity to cisplatin have shown that sensitivity often correlates well with interstrand cross-link formation (7,8,9). No similar correlation has been found for DNA-protein crosslinking and cytotoxicity in Chinese hamster (4) or mouse cells (6). In order to assess the possible importance of DNA cross-link formation we have studied the DNA excision repair characteristics of two lines of Walker rat cells sensitive and resistant to cisplatin and difunctional cytotoxic agents but not to monofunctional, cytotoxic agents. Additionally we have examined the biochemical responses of the two cell lines to DNA damage.

2. SENSITIVITY OF WALKER CELLS TO CYTOTOXIC AGENTS

The two lines of Walker cells possessed markedly different sensitiv-ities to chlorambucil, as predicted by the original selection procedure.

Similar differences were found in the sensitivities of the two cell
lines to cisplatin (Fig. 1) and mustard gas (Fig. 2). On the other
hand the two cell lines exhibited equal sensitivity to the monofunctional methylating agent N-methyl-N-nitrosourea and neither cell
line was uniquely sensitive to this agent as compared with the effect of
this compound on a variety of other rodent and human cell lines.

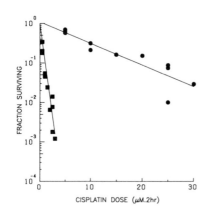 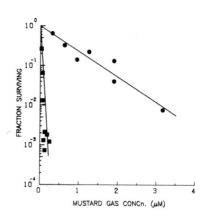

FIGURE 1.   FIGURE 2.

3. UPTAKE OF CYTOTOXIC DRUGS BY WALKER CELLS

The difference in the sensitivity of the two cell lines to the
difunctional cytotoxic agents was not due to a difference in drug uptake and in the subsequent reactions with target molecules as indicated
by essentially equal levels of reaction with the cellular macromolecules, DNA, RNA and protein of Walker sensitive and resistant cells
following their treatment with a range of concentrations of cisplatin.
Moreover equal levels of crosslinking of DNA were observed (by sucrose,
gradient sedimentation of labelled DNA) in the two cell lines following
a given dose of mustard gas.

4. LOSS OF PLATINUM ADDUCT FROM THE CELLULAR DNA OF WALKER CELLS

A difference in the response to DNA damage could result from differences in the way the two cell types process lesions on their DNA. More
specifically differences may exist in the way lesions on DNA are removed
by (a) DNA excision repair process(es).

4.1. Loss of total DNA bound adducts

Accordingly, we have examined the rate of loss of total DNA platinum adducts from cellular DNA with time after treatment with cisplatin. Least squares regression analysis of the data indicated half lives for the loss of platinum from DNA of 60 and 110 hours for Walker resistant and Walker sensitive cells, respectively.

4.2. Platinum-induced DNA interstrand and DNA protein crosslinks

The loss of DNA interstrand and DNA protein crosslinks were followed by means of alkaline elution analysis of labelled DNA at various times after treatment of Walker sensitive (Fig. 3) and resistant (Fig. 4) cells with cisplatin. The relatively small differences in either the

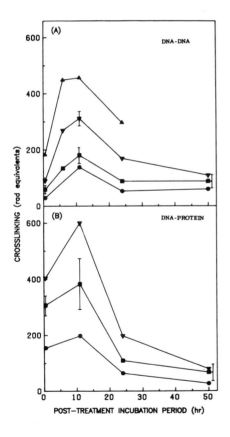

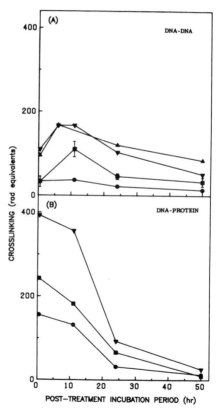

FIGURE 3.   FIGURE 4.

initial amounts formed or rates of loss of these lesions as between the two cell types was thought to be inadequate to account for the large difference in their sensitivity to cisplatin.

5. EFFECT OF DAMAGE TO DNA ON DNA SYNTHESIS IN SENSITIVE AND RESISTANT WALKER CELLS

The alternative possibility that the two cell lines might differ with respect to their abilities to replicate DNA on a damaged template was investigated. Since the cells responded in a similar relative manner to the toxic effects of cisplatin and sulphur mustard (SM), the latter agent was used in preference to cisplatin for studies of DNA synthesis since its very short half-life of reaction permitted a study of the effects on DNA synthesis of pulse treatments and under conditions that did not introduce additional perturbations of DNA synthesis in treated cells.

5.1. Effect on replicon initiation

DNA replicon initiation (10' pulse) was inhibited to a similar extent in both Walker sensitive and resistant cells immediately following treatment with SM.

5.2. Effect of SM on rate of DNA synthesis

The initial rate of DNA synthesis during a 4 hr. labelling period was inhibited to a similar extent in both cell lines following doses of SM up to 3 μM (0.48 μg/ml) (Fig. 5). A more detailed study of the effect of SM on DNA synthesis at later times after treatment, however, revealed possibly important differences as between the two cell lines. Again, both cell lines exhibited a comparable depression in rate of DNA synthesis (20' pulse) for up to 4 hours after treatment. Thereafter DNA synthesis was less depressed than previously in the resistant cell but continued to be further depressed in the sensitive cells (Fig. 6).

5.3. Effect of SM on elongation of DNA molecules

No differences were found as between the two cell lines in the rate of elongation (during 24 hours) of those nascent DNA molecules that had been synthesised, during 4 hours after treatment. These observations indicate that sensitive cells are not deficient in daughter-strand gap repair.

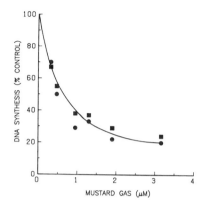

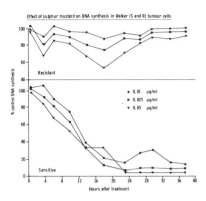

FIGURE 5.   FIGURE 6.

6. CONCLUSIONS

The small differences in the excision repair characteristics of
sensitive and resistant Walker tumour cells would seem to be inadequate
to account for the large differences in their sensitivities to
difunctional cytotoxic agents. On the other hand, their different
responses with regard to temporal effects on the inhibition of DNA
replication at late times after treatment would suggest that a particular
lesion(s), probably in chromatin, that affects the control of DNA
replication is either formed preferentially or repaired less
efficiently in the sensitive cell as compared with the resistant cell.

REFERENCES

1. Roberts JJ, Thomson AJ: The mechanism of action of antitumor platinum
   compounds. Progr Nucl Acid Res Mol Biol (22): 71-133, 1979.
2. Roberts JJ: Cisplatin in Cancer Chemotherapy. The EORTC Cancer
   Chemotherapy Annual 4. Pinedo HM (ed). Elsevier Medica Amsterdam,
   Oxford, 1982, pp.95-117.
3. Pascoe JM, Roberts JJ: Interactions between mammalian cell DNA and
   inorganic platinum compounds. I DNA interstrand crosslinking and
   cytotoxic properties of platinum II compounds. Biochem Pharmacol
   (23): 1345-1357, 1974a.
4. Zwelling LA, Bradley MO, Sharkey NA, Anderson T, Kohn KW: Cytotoxicity
   and DNA crosslinking in Chinese hamster cells treated with cis and
   trans Pt.II diammine dichloride. Mutation Res (67): 271-280, 1979.
5. Zwelling LA, Kohn KW, Ross WE, Ewis RAG, Anderson T: Kinetics of
   formation and disappearance of a DNA crosslinking effect in mouse

leukemia L1210 cells treated with cis- and trans-diamminedichloro platinum(II). Cancer Res (38): 1762–1768, 1978.

6. Zwelling LA, Anderson T, Kohn KW: DNA-protein and DNA interstrand crosslinking by cis- and trans-platinum(II) diamminedichloride in L1210 mouse leukemia cells in relation to cytotoxicity. Cancer Res (39): 365-369, 1979a.

7. Zwelling LA, Michaels S, Schwartz H, Dobson PP and Kohn KW. DNA crosslinking as an indicator of sensitivity and resistance of mouse L1210 leukemia cells to cis-diamminedichloro platinum (II) and L-phenylalanine mustard. Cancer Res (41): 640-649, 1981.

8. Erickson LC, Zwelling LA, Ducore JM, Sharkey NA, Kohn KW: Differential cytotoxicity and DNA crosslinking in normal and transformed human fibroblasts treated with cis-diamminedichloroplatinum(II). Cancer Res (41): 2791-2794, 1981.

9. Laurent G, Erickson LC, Sharkey NA, Kohn KW: DNA crosslinking and cytotoxicity induced by cis diamminedichloroplatinum(II) on human normal and tumor cell lines. Cancer Res (41): 3347-3351, 1981.

10. Meyn RE, Jenkins SF, Thompson LH. Defective removal of DNA cross-links in a repair-deficient mutant of Chinese hamster cells. Cancer Res (42): 3106-3110, 1982.

11. Ducore JM, Erickson LC, Zwelling LA, Laurent G, Kohn KW. Comparative studies of DNA crosslinking and cytotoxicity in Burketts lymphoma cell lines treated with cis-diamminedichloroplatinum(II) and L-phenylalanine mustard. Cancer Res (42): 897-902, 1982.

12. Strandberg MC, Bresnick E, Eastman A: The significance of DNA cross-linking to cis diamminedichloroplatinum(II)-induced cytotoxicity in sensitive and resistant lines of murine leukemia L1210 cells. Chem Biol Interactions (39): 169-180, 1982.

13. Shooter KV, House R, Merrifield RK, Robins AB: The interaction of platinum(II) compounds with bacteriophage T7 and R17. Chem Biol Interactions (5): 289-307, 1972.

14. Filipski J, Kohn KW, Bonner WM: The nature of inactivating lesions produced by platinum(II) complexes in phage γ DNA. Chem Biol Interactions (32): 321-336, 1980.

15. Tisdale MJ, Phillips BJ: Alterations in adenosine 3',5'-monophosphate-binding protein in Walker carcinoma cells sensitive or resistant to alkylating agents. Biochem Pharmacol (25): 1831-1836, 1976.

IS ALKYLATING AGENT "PRIMING" A DNA REPAIR PHENOMENON?

J.L.MILLAR, B.C. MILLAR, M. TILBY AND B.D.EVANS.

1. INTRODUCTION

   In the late sixties Jeney, Connors and Jones (1) showed
that a low dose of merophan could reduce the toxicity of a
second high dose of the same drug or melphalan. Similar
protection against radiation-induced death was also demonstrated
when mice were pretreated with colchicine or vinca alkaloids (2).
In 1975 Millar and coworkers showed that the recovery of bone
marrow CFUs, in mice receiving a small dose of cyclophosphamide
2 days before a high dose of busulphan, was enhanced (3).
The same group has since shown that the enhanced recovery of
normal tissue is not accompanied by a protective effect
towards the tumour (4,5). This phenomenon has been called
"priming" and has been demonstrated using a range of drugs
including cytosine arabinoside (AraC) as the "priming" (i.e.
small dose) agent. Notable exceptions are radiation and
busulphan (6).

2. PROCEDURE

2.1. Materials and methods

   2.1.1. In vitro. The routine handling of Chinese hamster
cells V79-753B and experimental design have been described
previously (7). Normal human bone marrow was aspirated via
illiac crest puncture. After washing cells were resuspended
at a concentration of 10^6/ml in RPMI containing 15% of either
normal or CY sera and 1.0 µCi/ml ^{3}H-TdR. All sera were
dialysed prior to use to remove inhibitors. 1.0 ml samples
were incubated overnight in an atmosphere of 5% CO_2 / 95% air
after which the cells were pelleted through oil (8) to remove

the media and the incorporated radioactivity counted. Each
patient's sera was examined at least twice.

2.1.2. In vivo. In the split dose experiments with cyclophosphamide (cy) C57 bl. male mice were used (9). In all
other experiments CBA mice were used.

2.1.3. Chemicals. Melphalan (Wellcome Laboratories) was
dissolved in 2% acid/ethanol; cy (Koch-Light Laboratories) and
4-hydroperoxycyclophosphamide (4-OOH cy) (kindly supplied by
Boehringer Ingelheim Hospital Division) were dissolved in
saline. 3-aminobenzamide was kindly supplied by Dr. S. Shall.
Chloroquine, cycloheximide and caffeine were obtained from
Sigma Chemical Company.

3. RESULTS AND DISCUSSION

Animals given a "priming" dose of 50 mg/kg cy survived a
challenge dose of 400 mg/kg cy, normally the LD_{50}. If this
challenge dose was increased to 500 mg/kg the animals died.
However, if the challenge dose was administered over 24 hours,
50% of "primed" animals survived a total dose of 600 mg/kg cy,
a dose lethal to control animals irrespective of the time
course of drug administration (9). These findings suggested
that repair enzymes may have been induced that require a finite
time for expression. However, attempts to block "priming" by
cy or melphalan in vivo using established inhibitors of DNA
repair, viz caffeine, chloroquine, cycloheximide and 3-amino-
benzamide, given over a variety of dosages and schedules have
proved ineffective. Additionally, "priming" does not affect
the dose response curve of bone marrow, in vivo, towards
alkylating agents (4,10). If repair enzymes are induced by
"priming" it would be predicted that the sensitivity of cells
would be reduced in "primed" animals compared with unprimed
controls.

Attempts to reproduce the "priming" phenomenon in vitro,
have proved negative. Using Chinese hamster cells a "priming"
dose of melphalan was administered 3.5 or 20 hours before
graded doses of melphalan. Examination of cell survival using
either drug schedule showed that such treatment did not enhance

the colony forming ability of these cells in vitro (Fig 1).
Similar negative results have been obtained using 4-OOH cy
"prime" prior to a challenge with melphalan (unpublished
observation).

Previous data has shown that the enhancement of recovery of
normal tissues after "priming" occurs in those tissues which
have an hierarchical structure (5,10), the stem cells undergo
several divisions during which time the progeny become committed
to differentiation resulting in an end cell which does not
divide further. Since Chinese hamster cells are a continuous
cell line and show no capacity for differentiation it is
arguable that this system is an inappropriate model for
comparison with events occurring in normal tissues, in vivo,
following a chemical insult. It seems more likely that the
results in vitro are analogous to the response of tumour cells
in vivo, which show no enhanced recovery following a "priming"
treatment (4,5).

An alternative explanation is that "priming" may induce the
release of some factor(s) which stimulates the stem cell
compartment of normal tissues to divide without the concomitant
commitment to differentiation. Such a model predicts that
when the challenge dose of drug is administered the survival
of animals is secured due to the expansion of this compartment
compared with that in control animals, even though the absolute
amount of cell killing may be the same in both groups. When
the stimulation of incorporation of ^{3}H-TdR into autologous
bone marrow was examined, using sera from patients taken at
different times after cy, there was marked stimulation of
^{3}H-TdR incorporation using 10 days post cy sera (Fig 2),
compared with that seen in cells exposed to normal serum;
followed by a decrease at later time intervals. This result
confirmed that some factor(s) is released into the blood stream
following treatment with an alkylating agent that is capable
of stimulating DNA synthesis (11) in bone marrow cells.
Experiments are now in progress to determine the nature of
this factor(s), and whether it is involved in the "priming"
phenomenon in vivo.

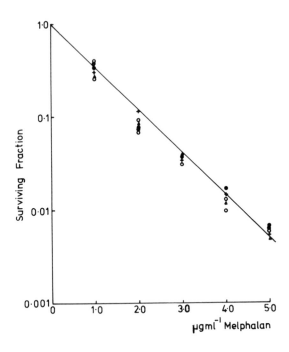

FIGURE 1. The effect of melphalan priming on V-79 cells
in vitro. O control cells, ● cells "primed" 20 hours before
challenge, + cells "primed" 3.5 hours before challenge, △
"primed" medium.

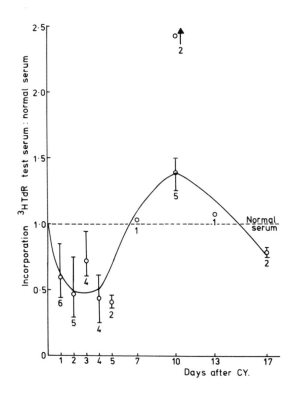

FIGURE 2. Stimulation of ^{3}H-TdR uptake into allogenic human bone marrow cells <u>in vitro</u> by sera from patients treated with cyclophosphamide. Numbers under the experimental points refer to size of each group.

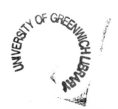

References
1. Jeney A jr, Connors TA, Jones M: The toxicity of merophan after treatment with subtoxic dose. Acta Physiol Acad Scien Hung Tomus (33):89-94,1968.
2. Smith WW, Wilson SM: Effects of vinblastine and vincristine on survival and haemopoiesis in irradiated mice. J Nat Can Inst (39):1055-1066,1967.
3. Millar JL, Hudspith BN, Blackett: Reduced lethality in mice receiving a combined dose of cyclophosphamide and busulphan. Br J Cancer (32):193-198,1975.
4. Millar JL, McElwain TJ: Combinations of cytotoxic agents that have much less than expected toxicity on normal tissues in mice. Antibiotics Chemother (23):271-282,1978.
5. Millar JL, Stephens TC, Wist EA: An explanation for the ability of cytotoxic drug pretreatment to reduce bone marrow related lethality of total body irradiation (TBI). Inc J Radiation Oncology Biol Phys (8):581-583,1982.
6. Millar JL, Blackett NM, Hudspith BN: Enhanced post-irradiation recovery of the haemopoietic system in animals pretreated with a variety of cytotoxic agents. Cell Tissue Kinet (II):543-553,1978.
7. Millar BC, Jinks S: The effect of dexamethasone on the radiation survival response and misonidazole induced hypoxic-cell toxicity in Chinese Hamster cells V-79-753B in vitro. Br J Radiol (54):505-511,1981.
8. Millar JL, McElwain TJ, Clutterbuck RD, Wist EA: The modification of melphalan toxicity in tumour bearing mice by S-2-(3-aminoprophylamino)-cyclophorothioic acid (WR 2721). Am J Clin Oncol (5):321-328,1982.
9. Evans BD, Smith IE, Clutterbuck RD, Millar JL: Prevention of acute deaths in mice after very high dose cyclophosphamide by a divided dose schedule. Br J Cancer (48):(In press).
10.Millar JL, Hudspith BN, McElwain TJ, Phelps TA: Effects of high-dose melphalan on marrow and intestinal epithelium in mice pretreated with cyclophosphamide. Br J Cancer (38): 137-142,1978.
11.Burke PJ, Diggs CH, Owens AH jr: Factors in human serum affecting the proliferation of normal and leukaemic cells Cancer Res (33):800-806,1973.

DTIC INDUCES DAMAGE IN MELANOMA DNA DURING SEMI-CONSERVATIVE DNA SYNTHESIS

U. LÖNN AND S. LÖNN

1. INTRODUCTION

   DTIC is an anti-neoplastic drug used in treatment of various malignant diseases such as lymphomas, sarcomas and melanomas. The mechanisms by which it exerts its cytotoxic effects is poorly understood although it is known that some of the metabolites formed from DTIC by liver microsomal enzymes exert cytotoxic functions (1-3).

   DTIC is a purine-analogue and should theoretically be able to interact with cellular DNA. Therefore we have analysed the effect of DTIC on the synthesis of DNA replication intermediates as well as the stability of steady-state labelled and pulse-labelled DNA during treatment with DTIC. To characterise the DNA we have used cell lysis in dilute alkali which releases small DNA fragments from bulk DNA (4,5). The DNA fragments can then be separated by agarose gel electrophoresis. Using this approach we have shown that DTIC induces damage in the DNA during semi-conservative DNA synthesis.

2. MATERIALS AND METHODS

   A human melanoma cell line (CRL 1424), obtained from Flow Laboratories was grown as monolayers at 37°C in 5% CO_2 in air. The culture medium was Eagle minimal essential medium with Earle's salt mixture, 2mM 1-glutamine, 10% foetal calf serum and antibiotics (5).

   For experiments, the cells were seeded in small culture dishes (35x10mm) with 3ml medium 24h before the addition of 100μCi tritiated thymidine (Amersham Center, UK) and the incubation performed for desired length of time. Aphidicolin was dissolved in ethanol before the addition to the cell cultures. DTIC-Dome (dacarbazine) was obtained from a local pharmacy. Fresh solutions were always made up immediately before starting experiments. All our experiments were performed in the dark since degradation of DTIC may occur in light.

   To lyse the cells the medium was drained from the culture dish and the cells rinsed twice in cold phosphate-buffered saline. Cell lysis was performed in the dark at 0°C by the addition of 2.25ml of 0.03M NaOH. After 30min the solution was neutralised by the addition of 0.9ml of 0.067M/0.02M NaH$_2$PO$_4$. Finally the solution was made 0.5% in SDS and after 30min at room temperature the DNA was analysed in 0.75% agarose gels (6).

The 0.75% agarose flat bed gels were made as decribed earlier (7). The labelled DNA was separated in the agarose gel using a LKB Multiphor electrophoretic system. The gels were gut into 1mm-thick slices that were assayed for radioactivity with a toluene-based scintillation fluid containing 3% Soluene 100 in a Packard scintillation counter.

3. RESULTS AND DISCUSSION

As biological material we use cultured human malignant melanoma cells. To analyse the DNA the cells are lysed in dilute alkali which removes macromolecules from the DNA and disrupts the base pair structure of the DNA. However, the DNA strands cannot separate before enough time has elapsed to allow unwinding of the DNA. The unwinding is initiated at gaps present in the DNA chains. Such gaps are known to exist e.g. during the process of synthesis of new DNA chains. When the alkaline solution is neutralised the high molecular weight DNA is renatured and forms double-stranded DNA. However, small DNA fragments generated by the action of drugs or small DNA replication intermediates will not renature and remain in the solution as single-stranded DNA molecules. The single-stranded DNA molecules can then be separated by agarose gel electrophoresis (5,6).

3.1 DNA replication intermediates formed in undisturbed cells

In steady-state labelled DNA one can detect only labelled high molecular weight DNA close to the trough of the agarose gel, and no labelled DNA fragments entering the gel. However in pulse-labelling experiments one can detect apart from the high molecular weight DNA also two well defined populations of DNA replication intermediates, Okazaki-fragments and a 10kb DNA population (5,6).

When cells released from hydroxyurea-block into the S-phase are examined, one can detect first labelled Okazaki-fragments and then also labelled 10kb DNA and high molecular weight DNA, indicating that the 10kb DNA fragmenmts are formed from the Okazaki-fragments (8). So far we have not been able to chase leabelled Okazaki-fragments into 10kb DNA molecules. The reason for our inability to do this experiment is probably that the Okazaki-fragments are joined together to larger molecules by DNA polymerase α whereas the 10kb DNA molecules are joined together to form high molecular weight DNA by another enzyme or set of enzymes. This is inferred from the finding that aphidicolin, which is a specific inhibitor of DNA polymerase α (9), prevents the joining of Okazaki-fragments but allows already formed 10kb DNA to give rise to high molecular weight DNA (5).

3.2 DTIC induces fragmentation of DNA

To examine the effect of DTIC on steady-state labelled DNA we performed the following experiments. Cells were labelled with tritiated thymidine for 24h and then cultivated for another 24h in fresh medium. DTIC (10μg/ml) was then added to the culture medium; after incubation for 60min in the dark the cells were lysed in dilute alkali and the labelled DNA separated in 0.75% agarose gels. Control cells that had not been treated with DTIC were analysed in parallel. The electrophoretic separation of DNA from DTIC-treated cells showed that apart from the high molecular weight DNA there is also a population of DNA fragments located at slices 23-20. The fragments are not present in control cells. Furthermore if the cells are lysed at neutral pH one cannot detect the fragments indicating that DTIC induces alkali-labile bonds in the DNA.

3.3 Aphidicolin prevents DTIC from fragmenting the DNA

DTIC is a purine-analogue and should therefore theoretically have the possibility to function as a DNA precursor. If so, it is possible that the induction of alkali-labile bonds in the DNA occurs during semi-conservative DNA synthesis. Aphidicolin is a specific inhibitor of DNA polymerase α and thereby inhibits DNA synthesis (9). We therefore examined whether aphidicolin may prevent DTIC from inducing damage in the DNA. Cells with steady-state labelled DNA were treated with aphidicolin for 60min before the addition of DTIC. The cells were subsequently lysed in dilute alkali and the DNA then analysed by agarose gel electrophoresis. The results showed that there is no fragmentation of the DNA by DTIC cells pretreated with aphidicolin. Hence it is not possible for DTIC to induce alkali-labile bonds in the DNA in cells without functioning DNA polymerase α. We have earlier shown that in cells treated with aphidicolin for 60min there is no movement of the replication fork (5).

3.4 DTIC preferentially damages newly synthesised DNA

To investigate whether DTIC interferes with the formation of DNA replication intermediates we performed pulse-labelling experiments in the presence of DTIC. First we analysed the DNA labelled during a 5min pulse with thymidine placed at the end of the drug-treatment period of 60min. The results showed that the label was incorporated into Okazaki-fragments but not into high molecular weight DNA or 10kb DNA, indicating that there is no movement of the replication forks in cells treated with DTIC for 60min. When cells were treated with DTIC for shorter time-periods we found that a treatment for 30min is needed to stop the movement of the replication forks. Therefore we analysed cells pulsed with tritiated thymidine during the first 5min of the treatment with DTIC, which was for 60min. When the DNA was separated by agarose gel electrophoresis the results showed that the majority of the labelled DNA was located at slices 23-30, i.e. the location of DNA fragments released from steady-state labelled DNA as described in 3.2. There was also some label in Okazaki-fragments but there was no labelled high molecular weight DNA or 10kb DNA. Hence the DNA synthesised during the first 5min of the treatment with DTIC is completely fragmented.

3.5 Conclusion

In conclusion, we have shown that DTIC induces damage in melanoma DNA. This can be detected as the formation of alkali-labile bonds in the DNA. The lesions are not induced in cells without functioning DNA polymerase α. Furthermore, DTIC preferentially induces damage in newly synthesised DNA. The results indicate that DTIC induces damage in melanoma DNA during semi-conservative DNA synthesis.

4. ACKNOWLEDGEMENTS

This work was supported by grants from the Swedish Cancer Society, T R Söderbergs Foundation, Magnus Bergvalls Foundation and Karolinska Institutet.

5. REFERENCES
1. Montgomery JA: Cancer Treat Rep (60): 125-134, 1976.
2. Bono V: Cancer Treat Rep (60): 141-148, 1976.
3. Loo TL, Housholder G, Gerulath AH, Saunders P, Farquhar D: Cancer Treat Rep (60): 149-152, 1976.
4. Ahnström G, Erixon H: In: Friedberg E, Hanawalt PM (eds) DNA Repair, A Laboratory Manual of Research Procedures, Part B. Marcel Dekker Inc, 1981, pp 403-418.
5. Lönn U, Lönn S: Proc Natl Acad Sci (USA) (80): 3996-3999, 1983.

6. Lönn U: Chromosoma (84): 663-673, 1982.
7. Lönn U: Cell (13): 727-733, 1978.
8. Lönn U: Cell Biology International Reports (6): 687-696, 1982.
9. Huberman J: Cell (23): 647-648, 1981.

THE NON-RANDOM BINDING OF CHLORAMBUCIL TO DNA IN CHROMATIN

A. JENEY, K.R. HARRAP AND R.M. ORR

INTRODUCTION

DNA is intimately associated with nuclear proteins in the highly organised chromatin structure. It is conceivable that the molecular pharmacology of drugs acting on DNA may be better elucidated if more attention is devoted to their overall reaction with chromatin. This view has been accepted in several laboratories where important data have emerged from studies on chromatin alterations induced by antitumour drugs (1-4). It is now becoming apparent that the constraints upon DNA in chromatin may be major determinants of drug access to and the ensuing damage of DNA (5-7). In this communication data demonstrating the relevance of the subunit structure of chromatin to the action of chlorambucil are presented.

PROCEDURES

The alkylating agent-sensitive and -resistant lines of the Walker 256 carcinosarcoma were used. Female Wistar rats were transplanted i.p. with 2 x 10^6 cells and chlorambucil treatments were given subcutaneously in dimethyl sulphoxide. $3H$-chlorambucil (936mCi/mmol) was prepared by the Radiochemical Centre (Amersham, Bucks, England). The technique applied for isolation of chromatin fractions was based on the observations that DNA wrapped around the core particle is much les easily digested by micrococcal nuclease than linker DNA. Purified nuclei were incubated for various times at 37°C with 2 or 50 units of micrococcal nuclease per 1 OD_{260} unit of nuclei, either in 50mM Tris-HCL, 25mM KCl, 1mM $MgCl_2$, 10mM $CaCl_2$, 0.25M sucrose, pH 7.5 (high salt medium), or in 1mM $CaCl_2$, 10mM NaCl, 3mM MgCl, 10mM Tris-HCl, pH 7.4 (low salt medium). Digestion was terminated by adding EDTA to 20mM final concentration. To estimate the efficiency of nuclease digestion, samples were taken at various intervals and DNA precipitated with 1M $HClO_4$ containing 1M NaCl. Digested DNA was measured optically in the supernatant after centrifugation. Nuclei were centrifuged at 1000g for 10min to remove the released chromatin segments (S_1 fraction containing digested linker DNA). The nuclei (P_1) were

407

lysed in 1mM EDTA and separated into oligonucleosomal (S_2) and polynucleosomal (P_2) fractions by centrifugation at 3000g for 20min. The oligonucleosomal fraction was sedimented on a 5-30% sucrose gradient in 1mM EDTA, 0.5M NaCl, 1mM sodium phosphate buffer, pH 7.4, in an MSE 65 Superspeed centrifuge at 29,000rpm for 16 hours. Oligonucleosomes of various lengths were characterised by measuring their template capacity for DNA polymerase activity and thermal denaturation profiles. The reaction mixture for the DNA polymerase assay contained 0.5 units of DNA polymerase (Micrococcus luteus), 50pmoles dATP, 200pmoles dGTP, dCTP and ^{3}H-TTP (0.1μCi), 2μmoles $MgCl_2$, 0.05M Tris-HCl, pH 7.4, 200μg bovine serum albumin and the relevant chromatin fraction corresponding to 10μg of DNA. Radioactivity was measured in DNA collected on Whatman G/F discs afer precipitation with 10% trichloracetic acid. The thermal denaturation of chromatin fractions were measured after dialysis against 0.25mM EDTA in a Cary 219 spectrophotometer.

RESULTS AND DISCUSSION

Chromatin structure was studied by digesting nuclei with micrococcal nuclease in low and high salt medium. Fig. 1 shows that in high salt medium condensed chromatin is much less sensitive to micrococcal nuclease digestion than in low salt medium. Chlorambucil treatment gives rise to changes in the limit digest of chromatin only in the low salt medium. In this case there was a definite enhancement of DNA digestion afer 6 hours treatment with chlorambucil.

Digestion of Walker tumour nuclei by M. nuclease after in vivo treatment with Chlorambucil

Fig 1

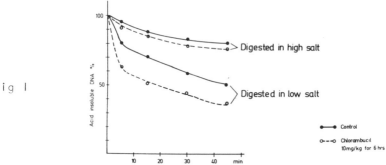

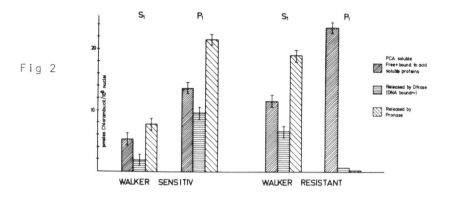

Detection of ^{3}H-Chlorambucil in chromatin fragments solubilized by M. nuclease (S_1) and polynucleosomal fraction (P_1)

F i g 2

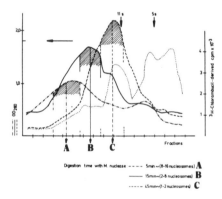

Separation of oligonucleosomes (S_2) in 5-20% sucrose containing 0,5M NaCl

F i g 3

Fig. 2 shows chlorambucil concentrations in chromatin fragments solubilised by micrococcal nuclease (S_1) and the polynucleosomal fraction (P_1) 6hr after treatment with 12.4mg/kg chlorambucil the Walker sensitive and resistant tumour nuclei contained simlar amounts of chlorambucil (and its metabolites), 59.2 and 64.2pmoles per 10^8 nuclei respectively. However, there was a remarkable difference in the distribution of the drug among the chromatin fractions and in drug binding to DNA and protein. In the S_1 fraction much more chlorambucil was recovered in the resistant than in the sensitive Walker tumour. In the sensitive line the majority of the drug could be released only with the pronase digestion, while a significant amount was present in the DNA of the polynucleosomal fraction. On the contrary, no chlorambucil could be detected in the polynucleosomal DNA of the Walker resistant tumour, in which the drug was associated primarly with acid soluble material (histones).

Fig. 3 shows the separation of oligonucleosomes by sucrose density gradient sedimentation. Chlorambucil-derived radioactivity appeared both in the monomer region and at the top of the gradient.

CHLORAMBUCIL ACTION ON NUCLEOSOMES

Fig 4

Characterisation of nucleosomes :		SDG FRACTIONS		
		A	B	C
Tm point (°C)	Control	77°C	76°C	70°C
	Chlorambucil	77°C	75°C	70°C
Hyperchromocity (%)	Control	21.5%	23.9%	30.0%
	Chlorambucil	24.3%	27.6%	28.7%
Template activity[+]	Control[++]	2.9	3.4	4.8
	Chlorambucil[+++]	83%	60%	50%

[+] = Incorporation of ³H-TTP in the presence of DNA polymerase
[++] = x 10⁴ cpm per mg DNA
[+++] = % of control

Digestion time with M. nuclease ---- 5min ~(8-16 nucleosomes) A
——— 15min ~(2-8 nucleosomes) B
---- 45min~(1-2 nucleosomes) C

Fig. 4 compares the analyses on the individual fractions. Tm, hyperchromocity, and template activity were related to the length of the oligonucleosome chain. The reduction of template activity induced by chlorambucil was most apparent in the mononucleosomal fraction.

These data indicate that chlorambucil binds to chromatin in a non-random fashion; certain core particles appear to be attacked preferentially by this drug. After removing non-histone-associated chlorambucil from chromatin by including 0.5M NaCl in the sucrose gradient, more radioactivity was measured in the monomer than in the longer oligonucleosomal fractions. This observation, together with the reduced template capacity of the monomer fractions, may be regarded as an indication of the uniqueness of drug binding within chromatin. The difference in binding between the sensitive and resistant Walker tumours is also worthy of note. It is possible that the antitumour properties of chlorambucil depend upon the alkylation of core-DNA and the modification of non-histones associated with the core-particle.

REFERENCES

1. Jeney A, Szabo I, Szabo J, Valyi-Nagy T, Institoris L: Pharmaco-biochemical studies on cytotoxic polyol-derivatives. II. The effect of biological alkyating agents on the thermal-denaturation properties of DNA. Eur J Cancer (6):297-303, 1970.
2. Harrap KR, Riches PG, Gascoigne EW, Sellwood SM, Cashman CC: The alkylating agent: Does a knowledge of its mode of action suggest leads for improving its therapeutic effectiveness? In: Davis W, Maltoni C (es) Biological Characterisation of Human Tumours. Excerpta-Medica Amsterdam-Oxford, 1976, pp 106-121.
3. Jeney A, Dzurillay E, Lapis K, Valko E: Chromatin proteins as a possible target for antitumour agents: Alterations of chromatin proteins in Dibromodulcitol treated Yoshida tumours. Chem-Biol Interactions (26): 349-361, 1979.
4. Wolf H, Raydt G, Puschendorf B, Grunicke H: Effect of the alkylating agent triethyleneiminobenzoquinone on the synthesis of DNA and on the incorporation of (^{3}H)-lysine into nuclear proteins of Ehrlich ascites tumour cells. FEBS Letters (35): 336-340, 1973.
5. Tew KD, Sudhakar S, Schein PS, Smulson ME: Binding of chlorozotocin and 1-(2-chloroethyl)3-cyclohexyl-1-nitrosourea to chromatin and nucleosomal fractions of HeLa cells. Cancer Res (38):3371-3378, 1978.
6. Jeney A, Harrap KR: Chromatin in normal and tumour cells. In: Letnansky K (ed) Biology of the Cancer Cell. Kugler Publications Amsterdam, 1980, pp 389-398.
7. Harrap KR, Jeney A, Thraves PJ, Riches PG, Wilkinson R: Macromolecular targets and metabolic properties of alkylating drugs. In: Sartorelli AC, Lazo JS, Bertino JR (eds) Molecular Actions and Targets for Cancer Chemotherapeutic Agents. Academic Press, New York, 1981, pp 45-84.

ALKYLATING ANTITUMOUR AGENTS DECREASE HISTONE ACETYLATION IN EHRLICH-ASCITES TUMOUR CELLS

H. GRUNICKE, H. ZWIERZINA, A. LOIDL, W. HELLIGER AND B. PUSCHENDORF

SUMMARY

Treatment of Ehrlich-ascites tumour cells with the alkylating agents triaziquonum, N-mustard (chlormethin, cyclophosphamide and 4-(2-sulfonatoethylthio)-cyclophosphamide decreases the acetylation of core histones. The effect is not due to an inhibition of acetyl CoA formation. Depression of histone acetylation occurs at all concentrations of the drug which cause a significant inhibition of cell proliferation.

INTRODUCTION

The detailed mechanism by which alkylating agents inhibit cell proliferation is still obscure. For more than two decades attention has been focused on the interaction of alkylating agents with DNA (for review see 1). However, if chromatin is assumed to be the essential target of alkylating drugs, alterations of other chromatin constituents may be equally important. Effects of alkylating agents on nuclear proteins have been reported (2-6).

In this paper it is demonstrated that alkylating agents depress the acetylation of histones - a postsynthetic modification which has gained special attention due to its possible role in the regulation of chromatin structure and function (7).

MATERIALS AND METHODS

Ehrlich ascites tumour cells were grown and harvested as described elsewhere (2). Determination of antitumour activity was performed as described previously (2). N-mustard (chlormethin) was obtained from Sigma Chemicals, Munich, Germany. Triaziquonum (2,3,5-trisethyleneiminobenzoquinone-1,4) was a gift from Bayer

413

A.G., Leverkusen, Germany. Cyclophosphamide and its derivative
4-(2-sulfonatoethylthio)cyclophosphamide were donated by ASTA-
Werke A.G., Bielefeld, Germany. Histones were labelled by i.p.
injection of either 2 mCi ^{3}H-acetate (specific activity 2.8 mCi/
mmol or o.o4 mCi ^{3}H-lysine (specific activity 68.4 Ci/mmol) per
animal as indicated. Cells were collected 3o min after administra
tion of the label. Histones were prepared as described previously (8) and fractionated by slab gel electrophoresis employing
either: Sodiumdodecylsulfate (SDS)-polyacrylamide gels (o.o75x14x
32 cm) according to Laemmli (9) or Triton-X-1oo containing polyacrylamide gels (o.o75x14x48 cm) as described by Cohen et al. (1o).
Gels were stained with Coomassie blue and scanned in a Beckman
DU 8 spectrophotometer. Protein was determined by the Lowry procedure (13). DNA was determined as described by Keck (14).

RESULTS AND DISCUSSION

Table 1 demonstrates that alkylating agents inhibit the incorporation of ^{3}H-acetate into histones of Ehrlich-ascites tumour
cells. Alkylating agents have been shown to inhibit the biosynthesis of histones and to reduce the histone/DNA-ratio (3,4).
However, the uptake of label from ^{3}H-acetate is independent of
protein synthesis as indicated by its resistance to puromycin.
Furthermore, the histone/DNA-ratio was found to be unchanged
during exposure to the drug (1.35±o.2 mg/mg in the controls
versus 1.32±o.1 mg/mg in cells 3 hrs after treatment with 1o^{-5}
moles/kg triaziquonum). One has to conclude, therefore, that the
alkylating agents reduce the acetylation of the histones. As can
be seen (table 2) acetylation of all core histones is reduced, but
H3 seems to be less affected compared to H2A, H2B and H4. Furthermore, not only the uptake of label from ^{3}H-acetate but also the
extent of acetylation is depressed. Table 3 demonstrates that
there is a slight but significant dose dependent decrease in the
relative acetylation of H4.

The depression of histone acetylation is not simply due
to a decrease in the number of living cells during exposure
to the drug. The cells maintain their capacity for phospholipid
synthesis (table 4). That vital functions are preserved for

at least 12 hr after treatment with triaziquonum (10^{-6} moles/kg) or cyclophosphamide (10^{-5} moles/kg) had been reported previously (3,15). Table 4 demonstrates that the depression of histone acetylation is not explained by an impaired synthesis of acetyl-CoA.

As can be seen from table 1 the reduction of histone acetylation is expressed at all concentrations of alkylating agents that cause a significant inhibition of cell multiplication. It is conceivable, therefore, that there is a causal relation between depression of histone acetylation and antitumour activity.

The detailed biological function of histone acetylation is still unknown. Numerous reports indicate a possible correlation of histone acetylation with the regulation of transcription (7). One might expect, therefore, that a depression of histone acetylation should affect RNA-synthesis. Reduced in vitro transcription of chromatin from cells treated with triaziquonum has been reported previously (16).

Tab. 1   Effect of alkylating agents on the incorporation of ^{3}H-acetate into histones and on cell multiplication of Ehrlich-ascites tumour cells.

Alkylating agents were applied in 0.2 ml 0.14 M NaCl i.p. Controls received the solvent only. Cells were collected 2 hr after administration of triaziquonum and N-mustard and 12 hr after exposure to cyclophosphamide and sulfidocyclophosphamide respectively. Puromycin was given 15 min before the ^{3}H-acetate label. This puromycin concentration reduces lysine incorporation into proteins to less than 5 % of the controls (data not shown).

	^{3}H-acetate incorporation (% of control)						Cell multiplication (% of control)				
Drug (moles/kg)	5.10^{-8}	10^{-7}	2.10^{-7}	10^{-6}	10^{-5}	10^{-4}	5.10^{-8}	10^{-7}	10^{-6}	10^{-5}	10^{-4}
Triaziquonum	97	83		57	41		93	45	3		
N-mustard				68	56	37		69	17	5	
Cyclophosphamide				88	75	66		80	30	21	
Sulfido-cyclophosphamide [+]				93	54	66					
Puromycin			112								

[+] 4-(2-sulfonatoethylthio)-cyclophosphamide

<u>Tab.2</u> ^{3}H-acetate incorporation into core histones after treatment with triaziquonum and N-mustard

Treatment with the alkylating agents was performed as described in legend to Tab.1. Histones labelled with ^{3}H-acetate in vivo were analysed by SDS-polyacrylamide electrophoresis as described under "Methods". Samples containing 1oo ug of protein were applied. The data represent the results of a quantiative evaluation of densito-metric scans from fluorographs. Fluorography was performed as described under "Methods". Total exposure time was 88 days at -7o°C. The data are given as % of the control, i.e. the value for the corresponding histone fraction of the control was set as 1oo%.

Drug

Histone fraction		% of control			
		H2A	H2B	H3	H4
Triaziquonum	1o^{-5} moles/kg	25.7	26.1	7o.3	32.1
N-mustard	1o^{-5} moles/kg	41.1	44.7	63.6	41.2

<u>Tab.3</u> Effect of N-mustard on the level of acetylation of histone H4

Tumour cells were collected 4 hr after exposure to the alky-lating agent. Histones were analysed on Triton-X-1oo containing polyacrylamide slab-gels as described under "Methods". Samples containing 1oo ug of protein were applied. This system separates the histone H4 subfractions differing in the level of acetylation. Relative acetylation of H4 was measured by scanning Coomassie blue-stained gels as described elsewhere (8).

N-mustard	Relative acetylation of H4 as % of the control
1o^{-6} moles/kg	98.3 $\pm$ 1.9
1o^{-5} moles/kg	86.7 $\pm$ 3.5
1o^{-4} moles/kg	76.5 $\pm$ 2.o

<u>Tab.4</u> Incorporation of ^{3}H-acetate into phospholipids of Ehrlich-ascites tumour cells after treatment with triaziquonum

Tumour-bearing mice received 2 mCi ^{3}H-acetate (specific activity 2.8 Ci/mmole) per animal i.p. 3o min later the cells were collected, washed in o.4 M NaCl 1o mM Tris-HCl, pH = 7.o. Trichloroacetic acid (TCA) was added to a final concentration of 1o% and the preci-pitate washed two times with cold 5% TCA. Phospholipids were extracted from the TCA-precipitate with chloroform methanol (2:1) and radioactivity determined in an aliquot of the chloroform methanol extract. Organic bound phosphate was determined according to Bartlett (17).

	cpm/umole P
Control	9165
+ Triaziquonum (1o^{-6} moles/kg)	11o25

417

References

1. Connors TA: Mechanism of action of 2-chloroethylamine derivatives, sulfurmustard, epoxides and aziridines. In: Sartorelli
   AC, Jones DG (eds)Antineoplastic and immunosuppressive agents,
   part 2.Springer Verlag,Berlin,1975,pp 18-34.
2. Grunicke H, Bock KW, Becher H, Gäng V, Schnierda J, Puschendorf
   B:Effect of alkylating agents on the binding of DNA to protein.
   Cancer Res(33):1o48-1o53,1973.
3. Wolf H, Raydt G, Puschendorf B, Grunicke H:Effect of the alkylating agent triethyleneiminobenzoquinone on the synthesis of
   DNA and the incorporation of ^{3}H-lysine into nuclear proteins
   of Ehrlich ascites tumour cells.FEBS-Letters(35):336-34o,1973.
4. Riches PG, Harrap KR:Some effects of chlorambucil on the
   chromatin of Yoshida ascites sarcoma cells.Cancer Res.(33):
   389-393,1973.
5. Thomas CB, Kohn KW, Bonner WM:Characterization of DNA-protein
   cross-links formed by treatment of L-121o cells and nuclei
   with bis(2-chloroethyl)methylamine(N-mustard).Biochem.(17):
   3954-3958,1978.
6. Yerushalmi A, Yaqil G:The interaction of chromatin with alkylating agents.Europ.J.Biochem.(1o3):237-246,193o.
7. Doenecke D, Gallwitz D:Acetylation of histone in nucleosomes.
   Mol.Cell Biochem.(44):113-128,1983.
8. Multhaup I, Csordas A, Grunicke H, Pfister R, Puschendorf B:
   Conservation of the acetylation pattern of histones and the
   transcriptional activity in Ehrlich-ascites tumour cells by
   Na-butyrate.Arch.Biochem.Biophys.(222):497-5o3,1983.
9. Laemmli UK:Cleavage of proteins during the structural assembly
   of the head of bacteriophage T4.Nature(227):68o-685,197o.
1o.Cohen LH, Newcock KM, Zweidler A:Stage specific switches in
   histone synthesis during embryogenesis of the sea-urchin.
   Science(19o):994-997,1975.
11.Bonner WM, Laskey RA:A film detection method for tritium
   labelled proteins and nucleic acid in polyacrylamide gels.
   Eur.J.Biochem.(46):83-88,1974.
12.Laskey RA, Mills AD:Quantitative film detection of [3]H- and
   [14]C in polyacrylamide gels by fluorography.Eur.J.Biochem.
   (56):335-341,1975.
13.Lowry OH, Rosebrough NI,Farr AL, Randall RE:Protein measurement
   with the Folin phenol reagent.J.Biol.Chem.(193):265-275,1951.
14.Keck K:An ultramicro technique for the determination of
   deoxypentose nucleic acid.Arch.Biochem.Biophys.(63):446-467,
   1956.
15.Fuith LC, Zwierzina H, Puschendorf B, Grunicke H:Comparative
   studies on the effect of alkylating antitumour agents on
   histone biosynthesis and histone acetylation of Ehrlich
   ascites tumour cells(abstract).Regards sur la biochemie(3):
   22,1981.
16.Puschendorf B, Wolf H, Grunicke H:The effect of the alkylating
   agent trisethyleneiminobenzoquinone(Trenimon) on the template
   activity of chromatin and DNA in RNA and DNA polymerase
   systems.Biochem.Pharmacol.(2o):3o39-3o5o,1971.
17.Bartlett GR:Phosphorous assay in column chromatography.J.
   Biol.Chem.(234):446-468,1959.

INFLUENCE OF THE NUCLEAR MATRIX ON NUCLEAR STRUCTURE AND RESPONSE TO ANTICANCER DRUGS

KENNETH D. TEW

1. STRUCTURAL AND FUNCTIONAL ASPECTS OF THE NUCLEAR MATRIX

The complexity of biochemical events in the nucleus predicates the existence of a non-stochastic organisation of the structural nuclear components. Such structural integrity has been well established for cytoskeletal elements. More recently, the emergence of the nuclear matrix (1) as a proteinaceous scaffold has been correlated with many functional aspects of nuclear integrity. The nuclear matrix is a composite structure of fibrillar nonhistone proteins, ribonucleoproteins, residual nucleolar RNA and small amounts of DNA, which possesses a basic spongelike structure when seen by electron microscopy (Fig. 1). Chromatin is attached at multiple sites on the inner nuclear membrane and the interchromatinic matrix (2). Such attachments must serve to organise chromatin in a non-random fashion within the nucleus. There is evidence that replication of DNA is initiated at these sites on the matrix (3). Other nuclear events which have been associated with matrix structure and function include synthesis, processing and transport of RNA, and steroid binding (3).

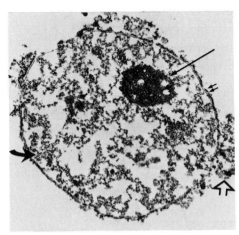

FIGURE 1. Electron micrograph (approx. print magn. x5000) of isolated nuclear matrix of Walker 256 rat carcinoma cell line. Isolation and microscopy procedures have been described (4-6). Curved arrow, interchromatininc fibrillar network which in some cases (open arrow) has "leaked" and become separated from the main matrix structure; small double arrow, residual nuclear membrane; long arrow, residual nucleolus. Nuclear matrix isolation: Triton extracted nuclei were treated with DNase I; 0.2mM MgCl$_2$ (x3); 2M NaCl (x3); 1% Triton; DNase I and RNase A. PMSF was present in all buffers.

In addition, it is clear that an intricate degree of order and reproducibility is required to ensure normal chromatid formation at mitosis.

Presumably a complex series of chromatin interactions with the nuclear matrix stabilise and organise nuclear structure prior to the onset of mitosis. Our recent studies (4) have suggested that a cell line with acquired resistance to alkylating agents has a modified karyotype when compared to its parent cell line. Coincident with this is a difference in the phosphorylation of the proteins of the nuclear matrix and it is possible that such post-translational modifications of matrix polypeptides control the condensation and separation properties of chromosomes during mitosis.

2. NUCLEAR MATRIX AS A DRUG TARGET

Treatment of cells in vitro with nitrosoureas or alkylating agents can result in electrophilic attack of cellular nucleophilic macromolecules by alkylating and carbamoylating species, produced by physiological decomposition of these drugs. The potential for a cell to survive treatment with nitrosoureas or alkylating agents may be determined severally by the type, number or diversity of drug lesions, their location within the nucleus and the rate and fidelity of their repair.

Levels of alkylation and carbamoylation of the matrix fraction are shown in Table 1. The matrix constitutes approximately 5% of the total nuclear protein (2.25pg/cell). Pulse labelling with ^{3}H-uridine or ^{3}H-thymidine demonstrated that 5% of the total nuclear RNA and 1-2% of the total DNA were associated with the matrix. Drug binding to the matrix of both CLZ and CCNU represented 30% of the total nuclear interactions, essentially all of which were covalent. Carbamoylation by CCNU was approximately twenty times greater than the corresponding alkylation, a value consistent with a similar ratio for the whole nucleus. The basic sponge-like structure of the nuclear matrix was unaltered by short term exposure to these drugs.

Table 1. COMPARATIVE NITROSOUREA INTERACTIONS WITH THE NUCLEAR MATRIX

| | pmol Drug Bound µg Matrix Protein | | % of Total Nuclear Drug Binding to the Matrix |
	Total	Acid Precipitable	
CLZ Alkylation	1.58+0.32	1.60+0.27	26.7+1.4
CCNU Alkylation	1.27+0.22	1.28+0.19	31.3+2.7
CCNU Carbamoylation	32.5+3.7	38.0+6.9	33.1+3.0

Each point is the mean + SD of at least 6 experiments. The matrix proteins constituted 4.7% to 5.0% of the total nucleoprotein constituents.

Using an _in vitro_ assay (5) to measure the potential for DNA to associate with proteins of the nuclear matrix it was found that approximately 80% of the DNA reassociated with the matrix at a protein:DNA ratio of 50:1. A linear reassociation was found until all reassociation sites were saturated (Fig. 2).

Direct alkylation or carbamoylation of the matrix proteins _per se_ did not affect these DNA-protein interactions. However, using alkylated DNA (1 alkylation per 10^2-10^4 base pairs), there was a significant reduction of alkylated nucleic acid bound to the matrix at the same protein:DNA ratio (Fig. 2). Further analysis revealed that the reduced binding of DNA to matrix was a composite function of interference with the base recognition sites and a release of some unstable alkylations during the reassociation procedure. Because of the role of the matrix in replication, transcription and chromatin organisation through loop attachments (2,3), the extent of drug modification may adversely influence the capacity of the matrix to mediate these nuclear functions.

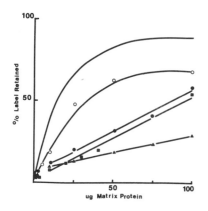

FIGURE 2. _In vitro_ reassociation assay of DNA and matrix proteins from HeLa cells (from Ref. 5). Varying concentrations of matrix proteins were added to 1µg of phenol extracted DNA in a total volume of 1.5ml TN buffer (0.1M NaCl, 0.1mM EDTA, 10mM Tris pH 7.4, 3mM $MgCl_2$, 0.1mM DTT and 1mM PMSF) and incubated for 1hr at 22°C. The samples were layered onto 25mm HAWP 0.45µM Millipore filters which had been presoaked in TN buffer. Suction was applied at a rate which required 5-10 seconds for sample filtration; this was followed by a single 5ml wash of TN buffer. Filters were transferred to glass vials and the DNA bases hydrolsed by boiling in 0.5ml of 0.5N HCl for 10 minutes. Vials were cooled, and filters dissolved in 1ml ethyl acetate prior to the addition of 10ml of scintillation fluid. Experimental results are a percentage reassociation of DNA expressed as a function of varying matrix protein concentrations. Top curve is DNA prelabelled with ^{3}H-thymidine; O = DNA alkylated with (^{14}C-ethyl) chlorambucil; ● = DNA alkylated with (^{14}C-chloroethyl) CCNU; ■ = DNA alkylated with (^{3}H-methyl) MNU; ▲ = DNA alkylated with (^{14}C-chloroethyl) chlorozotocin.

Electrophilic and hydrophobic drug modifications of the nuclear matrix have also been demonstrated (6). Estramustine, a conjugate of nitrogen mustard and estradiol, possesses cytotoxic properties which are independent of its steroid/mustard constituents. Non-covalent binding to the structural components of both the cytoskeleton (7) and the nuclear matrix (6) are responsible for the cytotoxic properties of estramustine in vitro. Resultant abnormalities in chromatid formation (see Hartley-Asp, this volume) could be the direct result of such drug binding and may influence its observed antimitotic effects (8).

3. THE MATRIX AND DNA REPAIR

Poly(ADP-ribose) polymerase is a nuclear enzyme which catalyses the synthesis of poly(ADP-ribose) units from the substrate, nicotinamide adenine dinucleotide (NAD), requiring DNA and acceptor histone and non-histone proteins for its catalytic activity (9). One of the primary acceptors for ADP ribosylation has been shown to be the enzyme itself (10). The enzyme has a putative role in DNA repair (11), but the mechanism(s) by which such a function is managed is indeterminate. Because of the role of the nuclear matrix in other aspects of nucleic acid synthesis and processing (3), we have considered how poly(ADP-ribose) polymerase might be associated with the nuclear matrix of Walker 256 mammary carcinoma cells.

Gel electrophoresis of (^{32}P) labelled, ADP-ribosylated matrix proteins is represented in the autoradiogram as shown in Fig. 3.

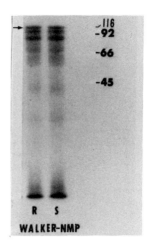

FIGURE 3. Autoradiogram of (^{32}P) ADP-ribosylated nuclear matrix protein bands. The isolated nuclei from WS and WR cells were incubated with (^{32}P) NAD as the substrate in the absence of exogenous NAD in the test buffer. The nuclear matrix was prepared (see Fig. 1 legend) and polypeptides separated on a 10% SDS polyacrylamide gel. Subsequent autoradiography revealed the presence of ADP-ribosylated matrix proteins. Lane 1 Walker 256 resistant to bifunctional alkylating agents; Lane 2 Walker 256 parent cell line. Numbers in right column are M.W. markers. Arrow shows putative 112kdal poly(ADP-ribose) polymerase (from 12).

The concentrations of NAD used in this analysis favoured the formation of limited ADP-ribose polymer chains, reflecting the ADP-ribosylation of matrix proteins by the utilisation of endogenous NAD. Ten distinguishable radiolabelled bands were apparent. The predominant ADP-ribosylated products were between 60 and 112 kdal. The major matrix lamins between 60-75kdal were ADP-ribosylated suggesting that these structural proteins were acceptors for ADP-ribosylation. Other major acceptor proteins on the autoradiogram included 45kdal, 90kdal and 112kdal polypeptides. Low molecular weight proteins, presumably residual histones, were ADP-ribosylated, but not as extensively as reported previously for total nuclear histones (10). To confirm the presence of poly(ADP-ribose) polymerase activity on the nuclear matrix, acid precipitable matrix material was obtained following an in vitro ($32P$) incubation assay Table 2. Data suggest that enzymatic activity was associated with the nuclear matrix and this would be consistent with the 112kdal polypeptide (Fig. 3) representing the automodified enzyme.

Table 2. POLY(ADP-RIBOSE) POLYMERASE ACTIVITY ASSOCIATED WITH THE NUCLEAR MATRIX

	WS	WR
	(($32P$)-NAD CPM incorp/μg Protein)	
Nuclear Matrix Proteins	4.7	5.6
+ 100 μM NAD	25.3	27.0

Since the enzyme was not removed by the high salt (2M NaCl) washes during the matrix isolation procedure, putative enzyme matrix interactions are presumably non-ionic in nature; possibly through covalent or hydrophobic bonding. Since the major matrix proteins act as acceptors for ADP-ribose units and the enzyme is matrix associated, this may suggest a role for the nuclear matrix in DNA repair. Similarity in polymerase activity in WR and WS may indicate that increased DNA repair potential is not important in the acquisition of alkylating agent resistance in WR cells.

REFERENCES

1. Berezney R and Coffey DS: Nuclear protein matrix: association with newly synthesised DNA. Science (189): 192-193, 1975.
2. Pardoll DM, Vogelstein B and Coffey DS: A fixed site of DNA replication in eucaryotic cells. Cell (19): 527-536, 1980.
3. Maul G: The Nuclear Envelope and the Nuclear Matrix. Alan R. Liss, New York, 1982.

4. Tew KD, Moy BC and Hartley-Asp B: Acquired drug resistance is accompanied by modification in the karyotype and nuclear matrix of a rat carcinoma cell line. Exp Cell Res. In press, 1983.
5. Tew KD, Wang AL and Schein PS: Alkylating agent interactions with the nuclear matrix. Biochem Pharmacol. In press, 1983.
6. Tew KD, Erickson LC, White G, Wang AL, Schein PS and Hartley-Asp B: Cytotoxicity of Estramustine, a steroid nitrogen mustard derivative, through non-DNA targets. Mol Pharm. (24): 324-328, 1983.
7. Stearns ME and Tew KD: Nuclear and cytoskeletal effects of an estradiol-nitrogen mustard conjugate, Estramustine (Abstract) J Cell Biol. (99): 1093, 1983.
8. Tew KD and Hartley Asp B: Cytotoxic properties of Estramustine are unrelated to its alkylating and steroid constituents. Urology. In press, 1983.
9. Chambon P, Weill JD and Mandel P: NMN activation of a new DNA dependent poly A synthesising nuclear enzyme. Biochem Biophys Res Commun. (11): 39-43, 1963.
10. Jump DB and Smulson ME: Purification and characterisation of the major non-histone protein acceptor for poly ADP-ribose in HeLa cell nuclei. Biochemistry (19): 1024-1030, 1980.
11. Durkacz BW, Onidiji O, Gray DA and Shall S: ADP-ribose participates in DNA excision repair. Nature (283): 593-596, 1980.
12. Moy BC and Tew KD: Nuclear matrix associated poly(ADP-ribose) polymerase and evidence of modified matrix proteins. Submitted.

CYTOTOXICITY OF A STEROID-LINKED MUSTARD (ESTRAMUSTINE) THROUGH NON-DNA
TARGETS

BERYL HARTLEY-ASP

Drug induced DNA alterations have for several years been accepted as
ultimately leading to cell death. Less attention has by comparison been
given to drug interactions with nuclear proteins. The nuclear protein matrix
has recently, however, come into focus as an extremely important structure
with regard to replication sites, hormone receptors, nuclear shape etc.
(see Tew, this volume).   Thus, drug interaction with the nuclear
matrix could lead to severe disturbances in cell growth.

Nitrosoureas have been shown to preferentially interact with the nuclear
matrix (1), but due to their high reactivity for DNA, discrimination of the
importance of matrix binding has proved difficult. Estramustine, estra-
diol-3-N-bis(2-chloroethyl carbamate), fig 1, a drug of use in the treatment
of advanced prostate carcinoma (2) appears to be a drug which preferentially
reacts with the nuclear matrix.

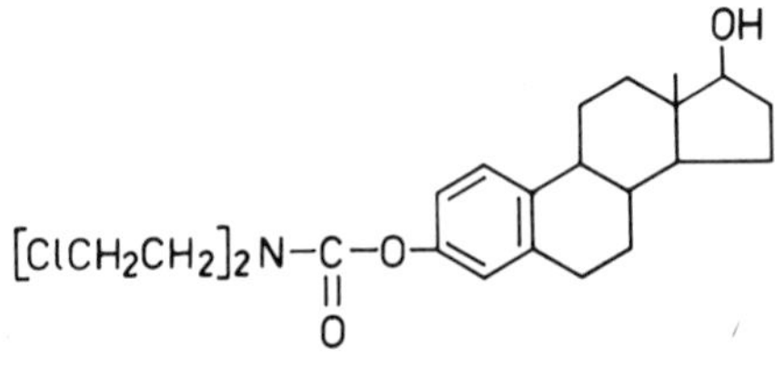

FIGURE 1.   Structural formula of estramustine.

Estramustine is cytotoxic to human prostate carcinoma cells in vitro, which
are unresponsive to hormones (3) but which can be killed at higher concentrations by the alkylating moiety, nor-nitrogen mustard (fig 2). It is also
as active against Walker 256 rat mammary carcinoma cells with aquired resistance to a wide range of nitrogen mustard derivatives as it is against the
sensitive line (4). Both these factors point to a different mode of action
for estramustine than that of either an alkylating agent or a steroid.

425

FIGURE 2.   FIGURE 3.

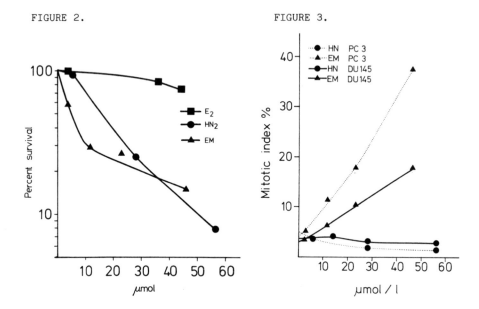

FIGURE 2. Human prostate cancer cells (DU 145) at $2x10^5$ cells/ml were treated for 24 h with estramustine (EM), nor-nitrogen mustard (HN_2), estradiol 17-β (E_2) and then incubated for a further 10 days to allow for colony formation. Survival is given as a percent of the control.

FIGURE 3. Human prostate cancer cells, PC-3 and DU 145, at $4x10^5$ cells/ml and $5x10^4$ cells/ml respectively, were treated for 24 h with estramustine (EM) or nor-nitrogen mustard (HN). Suspended and prepared for mitotic index analysis as described in ref 6. Colchicine was not used. Fig taken from ref 6.

Using HeLa cells an ID_{90} of approx 2.5 µg/ml was established for estramustine (4). Experiments to estimate the amount of DNA damage, using the alkaline elution technique, were carried out at concentrations above the ID_{50} and at various time points. In contrast to that found for nitrogen mustards (5), no differences between drug treated and controls were found for single stand breaks, DNA-DNA or DNA-protein cross-links at any of the concentrations or time points showing that no appreciable DNA-damage was produced by estramustine treatment (4).

The absence of DNA damage was confirmed by cytological methods as no chromosomal aberrations or increase in sister chromatid exchange (SCE) levels were found (6). However, cytology did reveal an unexpected action of estramustine, it was found to behave as an anti-mitotic agent. In agreement with that of the classical anti-mitotic agents, colchicine and vinca-alkaloids, estramustine caused an arrest of cells in the first metaphase of treatment, a disorientation of chromosomes from the metaphase plane, contraction of chromosomes (fig 4c) and lack of anaphase figures (fig 4a). This can be expressed qualitatively by an increase in mitotic index which does not occur after treatment with nor-nitrogen mustard (fig 3). Chromosomal aberrations were found at the highest concentrations after nor-nitrogen mustard treatment. As seen in fig 4d estramustine also affects second divisions, as spindle orientation is disrupted, but chromosomal contraction is not as strong as during the first division. Fig 4d also indicates the low level of SCE's found after estramustine treatment.

That the anti-mitotic and cytotoxic action of estramustine is an effect of the intact molecule was confirmed by using both radiolabelled drug and specific analytical methods for the determination of estramustine and its metabolites estromustine, estradiol and estrone (7). It was found that nuclear uptake in HeLa cells was approx. 1.5% of the available drug. Isolation of the nuclear protein matrix revealed that approx. 0.4% of the nuclear available drug was bound to this component (Table 1). Little drug binding was found in the nucleic acid fraction which is consistant with the lack of DNA-damage. Ethyl acetate extraction of the matrix preparation yielded 98% of the drug indicating non-covalent binding of drug to matrix. The matrix bound drug was found to be either estramustine or its oxidative metabolite estromustine (4).

The nuclear distribution of estramustine contrasts radically from that of colchicine (table 1), which does not bind in any high degree to the protein matrix, but does appear to react with the nucleic acid fraction indicating that colchicine's cytotoxic effect is perhaps not completely confined to its anti-mitotic effect. These results also indicate that even though estramustine and colchicine have very similar anti-mitotic effects there are other facets of their modes of action which differ. That estramustine cytotoxicity is not only based on its anti-mitotic effect is also

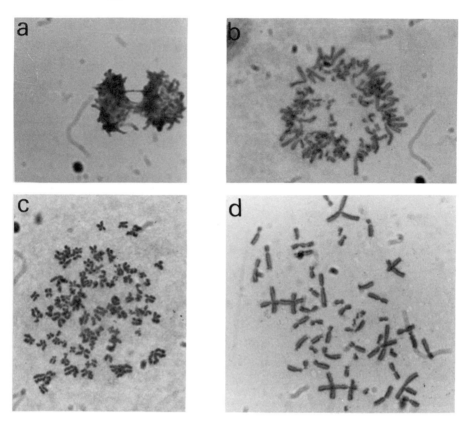

FIGURE 4. All photos are from human prostate carcinoma cell line DU 145.

4a. Normal anaphase
4b. Normal metaphase
4c. Estramustine treated (24 h 10 µg/ml) 1st division metaphase
4d. Estramustine treated (24 h 5 µg/ml) 2nd division: prepared
      for SCE analysis, see ref. 6.

TABLE 1

Cell fraction	% of available cellular estramustine	% of available cellular colchicine
Nucleus	1.5	2.5
Nucleic acids	2.3	73.0
Nuclear matrix	38.5	3.7

HeLa cells 5×10^6 ml were incubated for 24 h with 40 µl ^{3}H-estramustine
(102 Ci/m mol) or 125 µl ^{3}H-colchicine (57 Ci/m mol)/100 mls.
Nucleic acids and matrix are given as a percent of available nuclear drug.

indicated by the difference in sensitivity of the two prostate lines to estramustine; PC-3 showing the highest increase in mitotic index whilst being the least sensitive (6). Whether differences in drug uptake or distribution and binding to the protein matrix can resolve the difference is to be seen.

Thus, it appears that estramustine has a unique mode of action which differs from that of its alkylating moiety or steroid component. As 4 to 10 times higher levels of estramustine have been found in prostate cancer tissue contra plasma levels in the same patient (8), this could mean that the intact molecule can react as such at the tumour site killing hormone unresponsive cells, whilst the circulating plasma levels of estrogen are high enough to result in an action on hormone responsive cells providing a unique type of treatment for prostate cancer.

REFERENCES

1. Tew KD: A molecular rationale for nitrosourea induced cytotoxicity. In: Serrou B, Schein PS, Imbach JL (eds) Nitrosoureas in Cancer Treatment. INSERM Symp 19. Elsevier, 1981, pp 61-77.
2. Jönsson G, Högberg B, Nilsson T: Treatment of advanced prostatic carcinoma with estramustine phosphate (Estracyt^R). Scand J Urol Nephrol (11): 231-238, 1977.
3. Hartley-Asp B, Gunnarsson PO: Growth and cell survival following treatment with estramustine, nor-nitrogen mustard, estradiol and testosterone of a human prostatic cancer cell line (DU 145). J Urol (127): 818-822, 1982.
4. Tew KD, Erickson LC, White G, Wong AL, Schein PS, Hartley-Asp B: Cytotoxicity of a steroid-nitrogen mustard derivative through non-DNA targets. Molecular Pharmacol, (24): 324-328, 1983.
5. Ewig RAG, Kohn KW: DNA damage and repair in mouse leukemia L1210 cells treated with nitrogen mustard, 1,3-bis(2-chloroethyl)-1-nitrosourea, and other nitrosoureas. Cancer Res (37): 2114-2122, 1977.
6. Hartley-Asp B: Estramustine induced mitotic arrest in two human prostatic carcinoma cell lines DU145 and PC-3. The Prostate (5), in press.
7. Andersson SB, Gunnarsson PO, Nilsson T, Plym Forshell G: Metabolism of estramustine phosphate (Estracyt^R) in patients with prostatic carcinoma. Eur J Drug Metab Pharmacokin (6): 149-154, 1981.
8. Fritjofsson Å, Björk P, Gunnarsson PO, Norlén BJ: Binding and accumulation of active metabolites in tumours from prostatic cancer patients treated with Estracyt. In: Spitzy KH, Karrer K, Egerman H (eds) Proc 13th Int Congress Chemotherapy, Vienna, 1983.

POTENTIATION OF CYTOTOXICITY BY INHIBITORS OF NUCLEAR
ADP-RIBOSYL TRANSFERASE.

S.SHALL

1. INTRODUCTION

ADP-ribosylation of chromatin proteins is a component of
efficient DNA excision repair (1,2) probably because it regulates
DNA ligase II activity (3). The enzyme nuclear ADP-ribosyl
transferase or ADPRT, which synthesises $(ADP-ribose)_n$ uses
NAD^+ as a substrate and has an absolute requirement for DNA (4).

The enzyme seems to be capable of catalysing three
separate, related reactions which generate mono-(ADP-ribosyl)-
proteins, oligo- or poly- (ADP-ribosyl) proteins in which the
polymer may be linear or branched. Nuclear ADPRT has been
found in animals, plants and lower organisms; it is present in
almost all nucleated cells. Several terminally-differentiated
cells lack the enzyme activity.

2. Properties of nuclear ADPRT

Nuclear ADPRT is entirely dependent on DNA for its activity
because it has a specific requirement for ends of DNA strands;
closed circular DNA does not activate the enzyme but becomes
an activator when breaks are introduced.

The activity of ADPRT may be inhibited either by exogenous
inhibitors or by the nutritional deprivation of nicotinamide
which lowers the intracellular NAD level. A variety of inhibitors
of ADPRT are known including nicotinamide, 5-methylnicotinamide,
deoxythymidine, methylxanthines, benzamide, 3-aminobenzamide (3AB)
3-acetamidobenzamide and 3-methoxybenzamide. The related acid
analogues are not inhibitory.

DNA damage activates nuclear ADPRT, stimulates the synthesis
of $(ADP-ribose)_n$ and lowers cellular NAD levels (5). It seems

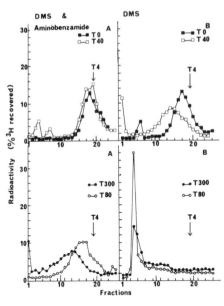

FIGURE 1. 3-aminobenzamide inhibits DNA excision repair. Sedimentation is from right to left. Control DNA bands in fractions 3 to 5.

that these consequences result from radiation and chemical damage in proportion to the number of sites in the DNA being repaired by strand-breakage. All the inhibitors of nuclear ADPRT will block the synthesis of poly (ADP-ribose) and therefore prevent the lowering of cellular NAD content.

3. Nuclear ADPRT is required for DNA excision repair (2)

The inhibitors of nuclear ADPRT retard DNA excision repair. For example, Fig. 1 shows the inhibition by 3mM 3AB of excision repair of DNA, measured by alkaline sucrose gradients. The cells were exposed to 100μM dimethyl sulphate (DMS) (about 7% cell survival) in the presence or absence of 3AB. In the absence of the enzyme inhibitor (B), the DMS reduced the molecular weight of the DNA considerably; 40 minutes after removal of the DMS the molecular weight had clearly increased, and by 80 minutes the DNA is at the bottom of the gradient. By contrast, when the ADPRT inhibitor is present (A), the DNA is degraded to about the same degree but the recovery (in the continuous presence of 3AB) is markedly slower; by 5 hours the DNA is still only partially repaired. Clearly, 3AB retards strand-rejoining, as do the other ADPRT inhibitors (6).

4. Inhibition of nuclear ADPRT synergistically potentiates the cytotoxicity of DNA-damaging agents

The synergistic potentiation of cytotoxicity was first demonstrated in mouse leukaemic L1210 cells using a soft-agar

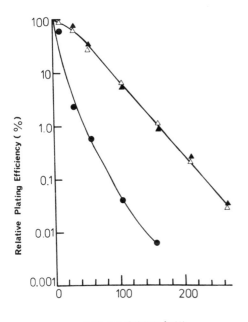

Dimethyl Sulphate (μM)

FIGURE 2. The synergistic
potentiation of cytotoxicity of
DMS by 2mM 3AB. Δ , exposed to
DMS for 1 hour, then washed and
plated in soft agar; ● ,
exposed to DMS and 2mM 3AB for
1 hour, then washed and plated
in soft agar containing 2mM
3AB; ▲ , exposed to DMS and
2mM 3-aminobenzoic acid for
1 hour, then washed and plated
in soft agar containing 2mM
3-aminobenzoic acid.

cloning assay to measure
cell survival; at the concentrations used, the enzyme
inhibitors were themselves
non-toxic (2,7). Fig. 2 shows
the potentiation of cytotoxicity
of DMS for L1210 cells induced
by the presence of 2mM 3AB.
Exposure of L1210 cells to
90μM DMS for 1 hour yields 10%
survival. When 2mM 3AB is
present during the subsequent
cloning assay, 22μM DMS is
sufficient to give only 10%
cell survival; this represents
a four-fold dose enhancement.
2mM 3-aminobenzoic acid which
does not inhibit ADPRT activity,
has no effect on the cytotoxicity of DMS.

Non-toxic concentrations of
5-methylnicotinamide potentiate
the cytotoxicity of
methylnitrosourea (MNU) with
dose-enhancement factors
between 3 and 10. The potentiation is dependent on the
concentration of 5-methylnicotinamide. The methylxanthines,
theobromine and theophylline also increase the toxicity of
MNU, as does deoxythymidine in the presence of sufficient
deoxycytidine to overcome the perturbation of deoxynucleotide
metabolism. Nicotinate which is not an inhibitor of ADPRT,
has no effect on MNU toxicity.

Both mouse and human cells are equally sensitive to this
potentiation of cell killing, but there are marked differences
amongst different cell types. For example, mouse L1210 cells

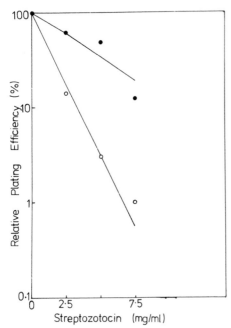

FIGURE 3. The synergistic potentiation of the toxicity of streptozotocin by 5-methyl-nicotinamide. ●, streptozo-tocin alone; o streptozotocin + 2mM 5-methylnicotinamide.

are very sensitive to the potentiation by 5-methyl-nicotinamide, while V79-A Chinese hamster lung fibroblasts are much less sensitive. 3-methoxybenzamide potentiates the killing in all cell types examined. The differences may be due to varying permeability to the inhibitors. $(ADP-ribose)_n$ participates in DNA repair in both lymphoid cells (L1210, K36-16, human T & B cells) and in fibroblasts (3T3, SV40 3T3, normal human fibroblasts), glial cells, glioma cells and sarcoma cells. It seems to be a general property of nucleated cells. There is also considerable variation in the potentiation with different damaging agents; monofunctional alkylating agents show a very large potentiation, by contrast in a few preliminary observations UV-irradiation and bifunctional cross-linking agents show little or no potentiation and ionizing radiation shows a moderate potentiation when exponentially-growing cells are irradiated.

Of special interest is the potentiation of the cytotoxicity of streptozotocin by 2 mM 5-methylnicotinamide (Fig. 3) because streptozotocin and its derivatives are used in the clinical treatment of pancreatic tumours. J.E. Trosko, C.C.Chang and P. Lui (personal communication) have shown that 2mM benzamide substantially enhances the cytotoxicity of streptozotocin towards Chinese hamster cells.

5. The potential of nuclear ADPRT inhibitors in cancer
   chemotherapy.

Nuclear ADPRT inhibitors and nicotinamide deprivation
synergistically increase the lethality of a variety of DNA-
damaging agents, including both nitrosoureas and ionizing
radiation. There is as yet no evidence for tumour specificity,
but there is some experimental data to encourage optimism.
Nonetheless, the enhanced cytotoxicity of streptozotocin, for
example, by innocuous ADPRT inhibitors may be of value in the
clinical use of streptozotocin in the treatment of certain
pancreatic tumours. In addition, chlorozotocin may also be
potentiated in its action by ADPRT inhibitors.

I would anticipate that the cytotoxicity of all small monofunctional alkylating agents would be potentiated by ADPRT
inhibitors. The response of bifunctional or bulky reagents and
of ionizing radiation is more difficult to predict, but recent
reports do encourage optimism and some further experimental
investigation would be warranted.

This work was supported by the MRC and the CRC.

REFERENCES

1. Shall S: In Hayaishi O, Ueda K (eds)ADP-Ribosylation
   Reactions. Academic Press, New York, 1982, pp 477-520.
2. Durkacz BW, Omidiji O, Gray DA, Shall S: Nature (283):
   593-596, 1980.
3. Creissen D, Shall S: Nature (296):271-272, 1982.
4. Hayaishi O, Ueda K: ADP-Ribosylation Reactions.
   Academic Press, New York, 1982.
5. Skidmore CJ, Davies MI, Goodwin PM, Halldorsson H, Lewis PJ,
   Shall S, Zia'ee A-A: Eur.Biochem. (101):135-142, 1979.
6. Gray DA, Durkacz BW, Shall S: FEBS Lett.(131):173-177, 1981.
7. Nduka N, Skidmore CJ, Shall S: Eur. J. Biochem. (105):525-530,
   1980.

CHAPTER VI

ENDOCRINE THERAPY

ADJUVANT TAMOXIFEN TREATMENT IN OPERABLE BREAST CANCER.
SHOULD THE TREATMENT CONTINUE FOR MANY YEARS?

A. Wallgren, K. Ideström, U. Glas, M. Kaigas, N-O Theve,
N. Wilking, L. Karnström, L. Skoog and B. Nordenskjöld.

Tamoxifen is an anti-estrogen with activity in advanced
breast cancer (1). It has few and usually mild side-effects.
Consequently, it should be an ideal agent for the treatment
of asymptomatic women. Preliminary results indicate that it
prolongs the disease-free interval (2,3,4,5,6). This is an
interim report of an ongoing trial of adjuvant tamoxifen. We
also report on the effect of discontinuation of therapy on
the failure rate.

MATERIALS AND METHODS

Postmenopausal patients less than 70 years old were,
after breast cancer surgery, stratified according to the
extension of the disease into two groups. The favourable
group consisted of patients with tumours smaller than 3 cm
in diameter and no axillary node metastases in the surgical
specimen. The unfavourable group had tumours larger than
3 cm and/or lymph node metastases.

Estrogen receptor assay by isoelectric focusing (7)
was performed with 80 per cent of the patients.

The patients with unfavourable tumour status were also
included in a previously described trial on postoperative
adjuvant cytotoxic chemotherapy (5). They were randomized
to receive either twelve courses of chemotherapy or post-
operative irradiation to the internal mammary, supraclavicu-
lar and axillary nodal regions and to the chest wall. These
areas were irradiated with 46 Gy in 4-5 weeks.

439

As seen in Table 1, 826 patients were in the trial by
January 1982. Tamoxifen 20 mg twice daily for two years was
given to 416 patients while 410 were randomized to serve as
controls.

Table 1.

| Treatment arm | Favourable group | Unfavourable group | | Total |
		Radiotherapy	Chemotherapy	
Tamoxifen	257	86	73	416
Controls	264	72	74	410
Total	521	158	147	826

All patients have been followed-up through December
1982. The mean time of follow-up was 44 months with a range
of 12-75 months. Compliance was estimated to be 86 per cent
at two years (5).

The time from randomization to failure was studied.
Failure was defined as recurrence of the disease anywhere in
the body or death from any cause.

The significance of differences between the treatment
groups was tested with the logrank test (8). In the analyses
the patients were stratified according to prognostic groups
and other treatment modalities. The p-values are, thus,
adjusted for any inequality of the distribution of such
varibles in the treatment groups. The analyses were
performed for the entire time of follow-up, and for two
separate periods viz. for the first three years and for the
years thereafter. The mean failure rate was calculated as the
number of patients who failed per woman year at risk during
each period.

RESULTS

The recurrence free survival rates for the patients of
the two treatment groups are given for the total material
in Fig. 1, for the patients of the favourable group in Fig.2
and for those in the unfavourable group in Fig. 3. The
numbers of patients at risk are shown along the X-axis.

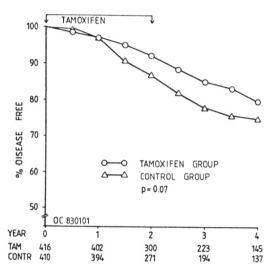

Fig 1. The recurrence free survival rates for the patients of the two groups for the total material. The numbers of patients at risk are shown along the X-axis.

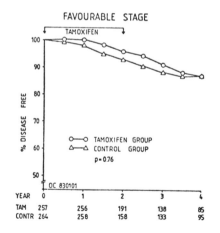

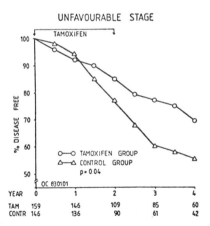

Fig 2. Little difference in the recurrence free survival rates was seen for the patients with favourable disease.

Fig 3. Among the unfavourable patients, those treated with tamoxifen fared better than the control patients (p=0.04).

Table 2 shows that during the first three years there was a significantly lower rate of failure among the tamoxifen treated patients (p=0.01). During the following years the failure rate was higher in the tamoxifen group than in the control group (p=0.06).

Table 2. Relative recurrence rates (control patients= 1.0) for tamoxifen treated patients by prognostic group and period of follow-up.

| Prognostic group | Years of follow-up | | |
	1-3	>3	all years
Favourable	0.70	2.10	0.92
Unfavourable	0.57	1.59	0.67
Total	0.61	1.82	0.75

The recurrence rates for the patients in the tamoxifen group compared to the control group by the level of estrogen receptors are given in Table 3. The failure rate was highest for patients with estrogen-receptor-poor tumours. Regardless of estrogen receptor level the rates were lower among the tamoxifen-treated patients than in the control group but the difference reached statistical significance only when the estradiol receptor concentration was > 0.1 fmoles/µg DNA (Table 3, p=0.02).

Table 3.

| ER fmoles/µg DNA | Patients and (failures) | | Ratio of recurrence rates |
	Tamoxifen	Controls	
< 0.1	81 (20)	92 (23)	0.92
0.11-0.69	85 (16)	79 (22)	0.57
> 0.7	158 (18)	154 (26)	0.62

DISCUSSION

Adjuvant tamoxifen treatment for two years reduced the failure rate in women with lymph node metastases or large tumours. Little benefit was demonstrated for patients without lymph node metastases and with tumour smaller than 3 cm; we need more patients to investigate this subset.

After the cessation of tamoxifen treatment, the mean failure rates for year four and following were higher in the tamoxifen group (Table 2).The recurrence-free survival curves of the two treatment groups run parallel to each other during the third year but seem to approach each other thereafter (Fig. 1). Apart from being a spurious result due to small numbers, this is what may be expected if tamoxifen delays the onset of a recurrence. The delay of the onset of tumour recurrence may be equivalent to the progression which occurs after a median time of 9 to more than 17 months during tamoxifen treatment for advanced disease (1). If so, the relapse is proably caused by the multiplications of resistant cells and further prolonged tamoxifen treatment may not increase the disease-free survival.

It is, on the other hand, possible that the tamoxifen as we have previously argued (9) assembles cells in a resting phase and that they start to regrow after the cessation of the treatment. In this case, the recurrences should be responsive to renewed tamoxifen. An increased failure rate after short term tamoxifen administration has been predicted from animal models (10).

In contrast to cytotoxic chemotherapy, tamoxifen has few and fairly mild side effects in most patients. This drug could therefore be considered of value as an adjuvant treatment even if it does not cure patients but only prolongs the disease-free survival. Therefore, prolonged medication over several years is presently studied in controlled studies in Sweden to assess if this will further postpone the recurrencies.

This work was supported by grants from The Swedish Cancer Society and King Gustaf V Jubilee Fund.

REFERENCES

1. Mouridsen H, Palshof T, Patterson J, Battersby L. (1978): Tamoxifen in advanced breast cancer. Cancer Treatm. Rev. 5, 131-41.

2. Hubay CA, Pearson OH, Marshall JS.et al. (1980): Anti-estrogen, cytotoxic chemotherapy, and bacillus Calmette-Guerin vaccination in stage II breast cancer. A preliminary report. Surgery 87, 494-501.

3. Palshof T, Mouridsen HT, Daehnfelt JL. (1980): Adjuvant endocrine therapy of breast cancer- a controlled clinical trial of estrogen and anti-estrogen:preliminary results of the Copenhagen Breast Cancer Trials. Recent Res. Cancer Res. 71, 185-89.

4. Fisher B, Redmond C, Brown A. et al. (1981): Treatment of primary breast cancer with chemotherapy and tamoxifen. N. Engl. J. Med. 305, 1-6.

5. Wallgren A, Baral E, Glas U. et al. (1981): Adjuvant breast cancer treatment with tamoxifen and combination chemotherapy in postmenopausal women. In Salmon SE, Jones SE, eds. Adjuvant therapy of Cancer III,pp 345-50.

6. Nolvadex Adjuvant Trial Organisation (1983): Controlled trial of tamoxifen as adjuvant agent in management of early breast cancer. Lancet, pp 257-61.

7. Wrange Ö, Nordenskjöld B, Gustafsson JÅ. (1978): Cytosol estradiol receptor in human mammary carcinoma: An assay based on isoelectric focusing in polyacrylamide gel. Anal. Biochem. 85, 461-75.

8. Peto R, Pike MC, Armitage P. et al.(1977): Design and analysis of randomized clinical trials requiring prolonged observation of each patient. II Analysis and examples. Br. J. Cancer 35, 1-39.

9. Nordenskjöld B, Löwhagen T, Westerberg H, Zajicek J.(1976): ^{3}H-Thymidine incorporation into mammary carcinoma cells obtained by needle aspiration before and during endocrine therapy. Acta Cytol. 20, 137-43.

10. Jordan VC, Naylor KE, Dix CJ, Prestwich G. (1980): Anti-estrogen action in experimental breast cancer. Recent Results Cancer Res. 71, 30-44.

ADJUVANT HORMONAL THERAPY OF BREAST CANCER

H A de HAAN & J DIVER

Breast cancer is rarely localised. Only when the need to treat occult micrometastases with systemic agents is appreciated and adjuvant therapy becomes widely adopted is it likely that our current treatments will have a major impact on the morbidity and mortality of this disease.

Theoretically, adjuvant therapy should begin perioperatively for this is the time during which metastases are smallest and the growth fraction is highest. Alternatively, it should be started as soon as possible after mastectomy. Chemotherapy trials have demonstrated clearly the advantages available especially to younger women with axillary lymph node involvement, but the sometimes appreciable acute toxicity and potential long-term complications limit the use of this therapy. Undoubtedly we need safer and more convenient alternatives.

Considering the natural history of the disease, relatively little time separates the various clinical stages of breast cancer and any agent of proven value for late disease should also be active in the earlier stages. Hormone and chemotherapy are equiactive in hormone-sensitive advanced breast cancer, but the former is to be preferred in such cases in view of the greater therapeutic index and ease of administration.

Adjuvant hormone therapy is not a new concept. In 1889 Schinzinger proposed that breast cancer recurrences might be delayed by prophylactic castration[1] but it was not until 1947 that results of this type of manoeuvre were first described.[2] Other retro-spective studies showing comparable benefits followed and later there were prospective randomised oophorectomy trials.[3] Whilst not all

445

were positive,[4] overall there was a strong trend in favour of castration and the excessive doubt cast on the validity of much of this work seems unjustified even though the numbers of patients involved were small. Three more recent large trials evaluating an irradiation-induced menopause post-mastectomy have each reported statistically significant superiority for this over mastectomy alone.[5-7] Furthermore, one randomised older women to either ovarian irradiation or the same treatment followed by long-term prednisone in order to inhibit oestrogen synthesis by the adrenal glands. The latter group did best suggesting that complete oestrogen suppression provides more effective treatment.[7] Other procedures such as adrenalectomy have been advocated but, for obvious reasons, adjuvant ablative manipulations have largely been confined to oophorectomy or ovarian irradiation. Nevertheless, it might be concluded that castration benefits have probably been underestimated.

Interest in additive hormone therapy to treat breast cancer has been stimulated by the introduction of the modern synthetic hormones. Animal models provide us with an indication of their efficacy in the adjuvant setting which can be mimicked by continuous administration of hormones before the appearance of experimentally-induced mammary tumours in rats. Both antioestrogens and gonadotrophin releasing hormones delay the detection and reduce the absolute numbers of emerging lesions.[8-10]

Most important of all, however, is the evidence accumulating from ongoing prospective, controlled clinical trials in many parts of Europe and North America involving the antioestrogen 'Nolvadex' (tamoxifen).[11-18] Definitive conclusions may still be premature but statistically significant interim results, both in terms of increased relapse-free interval and survival are emerging in those with adequate numbers of patients and periods of follow-up. The latest analysis of the NSABP B09 trial comparing L-phenylalanine mustard and 5-fluorouracil against their combination with 'Nolvadex' is showing some loss of effect using the combined chemohormonal therapy in younger patients but this is at discord with the majority of trials showing 'Nolvadex' to be of value either alone or in combination with chemotherapy, in premenopausal as well as postmenopausal women irrespective of lymph node status. Where statistical analyses across trials have been performed the benefits appear remarkably homogenous and a pooled overall effect of about 24% reduction in treatment failure rate has been described.[19] Surprisingly some studies are demonstrating usefulness independent of oestrogen receptor status but reasons for this have been postulated.[20]

Androgens, oestrogens and the aromatase inhibitor aminoglutethimide have been assessed but they would seem to offer little advantage over antioestrogens and are associated with increased toxicity. The new class of potent gonadotrophin releasing hormones in slow release formulations may be capable of inducing long-term effective castration whilst being the least toxic of all, but trials in breast cancer have not been instigated yet.

In contrast to cytotoxic agents, the general acceptability of hormones affords an excellent opportunity to explore the ultimate potential of adjuvant therapy. Optimal schedules whether as monotherapy, combination therapy or in sequence with chemotherapy, still need to be defined and the sensitivity to further therapy of ultimate relapses after adjuvant treatment is currently debated. However, cure may even be feasible in women with Stage I disease exposed indefinitely to adjuvant agents. These and other such issues will only be resolved after appraisal of many further clinical trials. In the meantime, the data that have accrued provide a strong scientific rationale on which adjuvant hormonal therapy can be justified clinically.

REFERENCES

1. Schinzinger: Uber carcinoma mammae. Zentralblatt fur Chirurgie (16): 29, 55, 1889.

2. Horsley GW: Treatment of cancer of the breast in premenopausal patients with radical amputation and bilateral oophorectomy. Ann Surg (125): 6, 703-717, 1947.

3. Treves N: An evaluation of prophylactic castration in the treatment of mammary carcinoma. Cancer (10): 393-407, 1957.

4. Ravdin RG, Lewison EF, Slack NH, Dao TL, Gardner B, State D, Fisher B: Results of a clinical trial concerning the worth of prophylactic oophorectomy for breast carcinoma. Surg Gyn Obst (131): 1055-1064, 1970.

5. Cole MP: A clinical trial of an artificial menopause in carcinoma of the breast. INSERM (55): 143-150, 1975.

6. Nissen-Meyer R: Ovarian suppression and its supplement by additive hormonal treatment. INSERM (55): 151-158, 34-40, 1975 Edition 1966.

7. Meakin JW et al: Ovarian irradiation and prednisolone therapy following surgery and radiotherapy for carcinoma of the breast. Can Med Assoc J (120): 1221-5, 1979.

8. Welsch CW et al: Effect of an oestrogen antagonist (tamoxifen) on the initiation and progression of gamma-irradiation-induced mammary tumours. Europ J Cancer Clin Oncol (17): 1255-1258, 1981.

9. Jordan VC: Use of the DMBA-induced rat mammary carcinoma system for the evaluation of tamoxifen treatment as a potential adjuvant therapy. Rev Endo-Rel Canc Suppl, 49-56, 1978.

10. Furr BJA, Vacaccia BE, Hutchinson FG: Effects of a biodegradable slow release formulation of the LHRH analogue, ICI 118,630, on growth of rat DMBA-induced mammary tumours. 3rd EORTC Conference, Amsterdam, Abstr IX: 23, 1983.

11. Ribeiro G, Palmer MK: Adjuvant tamoxifen for operable carcinoma of the breast. Br Med J (286): 827-830, 1983.

12. NATO: Controlled trial of tamoxifen as adjuvant agent in management of early breast cancer. Lancet 1: 257-261, 1983.

13. Palshof T: Adjuvant endocrine therapy of primary operable breast cancer. 3rd EORTC Conference, Amsterdam, Abs V.I, 1983.

14. Rose C et al: Antioestrogen treatment of postmenopausal women with primary high risk breast cancer. Breast Canc Res Treat (3): 77-84, 1983.

15. Fisher B et al: Treatment of primary breast cancer with chemotherapy and tamoxifen. N E J Med (305): 1-6, 1981.

16. Hubay CA et al: Adjuvant therapy of Stage II breast cancer. Breast Canc Res Treat (1): 77-82, 1981.

17. Tormey DC, Jordan VC: Adjuvant use of tamoxifen for at least five years in node positive cancer. IABCR Conference, Colorado, 1983.

18. Wallgren A et al: Adjuvant breast cancer treatment with tamoxifen and combination chemotherapy in postmenopausal women. In: Adjuvant Therapy of Cancer III Ed. Salmon SE & Jones SE. Grune & Stratton, New York, 1981.

19. de Haan, HA: A clinical review of 'Nolvadex' in the management of breast cancer. Rev Endo-Rel Canc Suppl (11), 15-24, 1983.

20. Patterson J et al: The biology and physiology of 'Nolvadex' (tamoxifen) in the treatment of breast cancer. Breast Canc Res Treat (2): 363-374, 1982.

NEW APPROACHES TO THE USE OF ENDOCRINE THERAPY IN BREAST CANCER

R. C. COOMBES, J. WILLIAMS, A. BRODIE, T.J. POWLES, A.M. NEVILLE

1. INTRODUCTION

Endocrine therapy has become more important in recent years in the management of breast cancer because of its lack of toxicity and consequent excellent remissions that it can sometimes provide. Furthermore, the oestrogen receptor assay can, to a certain extent, predict which patients will respond to therapy, thus reinforcing the need for a reappraisal of our strategy in selecting agents for clinical use and in defining their mechanism of action. Improved knowledge of mechanisms should lead to rational combinations which could lead to increased response rates and prolonged survival for patients with breast cancer.

This summary will consider a) the use of an experimental animal model for selecting agents for clinical testing, b) endocrine studies carried out in patients receiving various forms of hormone therapy and c) results of various endocrine therapies in patients with breast cancer.

2. THE NITROSOMETHYLUREA (NMU) INDUCED MAMMARY TUMOURS IN RATS

NMU, given intravenously to female W-ICRF inbred rats at a dose of 5mg/100g body weight, on three separate occasions over a 2 month period results in 70-80% of rats bearing mammary tumours which become palpable at 4-5 months. The tumours do not metastasise, but resemble human breast carcinomas in that they contain significant amounts of oestrogen receptor (ER) and regress on oophorectomy (1).

We have used this model to determine whether endocrine therapy is effective in causing tumour regression and whether it is possible to rank various therapies in this way.

451

3. OVARIECTOMY AND FACTORS INHIBITING REGRESSION

Table 1 shows that more than 50% of tumours regress following ovariectomy and can be stimulated by oestradiol. The ovariectomy effect can be inhibited by concomitant administration of oestradiol. Oestradiol alone causes marked stimulation of growth of the tumours. Unlike human breast cancer, however, perphenazine, which increases prolactin secretion also appears to overcome the effect of ovariectomy (2).

TABLE 1   Ovariectomy : factors inhibiting regression

Therapy	No. rats/ no. tumours	Response (tumours) Regression (50->100%)	Progression (>100%)
1. Ovariectomy	12:26	14(54%)	0
2. Ovariectomy and 17β-oestradiol (a)	12:31	4(13%)	3
3. Ovariectomy and perphenazine (b)	12:29	4(14%)	7
4. 17β-oestradiol alone	12:37	0	15

(a) 1μg/kg/day   (b) 5mg/kg/day   From Williams et al (2)

4. ENDOCRINE AGENTS

Table 2 outlines the results we obtained when using conventional endocrine therapy. Neither tamoxifen nor aminoglutethimide nor danazol produced marked tumour regression and no significant difference was seen between results using these agents and control animals.

TABLE 2   NMU Mammary Tumours : Regression rates using conventional endocrine therapy

Therapy	No. rats/ no. tumours	Response (tumours) Regression (50->100%)	Progression (>100%)
1. Ovariectomy	12:26	14(54%)	0
2. Tamoxifen (a)	12:26	5(19%)	0
3. Aminoglutethimide (b)	8:14	4(28%)	5
4. Danazol (c)	11:28	0 (0%)	2
5. Control	11:23	3(13%)	10

(a) 120μg/kg/day   (b) 75mg/kg/day   (c) 100mg/kg/day
From Williams et al (2)

In contrast, 4-OH-androstenedione, an aromatase inhibitor, produced marked tumour regression, particularly when compared to another new agent, trilostane, which was evaluated at the same time (Table 3).

TABLE 3   NMU Mammary tumours : regression rates using new agents

Therapy	No. rats/ no. tumours	Response (tumours) Regression (50->100%)	Progression (>100%)
1. Trilostane(a)	10:24	0 (0%)	2
2. 4-OH Androstenedione(b)	12:27	18(67%)	0

(a) 200mg/kg/day   (b) 50mg/kg/day

5.   4-HYDROXYANDROSTENEDIONE (4HAD) AND FACTORS INHIBITING REGRESSION

In view of its potency in this sytem, we decided to further evaluate 4 HAD and to determine which factors could influence its effect (Table 4).   The results that we obtained indicated that regression induced by 4HAD could, like that seen following oophorectomy, be abolished by concomitant oestrogen and perphenazine administration (Williams et al, in preparation).   Furthermore, when we combined it with the anti-oestrogen tamoxifen a reduced effect was seen (Table 4). Although more animals are needed to confirm this impression, Dr. A. Brodie has observed similar effects (3).

TABLE 4   4-OH Androstenedione : use in combination in NMU mammary tumours

Therapy	No. rats/ no. tumours	Response (tumours) Regression (50->100%)	Progression (>100%)
1. 4-OH-A (a)	12:27	18(67%)	0
2. 4-OH-A + 17β-oestradiol (b)	12:30	2 (6%)	5
3. 4-OH-A + perphenazine (c)	11:24	1 (4%)	5
4. 4-OH-A + tamoxifen (d)	11:23	9(39%)	0

(a) 50mg/kg/day   (b) 1μg/kg/day   (c) 5mg/kg/day   (d) 120μg/kg/day
From Williams et al (2)

These results in the rat indicate a) that using limited numbers of animals, minor effects will not be observed in this model and that only major manoeuvres such as oophorectomy or 4HAD administration significantly reduce the tumour size in these animals and b) unlike human breast carcinomas, but like DMBA tumours, these tumours are sensitive to alterations of prolactin levels.

6.   RESULTS IN PATIENTS WITH ADVANCED BREAST CANCER

Results of different therapies vary depending on whether the patient is pre- or post-menopausal. Table 5 summarises some of the studies we have recently carried out in premenopausal patients. Broadly, it appears that oophorectomy is still the most effective form of therapy. We have not formally evaluated tamoxifen in premenopausal patients, although ongoing studies suggest tamoxifen may be equivalent to oophorectomy.

TABLE 5   Endocrine therapy in premenopausal patients

Therapy	Total	Response (%)	Stable (%)
1. Ovariectomy	36	12 (33)	6 (17)
2. Danazol	14	1 (7)	3 (21)
3. Aminoglutethimide	12	0 (0)	1 (8)

Most patients with breast cancer are postmenopausal and thus better comparative studies can be carried out in this group. Table 7 outlines the experience of this unit with various therapies over the past 3-4 years. The results indicate that tamoxifen is equipotent to aminoglutethimide but danazol and trilostane have reduced effect. Medroxyprogesterone acetate has only been evaluated in heavily pre-treated patients as yet. Initial results using Buserelin indicate that this compound has minimal activity in these patients.

TABLE 6   Endocrine therapy in postmenopausal patients

Therapy	Total	Response (%)	Stable (%)
1. Tamoxifen*	65	22 (34)	14 (22)
2. Aminoglutethimide	278	81 (29)	55 (20)
3. Danazol	45	9 (20)	3 (7)
4. Trilostane	40	1 (2)	6 (15)
5. Medroxyprogesterone Acetate	34	4 (12)	5 (15)
6. Combined Tamoxifen*/ Aminoglutethimide/ Danazol	61	31 (51)	15 (25)

*   Difference in response rate significant $p = <0.01$.
From Harris et al (4); Coombes et al (5); Coombes et al (6); and Powles (7).

Our most significant observation has been to demonstrate that combination of therapies can lead to improved response rates. Thus, in a randomised study we compared the combination of tamoxifen, aminoglutethimide and danazol with tamoxifen alone. Using this combination we have obtained a 51% response rate, compared to 34% for tamoxifen alone (7). We now feel that this result is due to the fact that some patients who fail to respond to tamoxifen subsequently respond to aminoglutethimide and this is probably true also for danazol.

7. CONCLUSION

Our observations suggest that some of these new non-toxic endocrine agents may have a major role in breast cancer management. It is only comparatively recently that agents have been specifically designed for their use as hormone inhibitors in breast cancer and response rates may well increase as they are introduced into clinical use. The rat NMU-induced mammary tumour model, whilst having the limitations of being insensitive and possibly prolactin-dependent, may be a good screen for powerful antiendocrine therapy, particularly if 4HAD proves to have equivalent potency in patients. Ideally, drug handling should be examined in patients and in the rat model prior to using this rat to design combinations and scheduling etc.

Our results with combined endocrine therapy indicate that an approach directed at seeking agents with different sites of action may well be translated into improved response rates, and hopefully improved survival.

REFERENCES

1. Williams JC, Gusterson B, Humphreys J, Monaghan P, Coombes RC, Rudland P, Neville AM: N-Nitrosomethylurea-induced rat mammary tumours - hormone responsiveness but lack of spontaneous metastasis. J Natl Cancer Inst (66): 147-155, 1981.
2. Williams JC, Singh D, Brodie A, Coombes RC: Endocrine agents and their effect in rats bearing NMU-induced mammary tumours. (In preparation).
3. Brodie A: Personal Communication.
4. Harris AL, Powles TJ, Smith IE, Coombes RC, Ford HT, Gazet J-C, Harmer CL, Morgan M, White H, Parsons CA, McKinna JA: Amino-glutethimide for the treatment of advanced postmenopausal breast cancer. Eur J Cancer Clin Oncol (19): 11-17, 1983.
5. Coombes RC, Perez D, Gazet J-C, Ford HT, Powles TJ: Danazol treatment for advanced breast cancer. Cancer Chemother Pharmacol (10): 194-195, 1983.
6. Coombes RC, Powles TJ, Muindi J, Hunt J, Ward M, Perez D, Neville AM: Trilostane therapy for advanced breast cancer. In Press.
7. Powles TJ, Gordon C, Coombes RC: Clinical trial of multiple endocrine therapy for metastatic and locally advanced breast cancer with tamoxifen-aminoglutethimide-danazol compared to tamoxifen used alone. Cancer Res (42) (Suppl) 3458S-3460S, 1982.

THE PHARMACOLOGY OF A NEW ANTIESTROGEN

JAMES A. CLEMENS, LARRY J. BLACK AND ROBERT L. ZERBE

INTRODUCTION

Presently, attempts to pharmacologically antagonize estrogen action
are impeded by the weak estrogenic activity of the currently available
estrogen antagonists. Most antiestrogens, rather than being pure
antagonists, possess varying degrees of estrogen agonist activity. Thus,
the action of estrogens can be antagonized only to the point where the
agonist activity of the antiestrogen begins to be expressed.

Although a potent antiestrogen devoid of estrogenicity has yet to be
synthesized, significant progress has been made toward achieving this
objective. LY156758 has been found to be an effective antiestrogen with
a high affinity for estrogen receptors, and yet possess a very low degree
of estrogenicity (1). This report summarizes the studies on LY156758 and
its free base, LY139481.

PROCEDURE

Estrogen Antagonist Studies. Immature Sprague-Dawley rats (19-20 days,
40-45 g) were tested in groups of six. Compounds were injected
subcutaneously in a 0.1 ml corn oil vehicle, and controls received
vehicle injections. The rats were killed 24 hours after the last
treatment, uteri removed and the weight recorded. Relative binding
affinity was calculated as previously described (2).

Effects on Mammary Tumors. Rats with at least one measurable mammary
tumor were selected for further experimentation, and during the treatment
period, the tumor area was measured at weekly intervals. LY156758 or
tamoxifen were administered sc as a suspension in corn oil.

Effects on LH and Prolactin Release. Adult female rats were
ovariectomized (OVX), and 10 days later groups of rats received either
daily sc injections of 2 μg of estradiol benzoate (EB) or a combination

457

of EB and LY156758 or tamoxifen for 10 days. All compounds were
suspended in a corn oil vehicle. Groups of rats were decapitated between
1000 and 1200 h or between 1400 and 1600 h. Blood was collected and
assayed for prolactin and LH by radioimmunoassay.

RESULTS
    LY139481 had a higher relative binding affinity (RBA) than estradiol,
and the ratio increased in relation to temperature (Fig. 1). The mean
RBA was 1.43 ± 0.38 using a one hour incubation time at 4° C. At 30° C
an RBA 2.9 fold greater than that of estradiol was observed.

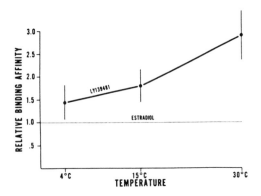

FIGURE 1. Relative binding affinity of LY139481 (estradiol=1.0).
Results are the mean ± standard error of eleven determinations. From
Black, Jones and Falcone (1).

    LY139481, but not tamoxifen, markedly antagonized low doses (0.03 and
0.05 µg) of estradiol (Fig. 2). The estrogen agonist activity of
tamoxifen was greater than the agonist activity of low doses of
estradiol. Both LY139481 and tamoxifen antagonized the higher doses of
estradiol (0.1 and 1.0 µg).
    In the mammary tumor model, administration of 1-10 mg/kg of LY156758
for 21 days inhibited tumor growth (Table 1). Tamoxifen also inhibited
tumor growth.
    The effects of LY156758 and tamoxifen on serum LH and prolactin
levels in EB-treated OVX rat are shown in Figures 3 and 4, respectively.
Interestingly, LY156758, but not tamoxifen, prevented the reduction in

459

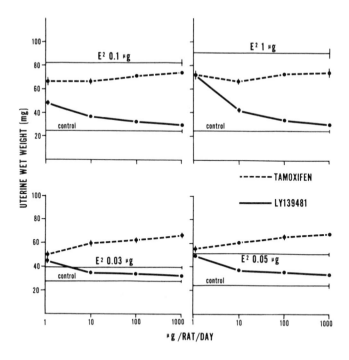

FIGURE 2. Antiuterotropic activity of LY139481 and tamoxifen. Daily sc injections of estradiol or antiestrogens in combination with estradiol were given for three days to immature rats. Rats were killed on the fourth day. Values are mean ± standard error.

Table 1. Effects of LY156758 on the growth of DMBA-induced mammary tumors.

Treatment	Duration of Treatment (days)	No. of Rats	Av. Tumor Area at Start (mm²)	Av. Tumor Area at Finish (mm²)
Control, corn oil	21	7	47.1 ± 7.5[a]	1614 ± 618
LY156758, 1 mg/kg	21	6	45.1 ± 13.2	343 ± 89
LY156758, 10 mg/kg	21	7	39.4 ± 9.0	217 ± 77[b]
Tamoxifen, 1 mg/kg	21	5	43.6 ± 11.8	105 ± 65[b]

[a]Mean ± SE; [b]$p < .05$ vs control.

morning serum LH levels by EB. In contrast, LY156758 did not alter afternoon LH levels, but tamoxifen blocked the afternoon rise. The after-noon rise in serum prolactin was blocked more effectively by tamoxifen.

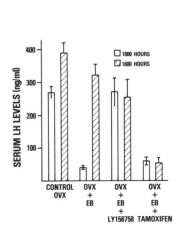

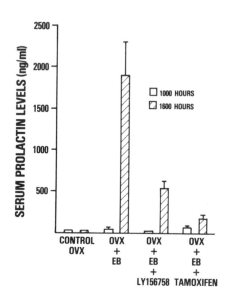

FIGURE 3. Effect of LY156758 on LH secretion in estradiol benzoate-treated OVX rats.

FIGURE 4. Effect of LY156758 on prolactin secretion in estradiol benzoate-treated OVX rats.

DISCUSSION

The results of this study demonstrate that LY139481 and its hydrochloride salt, LY156758, are potent antiestrogens. The low level of agonist activity and the ability to antagonize low levels of estradiol are highly desirable properties for a drug to be used to treat breast cancer in post-menopausal women where an estrogen deficient state exists. Perhaps the reason why antiestrogen therapy is of benefit in only about one-half of the patients with estrogen receptor positive tumors is that the antiestrogens fail to antagonize the low levels of circulating estrogens. This line of reasoning is supported by the observations that in patients who become refractory to tamoxifen therapy, a remission can be induced by adrenalectomy or aminoglutethimide treatment (3). These treatments remove the source of estrogens.

In contrast to the human breast cancer, where inhibition of prolactin release has little effect (4), the DMBA-induced tumor is highly prolactin dependent (5). This may be why LY156758 does not have a more dramatic antitumor effect in the rat (6) but may be more beneficial in treating human breast cancer.

461

In Phase I studies in normal male volunteers, LY156758 was well tolerated and produced minimal side-effects. No alterations in serum levels of LH, FSH, prolactin or testosterone were observed.

REFERENCES

1. Black LJ, Jones CD, Falcone JF: Antagonism of estrogen with a new benzothiophene antiestrogen. Life Sci (32): 1031-1036, 1983.
2. Black LJ, Jones CD, Goode RL: Differential interaction of antiestrogens with cytosol estrogen receptors. Mol Cell Endocrinol (22):95-103, 1981.
3. Gale K: Treatment of advanced breast cancer with aminoglutethimide Cancer Res suppl (42):3389-3396, 1982.
4. Heuson JC, Coume A, Stagnet M: Clinical trial of 2-Br-alpha-ergocryptine (CB154) in advanced breast cancer. Europ J Cancer (8):155-159, 1972.
5. Clemens JA, Shaar CJ: Inhibition by ergocornine of initiation and growth of 7,12-dimethylbenzanthracene induced mammary tumors in rats: effect of tumor size. Proc Soc Exp Biol Med (139):659-662, 1972.
6. Clemens JA, Bennett DR, Black LJ, Jones CD: Effects of a new antiestrogen, keoxifene (LY156758), on growth of carcinogen-induced mammary tumors and on LH and prolactin levels. Life Sci (32):2869-2875, 1983.

IN VITRO SYSTEMS FOR EVALUATING ANTI-ENDOCRINE AGENTS

G. LECLERCQ, N. DEVLEESCHOUWER AND J.C. HEUSON

1. INTRODUCTION

The value of tamoxifen in breast cancer treatment is now well established. However, the drug as most other antiestrogens of the triphenylethylene category, displays a weak estrogenic activity which may hamper its full therapeutic effectiveness. Search for new antiestrogens devoid of this undesirable activity has therefore been undertaken.

Several animal mammary tumor models are useful for evaluating the potential therapeutic effectiveness of anti-endocrine agents (i.e., DMBA and NMU - induced rat mammary tumors, MXT and GR tranplantable mouse mammary tumors...). However, in vivo screening requires large amounts of drug which cannot always be easily produced. This led to the development of in vitro systems for evaluating such compounds. In our laboratory, two cells lines either containing (MCF-7) or lacking (Evsa-T) estrogen receptors (ER) are routinely used for evaluating the cytotoxicity of new antiestrogens. This screening method combined with the measurement of the binding affinity of these drugs for ER appears extremely powerful for their preliminary characterization.

It is our purpose to overview some of our recent investigations to illustrate the efficency of our model in the selection of newly produced antiestrogens.

2. METHODS

2.1. Binding characteristics of the compounds to estrogen receptors

The binding affinity of the compounds was measured by a classical competitive inhibition test of the binding of ^{3}H-estradiol to a cytoplasmic ER preparation. The relative concentrations of un-labelled estradiol (control) and test-compounds required to

463

achieve a 50% inhibition of ^{3}H-estradiol binding gives the
binding affinity (BA = $\left[I_{50}\right]_{E2}/\left[I_{50}\right]_x$ x 100) (1).

The ability of ^{3}H-estradiol to displace bound unlabelled
estradiol, estrone (controls) or test-compounds from ER was used
for evaluating their binding stability (2).

The experimental details of these tests have been reported in
previous publications (3, 4). Crude cytosol or partially purified ER (ammonium sulfate precipitation) from rat uterus or
mouse mammary tumor were used.

2.2. Effect of the compounds on growth of the MCF-7 and Evsa-T cell lines

The effect of the compounds on cell growth was estimated by
measuring the amounts of DNA after 120 hours of culture in their
presence or absence (4,5). Fifty to 200 x 10^3 cells were plated in
35 mm Petri dishes containing MEM medium supplemented with L-glu-
tamine, antibiotics and 10% fetal calf serum. After 24 hours of
culture, the test-compound was added to the dishes. Forty-eight
hours later the medium was replaced by fresh medium containing
the compound. The cultures were then pursued for a 72-hours period
before final harvest. Total DNA of collected cells was estimated
at 24 (addition of compounds) and 144 hours (end of experiment).

3. RESULTS

3.1. Triphenylethylene antiestrogens

At concentrations ranging from 10^{-8} to 10^{-6}M, antiestrogens
of the triphenylethylene category usually produce a significant
inhibition of MCF-7 cell growth while they have no effect on
Evsa-T cells (5,6). Investigations of a series of compounds
revealed a close parallelism between their binding affinity for
ER and their ability to inhibit the MCF-7 cell growth (Table I).
This observation is consistent with the concept that antiestrogens
produce their antitumor activity through binding to the receptors.
This view is supported by the fact that the inhibition is suppressed by estradiol concentrations that are lower than, or equimolar
to those of the antagonist.

Hydroxylation of a phenyl ring of triphenylethylene antiestrogens leads to drugs with very high binding affinity for ER and

TABLE 1 : BINDING AFFINITY FOR ESTROGEN RECEPTORS AND INHIBITION OF MCF-7 CELL GROWTH.

	BA (E_2=100)	I_{50} (MOLARITY)
U - 23,469	0.1	No inhibition at 10^{-6}
ICI - 46,474 (Tamoxifen)	0.5 - 1	$10^{-6} - 10^{-7}$
U - 11,100 A (Nafoxidine)	5	$10^{-6} - 10^{-7}$
CI - 628	11	10^{-7}
U - 23,469 M	30	10^{-7}
CI - 628 M	$\geqslant$100	10^{-8}
ICI - 79,280 (Hydroxytamoxifen)	$\geqslant$100	10^{-8}

strong antiestrogenicity. Hydroxylation also increases the in vitro antitumor activity of the drugs as shown by their higher cytotoxicity on MCF-7 cells (Table I : ICI 46,474 vs. ICI 79,280; CI 628 vs. CI 628M and U 23,469 vs. U 23,469 M). Remarkably, the increase is related to the increase in binding affinity for ER produced by the hydroxylation.

Triphenylethylene antiestrogens contain a side-chain which is known to be essential for their physiological activity : without such a chain they lose their antiestrogenicity and ability to inhibit MCF-7 cell growth. Noteworthy, the grafting of a side-chain to a weak estrogen of the gem-diphenylethylene category (4,4-dihydroxy, 1,1-diphenyl-2,2-dichloroethylene) produced a compound able to inhibit MCF-7 cells (5). The inhibition was similar to that found with triphenylethylene antiestrogens since it was suppressed by estradiol. Moreover, the compound did not suppress the inhibition of U-11,100 A indicating an absence of estrogenicity.

That the grafting of an aminoethoxy side-chain on such a "symmetrical" diphenyethylene confers antiestrogenicity is of interest in view of the fact that triphenylethylene antiestrogens are in the trans configuration. When they are in the cis configuration, they usually display estrogenic activity. This geometrical isomerism also influences the MCF-7 cell growth : the trans isomer of tamoxifen shares the classical antitumor activity (inhibitory action suppressed by estradiol) while the cis isomer behaves as a weak estrogen (no inhibitory action; partial suppression of U 11,100 A inhibition) (5).

3.2. Suicide inhibitors

Efforts have been made to produce "suicide inhibitors" that irreversibly bind to ER. In principle, drugs that bind irreversibly to ER should display very strong estrogenic or antiestrogenic activity. Assessment of the biological activity of such compounds on breast cancer cell lines appears therefore as an appropriate test to evaluate which class they belong to. The study of a 11β-chloromethyl derivative of estradiol (ORG 4333) (4, 5, 7) and a 2-mesylate derivative of estrone which irreverbly bind to ER, demonstrated this fact (5). Thus, in MCF-7 cells the chloromethyl suppressed the growth inhibition of U-11,100 A as estradiol. In contrast, the mesylate inhibited growth at concentrations as low as the strongests antiestrogens ICI-79,280 and CI-628 M (Fig. 1). The inhibition was suppressed only by equimolar concentrations of estradiol. This contrasts with the behaviour of conventional antiestrogens such as tamoxifen, the inhibition of which is counteracted by lower concentrations (5, 6). Moreover, hydroxylated and methoxylated derivatives of estrone (2-OH, 2-OCH$_3$) did not inhibit growth suggesting that the cytotoxicity of the drug was associated with its mesylate residue. Remarkably, no growth inhibition occured in Evsa-T cells indicating that the drug has no major non-specific cytotoxicity.

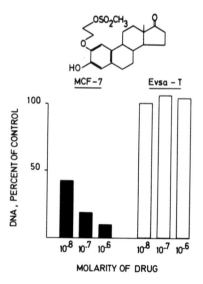

FIGURE 1. Effect of a mesylate derivative of estrone on MCF-7 and Evsa-T cell growth. For further details, see ref. 5. Origin of the compound: Dr. R.L. MORGAN; Louisiana State University, New Orleans.

4. DISCUSSION

The measurement of the binding affinity of antiestrogens for ER and the assessement of their in vitro antitumor activity on ER-positive and ER-negative breast cancer cell lines are two adequate tests for the establishement of structure-activity relationships. The data reported here are illustrative of this statement. Thus, in triphenylethylenes we have shown the importance of the side-chain, of the hydroxylation of a phenyl ring and of the configuration to produce a strong specific inhibitory activity. Data were also given suggesting that "suicide inhibitors" irreversibly interacting with ER may have a strong in vitro antitumor activity and thereby present a potential therapeutic activity.

The rapidity, the low cost and the small quantities of compounds required are the main advantages of our model. These advantages make it especially suitable for the screening of a large number of compounds. It is also a powerful complement for metabolic studies, since it easily provides informations on the biological activity of isolated metabolites (8, 9).

Data resulting from these in vitro tests appear therefore extremely powerful for the preliminary characterization of new drugs as well as for the proposition of guidelines for the design of compounds.

This work was supported by a grant from the Fonds Cancérologique de la Caisse Générale d'Epargne et de Retraite de Belgique.

REFERENCES

1. Korenman S.G. : Comparative binding affinity of estrogens and its relation to estrogenic potency. Steroids (13) : 163-177, 1969.
2. Katzenellenbogen J.A., Johnson H.J. and Carlson K.E. : Studies on the uterine cytoplasmic estrogen binding protein. Thermal stability and ligand dissociation rate. An assay for empty and filled sites by exchange. Biochemistry (12) : 4092-4099, 1973.
3. Leclercq G., Deboel M.C. and Heuson J.C. Affinity of estradiol mustard for estrogen receptors and its enzymatic degradation in uterine and breast cancer cytosols. Int. J. Cancer (18) : 750-756, 1973.

4. Leclercq G., Devleeschouwer N., Legros N. and Heuson J.C. : In vitro screening for cytotoxic estrogens of potential therapeutic activity. In : Raus J., Martens H. and Leclercq G. (eds) Cytotoxic estrogens in hormone receptive tumors. Academic Press, London, 1980, pp. 168-181.

5. Leclercq G., Devleeschouwer N. and Heuson J.C. : Guidelines in the design of new antiestrogens and cytotoxic-linked estrogens for the treatment of breast cancer. J. Steroid Biochem (10) : 75-85, 1983.

6. Lippman M.E., Bolan E. and Huff K. : The effect of estrogens and antiestrogens on hormone-receptive human breast cancer in long term tissue culture. Cancer Res. (36) : 4595-4601, 1976.

7. Van den Broek A.J., Leemhuis J., De Winter M.S., Zeelen F.J.: Org 4333, a potent, irreversibly binding estrogen agonist. Pharm. Weekblad Sc. Ed. (5) : 182-183, 1983.

8. Coezy E., Borgna J.L., Rochefort H. : Tamoxifen and metabolites in MCF-7 cells : Correlation between binding to estrogen receptors and inhibition of cell growth. Cancer Res. (42) : 317-323, 1982.

9. Bates D.J., Foster A.B., Griggs L.J., Jarman M., Leclercq G., Devleeschouwer N. : Metabolism of tamoxifen by isolated rat hepatocytes : antiestrogenic activity of tamoxifen N-oxide. Biochem. Pharmac. (31) : 2823-2827, 1982.

EXPERIENCE OF THE LHRH ANALOGUE, ICI 118,430, IN CARCINOMA OF THE PROSTATE

J.M. ALLEN, D.J. KERLE, G. WILLIAMS, S.R. BLOOM

INTRODUCTION

Over 40 years ago, the classic laboratory experiments of Drs. Huggins and Hodges (1) firmly established the androgen dependence of the prostatic cancer cell, and led to the concept of endocrine manipulation for adenocarcinoma of the prostate.

Eighty percent of tumours respond to lowering serum testosterone (2). The conventional means by which this is achieved however, encounter considerable objections. Orchidectomy is often rejected by patients and stilboestrol therapy is associated with significant cardiovascular morbidity and mortality.

Serum testosterone is controlled by the hypothalamic-pituitary axis. The hypothalamic decapeptide gonadotrophin releasing hormone (LHRH) controls release of luteinising hormone (LH) and follicle stimulating hormone (FSH) from the anterior pituitary which in turn controls testicular production of testosterone. Secretion of LHRH is pulsatile; this being a pre-requisite for normal gonadal function (3). Substitution of amino acids in the sixth and tenth positions of LHRH sequence results in agonists with increased potency and prolonged activity. Continuous stimulation of gonadotrophs by these superactive analogues of LHRH results in a paradoxical fall in LH and FSH and hence in testosterone (4). These agonists are therefore currently under evaluation in patients with endocrine responsive tumours such as adenocarcinoma of the prostate (5,6) and we report here the early clinical experience with the analogue ICI 118,630.

Patients and Methods

All patients gave written informed consent to participate in the study which had prior approval of the Royal Postgraduate Medical School Ethics

Committee. Patients had biopsy proven carcinoma of the prostate and had progressive disease.

A total of 35 patients have been entered into the trial and all have received a minimum of two months treatment. The longest period of treatment being eighteen months. Of these, 18 received the analogue as first choice whereas 17 had relapsed or failed to respond to conventional endocrine therapy (Table 1). The analogue was given subcutaneously daily and patients were encouraged and taught to give their own injection.

Table I

Previous endocrine treatment of 17 patients

6 - Orchidectomy + Oestrogens

6 - Oestrogens alone

3 - Orchidectomy alone

2 - Antiandrogens

Subjective response was determined by assessing the effect on the patients analgesia requirements and by the patients own appraisal of interference of the disease on their daily life. Objective response was determined by assessment of tumour characteristics by consultant urologist, acid phosphatase measurement and where possible bone scans. The endocrine response to treatment was monitored by measuring serum LH, FSH and testosterone over the course of treatment.

RESULTS

All patients who received the analogue as first line of treatment have shown a response. Five patients have subsequently relapsed after this initial response; two patients after one year complete remission and three patients who only showed an initial partial response have relapsed after three months. Of the patients who had relapsed on conventional endocrine therapy, six showed no response to treatment and have died within one month. Of the eleven patients still living, four patients who had progressive disease before starting the analogue now have stable disease,

whereas seven continue to progress. Of these 11 patients, eight patients
had severe pain, requiring narcotic analgesia prior to starting the
analogue. Seven patients have been able to withdraw or markedly reduce
their narcotic requirements, despite evidence of disease progression.

Endocrine assessment has shown that this analogue is a potent agonist
with a prolonged biological activity. The first dose results in a prompt
rise in serum LH which is sustained up to twelve hours after the dose.
Regular treatment with the analogue results in a loss of this acute response
(Fig. 1). A characteristic response is observed over three months of
treatment with the analogue. Serum testosterone rises in the first week,
but levels have returned to pretreatment values by the end of the first week
and are significantly supressed after two weeks. Serum testosterone
continues to fall until the end of the first month, levels are below those
achieved by stilboestrol and are equivalent to castrate levels (Fig. 2).

FIGURE 1

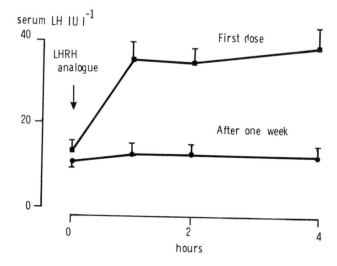

Figure 1 legend

Serum LH response (iu/l) over 4 hours to the first dose of ICI 118,630 (250
micrograms subcutaneously) and to an identical dose of the analogue after
one week of regular treatment.

FIGURE 2

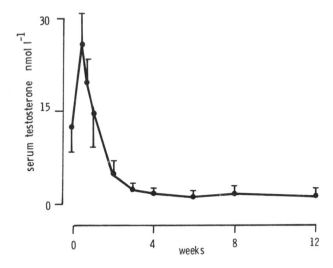

Figure 2 legend

Serum testosterone (nmol/l) over first three months of regular treatment with the analogue, ICI 118,630 in 18 patients who had not previously received endocrine therapy.

Over three months, there is no overall change in serum prolactin.

Side effects

Fifty per cent of new patients have described "hot flushes" and about one third of the "new" patients have reported a marked reduction in sexual activity since starting treatment.

DISCUSSION

In previously untreated patients, treatment with a superactive analogue of LHRH results in serum testosterone values that are equivalent to those achieved after orchidectomy. The clinical response to the analogue in this group of patients would appear to be similar to the predicted outcome after orchidectomy. Treatment with the agonist however is more acceptable to patients and additionally supresses serum gonadotrophins which are considered to be trophic to the prostate, without necessitating oestrogen therapy with the associated cardiovascular risk. Additionally, in contrast to conventional management, treatment with the analogue does not alter the serum prolactin. This may have additional benefits as prolactin is also considered to play a trophic role in prostate cancer. The results from this study compare favourably with those from other centres using different LHRH analogues.

However, in this study, the analogue was also used in the management of patients who had relapsed on conventional endocrine therapy. Despite evidence of further progression, about half of these patients experienced considerable relief of their bone pain, in some cases being able to withdraw from narcotic analgesia. The mechanism by which this is achieved is undetermined.

It would seem that the use of these superactive agonists could provide a safe and more effective treatment for adenocarcinoma of prostate although obviously longer term trials are needed.

REFERENCES

1. Huggins C, Hodges CV: Studies on prostatic cancer. The effect of castration, of oestrogen and of androgen on serum phosphatases in metastatic carcinoma of the prostate. Cancer Res (1): 293-297, 1941
2. Whitehead ED: Management of prostate carcinoma. N Y State J Med (81): 1481-5, 1981
3. Yen SSC, Tsai CC, Naftolin F, Vendenberg G, Ajabor L: Pulsatile patterns of gonadotrophin release in subjects with and without ovarian function. J Clin Endocrinol Metab (34): 641-5, 1972
4. Linde R, Doelle GC, Alexander N, Kirchner F, Vale W, Rivier J, Rabin D: Reversible inhibition of testicular steroidogenesis and spermatogenesis by a potent gonadotrophin-releading agonist in normal men. N Engl J Med (305): 663-7, 1981
5. Tolis G, Ackman D, Stellos A, Mehta A, Latorie F, Fazekas ATA, Cornam-Schally M, Schally AV: Tumour growth inhibition in patients with prostatic carcinoma treated with luteinising hormone releasing hormone agonists. Proc Natl Acad Sci USA (79): 1658-1662, 1982
6. Allen JM, O'Shea JP, Mashiter K, Williams G, Bloom SR: Advanced carcinoma of the prostate: treatment with a gonadotrophin releasing hormone agonist. Br Med J (286): 1607-09, 1983

COMPLETE ANDROGEN NEUTRALIZATION IS MOST IMPORTANT IN THE TREATMENT OF PROSTATE CANCER

F. LABRIE, A. DUPONT and A. BELANGER

1. INTRODUCTION

The unexpected finding that LHRH (luteinizing hormone-releasing hormone) agonists block testicular testosterone secretion and induce a marked loss in ventral prostate weight in the adult rat (1-3) opened the possibility of a new approach in the treatment of androgen-dependent diseases, especially cancer of the prostate. Fortunately, among all species studied, man is the most sensitive to the inhibitory effect of LHRH agonist treatment on testicular androgen formation and medical castration can be easily achieved without any side effects other than those related to hypoandrogenicity (3-5).

Following the pioneering studies of Huggins and collaborators (6), neutralization of testicular androgens has been usually achieved during the last 40 years by surgical castration or treatment with high doses of estrogens, two approaches which lead to subjective and/or objective improvement in 60 to 70% of cases for various time intervals (7, 8). However, surgical castration presents psychological limitations for many patients while high doses of estrogens frequently cause lethal cardiovascular complications (7). LHRH agonists thus offer an advantageous alternative for neutralization of testicular androgens.

Since man is unique among species in having a high secretion of weak adrenal androgens which can be converted into active steroids in the prostate as well as at the periphery (9), it is quite possible that reactivation of the cancer is due to the androgens of adrenal origin. We thus felt important to include neutralization of adrenal androgens in our antihormonal treatment regime.

The present report summarizes the results obtained in 68 patients having metastatic (stage D2) prostatic cancer, 44 of which had received no previous treatment while 24 had been treated with diethylstilbestrol (DES). Complete androgen neutralization has been achieved by the combined use of an LHRH agonist (to cause medical castration) and a pure antiandrogen (to neutralize adrenal androgens) in 59 patients while LHRH agonist treatment was substituted by surgical castration in 9 cases. The results obtained clearly demonstrate the need for complete neutralization of all androgens of both testicular and adrenal origin at the start of treatment of patients with advanced prostate cancer.

2. RESULTS AND DISCUSSION

Serum prostatic acid phosphatase (PAP) was rapidly reduced to 45% of pretreatment values as early as 5 days after starting the combined antihormonal therapy using the LHRH agonist and the antiandrogen in previously untreated patients. The serum PAP values progressively decreased and normal values were reached within two months in all except 4 patients who all showed normal serum PAP levels at 4 months. A similar pattern was seen in 9 previously untreated patients who were surgically castrated and received the same dose of the antiandrogen (data not shown). A striking difference is observed when the same treatment is applied to patients previously treated with DES. In fact, although serum PAP levels decreased to normal values in some patients, the concentration of serum PAP continued to increase in 11 out of 24 patients.

In 32 previously untreated patients, the combined therapy led to at least a 50% decrease in bone uptake accompanied by a normalization of serum PAP and no appearance of new lesions. The important finding is the absence of any progression of the disease in any of the patients previously untreated.

It can be seen in Table 1 that a markedly different response is observed in patients previously treated with DES

and receiving the same combined treatment where progression
of the disease continued in 42% of cases.

In the previously untreated patients, a rapid and complete
relief of pain was observed in all patients presenting this
symptom before treatment. Disappearance of bone pain was seen
within a few days. In patients previously treated with DES,
complete removal of androgens also led to a disappearance of
pain in all patients.

The most important conclusion which becomes apparent in
this study is that previously untreated prostate cancer in
man is extremely sensitive to androgens. In fact, when complete androgen neutralization is achieved in patients previously untreated, a positive objective response assessed
according to the criteria of the National Prostatic Cancer
Project is observed in more than 95% of patients. In fact, in
44 patients who received the combined therapy no progression
of the disease was observed in any patient and relapse has
been observed in only 2 cases up to 18 months of treatment.

Comparison of the positive responses observed in the
present study with those found following standard hormonal
therapy with DES or surgical castration (NPCP protocol 500)
(10) is important. In the latter study, a positive response
was observed in 67 out of 83 patients while, in the present
study, all 44 patients showed a positive response after
complete androgen neutralization (Fisher's test, $p < 0.001$).
Moreover, after 40 weeks of treatment, only 53 out of 83
patients were still in remission after surgical castration or
DES treatment (10) as compared to 23 out of 25 patients using
the present approach ($p < 0.001$.).

Since patients at stage D2 have an average of at least
ten metastases each, for a total of at least 460 metastases,
and only two tumors were apparently hormone-insensitive (or
became insensitive), the present data indicate that even at
the late metastatic stage, more than 99% of prostatic tumors
are androgen-sensitive. This finding has major implications
for therapy.

Another important finding in the present study is that con-

TABLE 1. Comparison of the objective response to the complete neutralization of androgens assessed according to the crite- ria of the USA National Prostatic Cancer Project (NPCP) achieved by the combined treatment with an LHRH agonist (D- Ser(TBU)[6] LHRH-ethylamide or D-Try[6]-LHRH-ethylamide) or sur- gical castration and a pure antiandrogen (Anandron) in pa- tients having advanced prostate cancer at stage D2 who were previously untreated or had previously been treated with DES (diethylstilbestrol).

Pre- vious treat- ment	Mths of treatment (average & limits)	Treat- ment	No of pts	% objective response				
				Com- plete	Par- tial	Sta- ble	Pro- gres- sion	Escape
None	10.9 (5-19)	LHRH-A + antiandr.	35	11% (4)	69% (24)	20% (7)	0% 0%	2/35 4.5%
None	8.3 (5-12)	castr. + antiandr.	9	11% (1)	33% (3)	56% (5)	0% 0	2/44 0/9
DES	9.5 (4-15)	LHRH-A + antiandr.	24	4% (1)	37% (9)	17% (4)	42% (10)	4/14 29%

comitant treatment with the pure antiandrogen completely pre- vents disease flare, a complication unfortunately observed in a significant proportion of patients treated with LHRH ago- nists alone (5, 11). With the present knowledge, there remains no rationale for the unethical use of LHRH agonists alone since the adverse effects of the initial rise in serum andro- gens can be so easily prevented, thus eliminating any unneces- sary risk to the patients.

Another most important conclusion which derives from this study is that a large proportion of prostatic cancer cells which continue to grow under the influence of androgens of adrenal origin become androgen-insensitive in this "androgen- poor" milieu. This is clearly demonstrated by the finding that complete androgen neutralization in patients previously treat- ed with estrogens leads to only a 58% positive/objective res- ponse as compared to 100% in previously untreated patients. The much lower rate of response observed in previously treated patients indicates a corresponding increase in the proportion of androgen-insensitive cancer cells in these patients. It is also hoped that the present findings and principles of antihormonal treatment could apply to other hormone-sensitive cancers, especially breast cancer.

REFERENCES

1. Auclair C, Kelly PA, Coy DH, Schally AV, Labrie F: Potent inhibitory activity of [D-Leu^6, des-Gly-NH$_2$^{10}]LHRH ethylamide on LH/hCG and PRL testicular receptor levels in the rat. Endocrinology (101): 1890-1893, 1977.
2. Labrie F, Auclair C, Cusan L, Kelly PA, Pelletier G, Ferland L: Inhibitory effects of LHRH and its agonists on testicular gonadotropin receptors and spermatogenesis in the rat. In: Hansson V (ed) 5th Ann Workshop on the Testis: Endocrine Approach to Male Contraception, Int J of Andrology, suppl 2, 1978, pp. 303-318.
3. Labrie F, bélanger A, Cusan L, Séguin C, Pelletier G, Kelly PA, Lefebvre FA, Lemay A, Raynaud JP: Antifertility effects of lHRH agonists in the male. J Androl (1):209-228, 1980.
4. Labrie F, Dupont A, Bélanger A, Cusan, L, Lacoursière Y, Monfette G, Laberge JG, Emond JP, Fazekas ATA, Raynaud JP, Husson JM: New hormonal therapy in prostatic carcinoma: combined treatment with an LHRH agonist and an antiandrogen. J Clin Invest Med (5): 267-275, 1982.
5. Santen RJ, Warner B, Demers LM, Dufau M, Smith J: Use of GnRH hormone agonists analogs. In Vickery B, Nestor JR JJ, Hafez ESE (eds) LHRH and its analogs - a new class of contraceptive and therapeutic agents. MTP Press, Lancaster-Boston, 1983, in press.
6. Huggins C, Stevens RE, Hodges CW: Studies on prostatic carcinoma. II. The effect of castration of advanced carcinoma of the prostate gland. Arch Surg (43):209-223, 1941.
7. Byar DP: The Veterans Administration Cooperative Urological Research Group's Studies of Cancer of the Prostate. Cancer (32):1126-1130, 1973.
8. Murphy GP, Slack NH: The questionable use of hormone therapy in advanced carcinoma of the prostate. Urol Clin North Amer (7):631-638, 1980.
9. Acevedo HF, Goldziecker JW: Further studies on the metabolism of 4-[4-^{14}C]androstane-3,17-dione by normal and pathological human prostatic tissues. Biochim Biophys Acta (97):564-570, 1965.
10. Murphy GP, Beckley S, Brady MF, CHU M, DeKernion JB, Dhabuwala C, Gaeta JF, Gibbons RP, Loening SA, McKiel CF, McLeod DG, Pontes JE, Prout GR, Scardino PT, Schlegel JU, Schmidt JD, Scott WW, Slack NH, Soloway M: Treatment of newly diagnosed metastatic prostate cancer patients with chemotherapy agents in combination with hormones versus hormones alone. Cancer (51)1264-1272, 1983.
11. Trachtenberg J: The treatment of metastatic prostatic cancer with a potent luteinizing hormone-releasing hormone analogue. J Urol (129):1149-1152, 1983.

AMINOGLUTETHIMIDE (ORIMETEN[R]): THE PRESENT AND THE FUTURE

I.M. JACKSON

INTRODUCTION

Aminoglutethimide (Orimeten[R]) was first introduced as an anticonvulsant (Elipten[R]) in the United States in 1960. It was withdrawn in 1966 following reports of a small number of adverse effects in children including adrenocortical insufficiency, which appeared to be associated with the experimental evidence of an inhibitory effect of the drug on steroid synthesis in the adrenal cortex. It was not until 1969 that the use of the compound in metastatic breast cancer was first reported and the purpose of this review is to describe the current position of aminoglutethimide in the management of this condition and other hormone-dependent tumours, and to outline possible future developments based on the outcome of ongoing and proposed research.

AMINOGLUTETHIMIDE AND CANCER THERAPY

Recent studies have shown an objective response rate of 28-37%, in unselected postmenopausal patients with advanced breast carcinoma, with a median duration of response of 14 months and an increase in survival time in those patients responding to the treatment. An increased response rate has been reported in patients with oestrogen-receptor positive tumours. Until recently, it was believed that this clinical effect was principally associated with a reduction in androgen production by the adrenal cortex, the main source of oestrogen precursors in the postmenopausal patient, and that the major action of aminoglutethimide was to inhibit steroid synthesis in the adrenal cortex at a number of stages. This 'medical adrenalectomy' was compared to surgical adrenalectomy in a randomised study with similar outcome in the two treatment groups. Recent work, however, has demonstrated an additional action of the compound, which is an inhibition of the aromatization of androgens to oestrogens occuring in several peripheral sites and in the tumour itself.

481

Available data suggest that the dose of aminoglutethimide required to significantly inhibit aromatization and reduce circulating endogenous oestrogen levels in the postmenopausal patient is less than the dosage currently recommended with concomitant glucocorticoid replacement therapy. Further work is in progress to define whether lower doses of the compound will be as clinically effective as the currently recommended dosage regimen, and also whether concomitant steroid therapy is indeed necessary at this reduced dosage level. In addition, since a proportion of the well documented toxicity of aminoglutethimide appears to be dose dependent e.g. effects on the central nervous system, it may be that the use of such reduced doses of the compound will be associated with improved tolerability.

ROLE OF AMINOGLUTETHIMIDE IN ADVANCED BREAST CANCER

1. Monotherapy

At the present time, the use of aminoglutethimide in patients with advanced disease is confined to postmenopausal patients or to patients who have undergone oophorectomy. In these patients the principal indication is as an alternative endocrine treatment following the use of tamoxifen, where a number of studies have reported a useful objective response rate to aminoglutethimide in previous responders to tamoxifen. In patients with primarily bony metastases there is now evidence of an increased response rate to aminoglutethimide compared to tamoxifen, and it may be that in these patients, earlier use of the compound should be considered.

2. Combination therapy

A number of studies have been carried out using aminoglutethimide in combination with other endocrine agents with to date minimal evidence of an increase in objective response rate compared to the use of single agents alone, and no evidence of a beneficial effect on survival time. No data are available on the use of the compound in combination with chemotherapy.

ROLE OF AMINOGLUTETHIMIDE IN EARLY BREAST CANCER

This question is currently being investigated in a multicentre double blind placebo controlled study in this country in postmenopausal patients at high risk of recurrence, who following primary treatment are randomised to receive either aminoglutethimide and hydrocortisone, or placebo, for 2 years or until relapse if this be earlier. To date, nearly 300 out of the proposed 400 patients have been entered into this trial.

ROLE OF AMINOGLUTETHIMIDE IN OTHER ENDOCRINE DEPENDENT TUMOURS

A number of studies have been carried out in advanced prostatic carcinoma and advanced endometrial cancer with evidence of objective and subjective benefit. Recent findings suggest a possible rationale for clinical evaluation in other conditions including ovarian and pancreatic carcinoma.

CONCLUSIONS

The current use of aminoglutethimide in advanced breast carcinoma is reviewed with a description of the contributory pharmacological effects relating to this current use. Current and proposed studies are outlined which are expected to define more fully the role of aminoglutethimide in the treatment of this condition and other hormone-dependent tumours.

THE DEVELOPMENT OF NEW ANTI-ENDOCRINE TYPE DRUGS

M. JARMAN, A.B. FOSTER, M.H. BAKER, P.E. GOSS, C-S. LEUNG, O-T. LEUNG,

R. McCAGUE, M.G. ROWLANDS, R.C. COOMBES and G. LECLERQ

I.   INTRODUCTION

Studies of the metabolism of agents used to treat hormone-dependent
breast cancer in post-menopausal women have guided the design of second-
generation analogues. We report here on the metabolism-directed design of
analogues of aminoglutethimide and tamoxifen. We also describe some new
chemistry we developed for assaying the potent experimental aromatase inhibitor
4-hydroxyandrostenedione in the plasma of rats prior to its introduction into
the clinic.

2.   AMINOGLUTETHIMIDE

2.1. Analogues with selective action against desmolase and aromatase

Of the two major inhibitory actions of aminoglutethimide (I) towards
steroidogenesis, namely towards the cholesterol side-chain cleavage enzyme
complex desmolase and towards aromatase, which respectively converts the
androgens androstenedione and testosterone into oestrone and oestradiol, it
is the latter which probably contributes principally to the therapeutic action
of I against hormone-dependent breast cancer.   Since inhibition of desmolase
also depletes corticosteroids, elimination of this action, whilst retaining
the effect on aromatase, is a desirable goal in analogue design. However the
inhibition by I of desmolase may, by depleting androgens, contribute to its
therapeutic effect against prostatic carcinoma (1). Hence a selective
inhibitor of desmolase could in this context be of potential therapeutic
benefit.

A selective inhibitor of desmolase was obtained by relocating the amino
function in I. N-Aminoglutethimide (II) (K_i = 4.6 μM) did not inhibit
aromatase and was a stronger inhibitor of desmolase than was I (K_i = 14 μM)
(2). In a collaborative study presented in more detail elsewhere (3)
several analogues of I were synthesised in which the glutarimide moiety was
replaced by succinimide, and which were strong inhibitors of aromatase but

485

which hardly inhibited desmolase. The most active of these, III, was as inhibitory towards aromatase as was I.

I; $R^1 = NH_2$, $R^2 = H$
II; $R^1 = H$, $R^2 = NH_2$
IV; $R^1 = NHAc$, $R^2 = H$
V; $R^1 = NHOH$, $R^2 = H$

III

2.2. Metabolism of aminoglutethimide and its relevance to analogue design

Acetylaminoglutethimide (IV) is the only major metabolite of I so far described in humans (4). It is non-inhibitory towards desmolase and aromatase (2) and is therefore an inactivation product. It may be noted that both II and III contain amino functions and hence would probably be inactivated by this pathway. Regarding other human metabolites, Santen et al. (5) have noted that I induces its own metabolism during chronic therapy, the mean plasma $t_{\frac{1}{2}}$ in 6 patients falling from an initial value of 13.2 h to 7.3 h after 3-5 weeks. Using reverse-phase thin-layer chromatography and HPLC we have detected a new major metabolite in patients' urine which appears to be an induced metabolite, and have identified it, using mass spectrometry, as hydroxylaminoglutethimide (V) (6). Like IV, V is also an inactivation product. The percentage inhibition of desmolase (substrate concn. 50 µg/ml) and aromatase (20 µg/ml) by I and V was respectively 85 and 90%, and 53 and 36% (7).

In summary, whereas the aim of segregating the desmolase and aromatase inhibitory actions has been achieved in these studies of analogues of aminoglutethimide there is scope for further improvement, especially with a view to avoiding induced metabolism by giving lower doses of a more potent analogue.

3. TAMOXIFEN

3.1. Metabolism of tamoxifen and biological activity of metabolites

Tamoxifen (VI) is converted both in vitro and in vivo into, inter alia, the N-desmethyl derivative (VII), the N-oxide (VIII) and the 4-hydroxy derivative (IX). Both VII and VIII have similar relative binding affinities (RBAs) for the estrogen receptor and antitumour activities against the MCF7 human tumour cell line in vitro whereas IX is ca. 100 times more potent than VI in both respects (8). However the antitumour activity of IX in vivo, for example against the DMBA-induced mammary carcinoma in rats (9), was less than that of VI, suggesting that IX may be converted in vivo into an inactive or rapidly excreted metabolite. In this context there is evidence that the glucuronic acid conjugate of IX is a metabolite of VI in vivo (10) although we have been unable to demonstrate this conversion using rat hepatocytes (8).

VI; $R^1 = NMe_2$, R^2, $R^3 = H$

VII; $R^1 = N(O)Me_2$, R^2, $R^3 = H$

VIII; $R^1 = NHMe$, R^2, $R^3 = H$

IX; $R^1 = NMe_2$, $R^2 = OH$, $R^3 = H$

X; $R^1 = NMe_2$, $R^2 = H$, $R^3 = OH$

3.2. Metabolism of tamoxifen and analogue design

In attempting to control the putative glucuronidation pathway we have investigated the novel ortho analogue (X) in the hope that the steric requirements for glucuronide formation and binding to the oestrogen receptor may differ, and that binding affinity might be retained whilst conjugation is impaired. This hope was not realised. The RBA values for X, its meta analogue (11), IX and VI were respectively 0.1, 2.5, 100 and 0.9. Glucuronide formation from X was not therefore studied.

4. 4-HYDROXYANDROSTENEDIONE

In addition to our approaches to second generation analogues we are introducing into the clinic 4-hydroxyandrostenedione (XI), a potent and specific inhibitor of aromatase (12). As part of this study we are developing a novel method for assaying the drug in plasma, based on gas chromatography and mass spectrometry. The major problem in quantifying XI using this methodology is protection of the enolic hydroxy group. Derivatives tend to be thermally labile. Thus the trimethylsilyl (XII) and trifluoroacetyl (XIII) derivatives

XI; R = H

XII; $R = Me_3Si$

XIII; $R = CF_3CO$

XIV; R = Me

XV; $R = C_6F_5CH_2$

XVI; $R = C_6F_5$

XVII; $R = C_7F_7$

$R = C_7F_7$

XVIII

XIX

decomposed on chromatography whereas the more stable methyl derivative (XIV) had poor gas chromatographic properties. Turning to protecting groups which could enable the use of specific detectors we first unsuccessfully investigated the electron-capturing pentafluorobenzyl ether (XV), and, following a published suggestion (13), the pentafluorophenyl ether (XVI). Success came finally with the heptafluorotolyl ether (XVII) which was made (Scheme) by phase transfer reaction (14) of XI with octafluorotoluene and characterised by mass spectrometry. The reaction proved selective for hydroxyl groups attached to unsaturated carbon, phenolic functions also reacting rapidly but alcohols reacting much more slowly. Thus oestrone which gave XVIII could be used as the internal standard for an assay of XI. Dichloromethane extracts of plasma from treated rats were subjected directly to the reaction in the Scheme and the products, in hexane, injected onto a column (1.6 m x 4 mm i.d.) of 3% OV 1 on Gas Chrom Q at 270°C, N_2 flow rate 27 ml/min. Cholesterol is also detected as its derivative (XIX) since, although slowly reacting, it is present in high concentration (ca. 2 mg/ml). Retention times for XVII, XVIII and XIX were respectively 12.0, 9.1 and 24.0 min. Preliminary results showed that only low levels (ca. 1 μg/ml)of XI were attained 24 h after subcutaneous injection of 50 mg/kg.

SCHEME. Reaction of 4-hydroxyandrostenedione with octafluorotoluene under phase transfer conditions.

Summarising, heptafluorotolyl is a novel and selective protecting group which has potential not only for solving the present problem of assaying XI but, more widely, for quantifying phenolic steroids. These clinical and preclinical studies of XI are complementary to the studies of its metabolism which are presented elsewhere (15).

REFERENCES

1. Worgul T, Santen RJ, Samojlik E, Veldhuis JD, Lipton A, Harvey HA, Drago JR, Rohner T.J: Clinical and biochemical effect of amino-glutethimide in the treatment of advanced prostatic carcinoma. J Urol(129): 51-55, 1983.
2. Foster AB, Jarman M, Leung C-S, Rowlands MG, Taylor GN: Analogues of aminoglutethimide: selective inhibition of cholesterol side-chain cleavage. J Med Chem(26): 26-54, 1983.
3. Rowlands MG, Bunnett MA, Daly MJ, Nicholls PJ, Smith HJ: Enzyme inhibition studies with derivatives of aminoglutethimide. (These Proceedings)
4. Douglas JS, Nicholls PJ: The partial fate of aminoglutethimide in man. J Pharm Pharmacol(24): 150P, 1972.
5. Murray FT, Santer S, Samojlik E, Santen RJ: Serum aminoglutethimide levels: studies of serum half-life, clearance and patient compliance. J Clin Pharmacol(19): 704-710, 1979.
6. Jarman M, Foster AB, Goss PE, Griggs LJ, Howe I, Coombes RC: Metabolism of aminoglutethimide in humans: identification of hydroxylaminoglutethimide as an induced metabolite. Biomed Mass Spectrom: in press.
7. Chohan PB, Coombes RC, Foster AB, Harland SJ, Jarman M, Leung C-S, Rowlands MG and Taylor GN: Metabolism of aminoglutethimide in man: desmolase and aromatase inhibition studies. In: Elsdon-Dew RW, Jackson IM, Birdwood GFB (eds) Aminoglutethimide: an alternative endocrine therapy for breast carcinoma. Academic Press, London, 1982 pp 19-21.
8. Bates DJ, Foster AB, Griggs LJ, Jarman M, Leclerq G, Devleeschouwer N: Metabolism of tamoxifen by isolated rat hepatocytes: anti-estrogenic activity of tamoxifen N-oxide. Biochem Pharmacol(31): 2823-2827, 1982.
9. Jordan VC, Allen KE: Evaluation of the antitumour activity of the non-steroidal anti-estrogen monohydroxytamoxifen in the DMBA-induced rat mammary carcinoma model. Eur J Cancer(16): 239-251, 1980.
10. Fromson JM, Pearson S, Bramah S: The metabolism of tamoxifen (I.C.I. 46, 474) Part I: In laboratory animals. Xenobiotica(3): 693-709, 1973.
11. Ruenitz PC, Bagley JR, Mokler CM: Estrogenic and anti-estrogenic activity of monophenolic analogues of tamoxifen, (Z)-2-[p-(1,2-diphenyl-1-butenyl)phenoxyl]-N,N-dimethylethylamine. J Med Chem(25): 1056-1060, 1982
12. Brodie AMH, Schwarzel WC, Shaikh AA, Brodie HJ: The effect of an aromatase inhibitor, 4-hydroxy-4-androstene-3,17-dione, on estrogen-dependent processes in reproduction and breast cancer. Endocrinology(100): 1684-1695, 1977.
13. Kovac P, Anderle D: Protective alkylation. In: Blau K, King G (eds) Handbook of derivatives for chromatography. Heyden, London, 1977, pp 223-224.
14. Starks CM: Phase-transfer catalysis. I. Heterogenous reactions involving anion transfer by quaternary ammonium and phosphonium salts. J Am Chem Soc(93): 195-199, 1971.
15. Parr IB, Rowlands MG, Foster AB, Jarman M: Metabolism of 4-hydroxy androstenedione by rat hepatocytes (These Proceedings).

ANTIESTROGENIC ACTION OF TAMOXIFEN DERIVATIVES IN THE HUMAN MAMMARY CARCINOMA CELL LINE MCF-7

U. EPPENBERGER, R. LÖSER*, W. KÜNG and W. ROOS

1. INTRODUCTION

Non-steroidal antiestrogens, whose chemical structure is based on triphenylethylene, have considerable potential for the treatment of hormone-dependent breast cancer. The application of Tamoxifen (trans-1-(4-β-dimethylaminoethoxyphenyl)-1.2-diphenyl but-1-ene) as an antiestrogen is now used routinely for the treatment of advanced breast cancer in women (1). The therapeutic response to Tamoxifen is correlated with the presence of estrogen receptors in mammary tumours (2). In addition, these non-steroidal compounds have been successfully applied to suppress the growth of human breast cancer cell lines containing estrogen receptors (3) and to elicit the regression of hormone-dependent mammary tumors in experimental animals (4). It is assumed that antiestrogens bind to the estrogen receptor in the respective target cells (5). However, the precise mechanism of antiestrogen action is not fully understood. Since the MCF-7 cell line proved to be a useful in vitro system to screen for antiestrogenic drugs (6, 7), the present study describes the antiestrogenic character of the following compounds in comparison with Tamoxifen and K-060: 3-hydroxytamoxifen, K-089: trans-1-/4'-(2-diethylaminoethoxy)-phenyl/-1-(3'-hydroxyphenyl-2-phenyl-1-buten, K-106: trans-1-/4'-(2-methylaminoethoxy)-phenyl/-1-(3'-hydroxyphenyl)-2-phenyl-1-buten, K-122: trans-1-/4'-(2-dimethylaminoethoxy)-phenyl/-1-(3'-hydroxyphenyl)-2-(p-tolyl)-1-buten, K-135: trans-1-/4'-(dimethylaminoethoxy)-phenyl/-phenyl/-1-(3'-hydroxyphenyl)-2-(4'methoxyphenyl)-1-buten.

The following aspects were investigated:
1) Binding to the cytosolic estrogen receptor of MCF-7 cells and human mammary carcinoma tissue
2) Growth inhibition in estradiol-stimulated MCF-7 cell cultures

491

3) Effect on the induction of progesterone receptor in the presence and absence of estradiol.

2. PROCEDURE

2.1 Material and methods

2.1.1 MCF-7 cells. The cells (passage 123) were cultured in IMEM-ZO medium (8) containing 50 IU penicillin/ml, 50 µg streptomycin/ml, 60 µg tyclocin/ml, 50 µg gentamycin/ml, 0.2 µg insulin/ml and 10 % (vol:vol) of heat-inactivated FCS, and processed as described (7).

2.1.2 Binding studies of the respective antiestrogenic drugs with MCF-7- and human mammary carcinoma cytosols were carried out as previously reported (7).

2.1.3 Growth experiments. MCF-7 cells were plated at a density of 5×10^4 cells per well containing 0.5 ml medium. 2 to 4 days later, the cells were incubated twice in serum-free medium to reduce endogenous steroid levels, followed by the incubation in media containing antiestrogens $\pm$ 10^{-10} M 17β-estradiol, which were changed every two days. After 5 days cells were trypsinized and enumerated in a Sysmex CC 108 cell counter.

2.1.4 Progesterone receptor assay. Cells were grown as described (7), the medium was changed to 5 % DC-FCS with the respective concentrations of estradiol and cytosols prepared as described, except that 10 mM sodium molybdate was included in the buffer to stabilize the receptor. A dextran-charcoal single-point assay was performed with 5 nM $/^3H/R5020^8$ (87 Ci/mmol; New England Nuclear Corp.) and 500 nM radioinert progesterone to measure unspecific binding.

2.2 Results

The dependency of the MCF-7 cells on 17-β-estradiol for the proliferation makes it a useful model to study the action of antiestrogens. After withdrawal of endogenous steroids by appropriate medium conditions (DC-FCS), the growth of these cells can be stimulated more than 3-fold by physiological doses of 17-β estradiol (10^{-10} M) as shown previously (6).

2.2.1 In competition-binding experiments using MCF-7 cytosol (Fig. 1 A) and human mammary carcinoma cytosol (Fig. 1 B) all compounds (K-089, K-106, K-122, K-135) inhibited binding of 17-β-estradiol. The relative binding affinities (Table 1) are in the same range as for 3-hydroxyfamoxifen

FIGURE 1. A) Competitive inhibition of estradiol binding by antiestrogens in MCF-7-cytosol; B) ... in human mammary carcinoma cytosol.

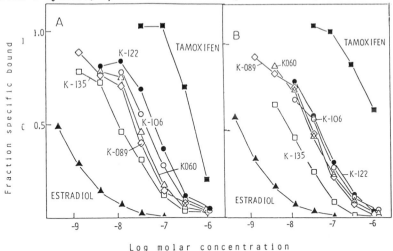

Log molar concentration

(K-060), at least 10-fold better than the affinity of Tamoxifen. Similar results could be obtained by competition experiments in human mammary carcinoma cytosol (Table 1).

Antiestrogen	MCF-7 Cells			Human Mammary Carcinomas		
	n	log Concentration at 50% Inhibition	Relative Binding Affinity (%)	n	log Concentration at 50% Inhibition	Relative Binding Affinity (%)
Tamoxifen	3	-6.25 ± 0.26	0.18	4	-5.87 ± 0.41	0.07
K060	4	-7.45 ± 0.36	2.82	6	-7.27 ± 0.19	1.86
K089	2	-7.54 ± 0.46	3.47	2	-7.55 ± 0.17	3.54
K106	4	-7.29 ± 0.29	1.95	6	-6.98 ± 0.29	0.95
K122	4	-7.29 ± 0.34	1.95	6	-7.14 ± 0.28	1.38
K135	4	-7.88 ± 0.23	7.59	6	-7.51 ± 0.36	3.23

Competitive binding assay of Tamoxifen and the respective antiestrogens (K060, K089, K106, K122 and K135) to cytosolic estrogen receptor of MCF-7 cells and human mammary carcinomas. MCF-7 cytosol and human mammary carcinoma tissue cytosol were incubated with 1 x 10^{-9}M /^{3}H/ 17 β-estradiol and the respective radioinert competitor ligand as shown in Fig. 2. The log concentrations at 50% inhibition were used to calculate the relative binding affinity which is defined as the ratio of the concentrations of radioinert estradiol to the competitor, which are necessary to achieve a 50% inhibition of the specific /^{3}H/-estradiol binding. n represents the number of experiments carried out.

2.2.2 The antiestrogenic action of these compounds is also demonstrated by their ability to reverse the estradiol-induced growth stimulation of MCF-7 cells (Fig. 2A). The dose-response curves reflect the affinities of the different antiestrogens to the estrogen receptor. The concentrations which inhibit proliferation are one to two orders of magnitude lower than those which are necessary with Tamoxifen. In the absence of exogenously added estradiol (Fig. 2B) a residual inhibitory effect is obvious, which max be caused by insufficient withdrawal of estrogen from the dextran

FIGURE 2. Influence of antiestrogens on the proliferation of MCF-7 cells in the presence (A) and in the absence (B) of estradiol (10^{-10} M).

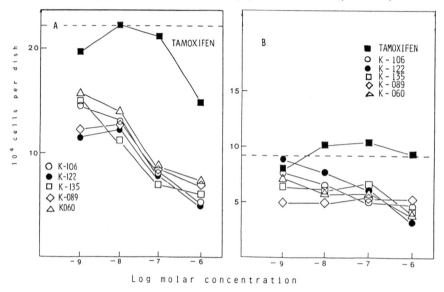

Log molar concentration

charcoal-treated fetal calf serum. Occasionally, under these conditions, we even find a moderate growth stimulation by the antiestrogens revealing their partially estrogenic nature.

2.2.3 The induction of the progesterone receptor by estradiol (Fig. 3A) is inhibited by 3-hydroxytamoxifen and its derivatives. Again the effect seems to be related to the affinity for the estrogen receptor. At a concentration of 10^{-7} M Tamoxifen was the weakest, K-135 the most effektive ligand. In the absence of estradiol (Fig. 3 B) the partially estrogenic action of Tamoxifen becomes evident, in contrast to the other antiestrogens which are not able to increase progesterone receptor levels at the given concentration.

2.3 Discussion

There are good evidences that the development of new and better antiestrogens than Tamoxifen is possible since the recurrence of mammary carcinomas

after successful endocrine therapy can be stopped again by the application
of an additional antihormonal drug such as medroxyprogesteroneacetate (MPA)
or aminoglutethimide. In these cases the hormone dependency of the tumour
cells persîsts and the degree of growth suppression by Tamoxifen seems to
be insufficient. In MCF-7 cells the newly developed triphenylethylene
derivatives K-060, K-089, K-106, K-122 and K-135 proved to be better ligands
for the cytosolic estrogen receptor of MCF-7 cells and human breast carcinoma biopsies by their ability to compete for the estrogen receptor, by
their inhibitory action on the proliferation of MCF-7 cells and the progesterone receptor induction than Tamoxifen. The inhibitory effect of the
compounds, measured as ability to reverse the growth stimulation exerted
by 10^{-10} M 17-β-estradiol closely reflects their affinity for the estrogen
receptor. In the absence of 17-β-estradiol all antiestrogens are able

FIGURE 3. Influence of antiestrogens (10^{-7} M) on progesterone receptor
concentration.

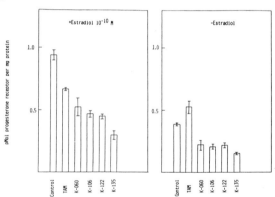

to stimulate the growth of MCF-7 cells at concentrations which were not
sufficient to inhibit 17-β-estradiol-induced proliferation. Therefore,
a complete characterization of such compounds has to comprehend both aspects
growth inhibition as well as agonistic activity. Further research dealing
with toxicological and pharmacocinetical studies of these compounds should
reveal whether clinical applications are possible.

REFERENCES

1. Smith IE, Harris AL, Morgan M, Ford HT, Gazel JC, Harmer CL, White H, Parsons CA, Villardo A, Walsh G, McKinna JA (1981): Tamoxifen versus aminoglutethimide in advanced breast carcinoma: a randomized cross-over trial. Br Med J 283: 1432-1434.
2. McGuire WL, Zava DT, Horwitz KB, Chamness G (1978): Steroid receptors in breast tumours: Current status. Curr Top Exp Endocrinol 3, 93-129.
3. Lippman ME, Bolan G, Hiff K (1976): The effect of estrogens and anti-estrogens on hormone-responsive human breast cancer in long-term tissue culture. Cancer Res 36: 4595-4601.
4. Rorke EA, Katzenellenbogen BS (1981): Antitumor activities and estrogen receptor interactions of the metabolites of the antiestrogens C1628 and U23,469 in the 7.12-dimethylbenz(a)anthracene-induced rat mammary tumor system. Cancer Res (41): 1257-1262.
5. Horwitz KB, McGuire WL (1978): Antiestrogens, mechanism of action and effects in breast cancer. In: McGuire WL (ed) Breast cancer: Advances in research and treatment. Vol. 2, New York: Plenum Publishing Corp. 22 155-204.
6. Roos W, Huber P, Oeze L, Eppenberger U (1982): Hormone dependency and the action of Tamoxifen in human mammary carcinoma cells. Anticancer Res 2: 157-162.
7. Roos W, Oeze L, Löser R, Eppenberger U (1983): Antiestrogenic action of 3-Hydroxytamoxifen in the human cancer cell line MCF-7. J Nat Cancer Inst. 71: 55-59.
8. Richter A, Sanford KK, Evans VJ (1972): Influence of oxygen and culture media on plating efficiency of some mammalian tissue cells. J Natl Cancer Inst 49: 1705-1712.

These studies were supported by the Swiss National Science Foundation grant No. 3.557.0.79, and by the Swiss Cancer League FOR.197.AK.81(5).

NUCLEAR ESTROGEN RECEPTORS IN HUMAN TUMOURS OF BREAST AND UTERUS

B. KONOPKA, S. CHRAPUSTA, Z. PASZKO AND H. PADZIK

INTRODUCTION

A substantial part /30-45%/ of tumours containing the cytoplasmic estrogen receptor /ERc+/ fail to respond to endocrine therapy. Presumably this may be due to a defect in receptor structure or to disturbances in translocation of the receptor to the nucleus. Therefore the presence of the nuclear estrogen receptor /ERn/ and cytoplasmic progestagen receptor /PRc/ may - in addition to the presence of ERc - be a more reliable index of the tumour's reactivity to hormones; namely, these factors represent the initial, intermediate and final manifestation of the intracellular changes specific for the estrogen ection.

Many studies deal with the problem of simultaneous occurrence of ERc and PRc in breast and uterine tumours, whereas less attention has been given to ERn, and in particular to its occurring jointly with ERc. Therefore further work on this subject seemed worthwhile.

MATERIALS AND METHODS

All tissues were stored in liquid nitrogen, till analysed /1-3 weeks/. ERn was determined according to Garola and McGuire /1/. Cytoplasmic receptors were assayed by the modified method of Korenman /2/.

RESULTS AND DISCUSSION

Salt extracts /0.6 M KCl in TEDG buffer/ of the nuclear fraction /860xg/ of breast cancer, myoma and myometrium homogenates were treated by saturation analysis, ultracen-

trifugation and electrophoresis in agar-agarose gel. An
analysis of ^{3}H-estradiol /^{3}H-E$_2$/ binding with the extracts
of these tissues /0.5-10 nM/ showed that under these conditions
one class of the specific binding sites was determined,
because of linear correlation coefficients of Scatchard's
curves were close to one /0.92-0.97/.

The affinity of ^{3}H-E$_2$ to the specific binding component
of the nuclear extracts of breast cancers /assayed at +30
and 0°C/ and of myomas /+30°C/ was typical of receptor binding
/K_d=0.3-0.9 nM/; only the specific binding component of the
nuclear extracts of myometrium exhibited a somewhat lower
affinity /K_d=3-4 nM/. Dissociation constants determined by
the DCC or HAP method did not differ. On the other hand,
the number of specific E$_2$-binding sites /determined by the
DCC method, as compared with the HAP method/ was as a rule
greater. Ultracentrifugation of the nuclear extracts saturated
with ^{3}H-E$_2$ /or, in the case of the uterus, with either ^{3}H-E$_2$
or ^{3}H-moxestrol /^{3}H-R 2858// in sucrose gradients containing
0.4 M KCl showed that bound estrogens migrate within the
3 S region. However, electrophoretic analysis of the components of nuclear extracts of myoma or myometrium, specifically binding ^{3}H-E$_2$ and ^{3}H-R 2858, testified to their
heterogeneity. Only a part of specifically bound ^{3}H-E$_2$
/5-10%/ migrated towards the anode and the remaining part
/90-95%/ - towards the cathode. In contrast, in case of
extracts of the nuclear fraction of breast cancers, the
major part of the specific complexes migrated towards the
anode. The cathodic fraction was shown not to bind dihydro-
testosterone, whereas it bound ^{3}H-R 2858. This indicates
that this fraction is not sex hormone binding globulin (SHBG).

The contents of "free" /ERnf/ and estrogen-bound /ERnb/
estrogen receptor detected in the nuclear extracts of breast
cancers varied between 0-1220 fmoles/mg of DNA. The mean
content of ERnf exceeded that of ERnb /Table 1/. When accep-
ting the value of 10 fmoles/mg of DNA as an arbitrary limit
between ERn+ and ERn- tumours, it was found that 50% of the

investigated tumours were ERnf-positive /only 38% in premenopausal patients/, and 67% were ERnb-positive. In 75% of
tumours either ERnb or ERnf or else both of them /ERnt/ were
present. There was a significant correlation /p=0.01/ between
the contents of ERnf and ERnb.

On account of the functional interrelation of the above
three receptors, their occurrence was analysed in detail
/Table 2/. ERc+ ERn+ tumours accounted for an average of
50% of breast cancers /in women up to 50 years old - 38%,
and in older ones - 59%; no age-concerning data are shown
in Table 2/. In case of ERc- ERn+ tumours, the respective
percentages were 23% /28% and 20%/, and in case of ERc+ ERn-
tumours, 15% /11% and 21%/. For both localisations /nucleus,
cytoplasm/ jointly, ER was found in 88% of breast cancers.

Evaluation of the correlations between the contents of
various ERc, PRc and ERn /ERnf and ERnb/ pair combinations
pointed to a significant positive correlation within all
pairs, except for the pair ERnb and PRc. Breast cancers
containing all three receptors were most frequent /28%/.
The frequency of tumours containing only ERc and ERn was
closely similar /23%/. Only 3.8% of tumours contained ERc alone.

Tumours containing neither one of the three receptors
accounted for 10% of the total number of tumours. Tumours
showing the presence of only PRc were extremely rare. Each
of the remaining combinations, i.e. tumours only containing
either PRc or PRc and ERn, accounted for 10% of all tumours
studied.

The frequency of occurrence of ERn /"free" or estrogen-
bound/ in breast cancers, found in the present studies,
exceeds the values reported by some authors /3,4/, whereas
it is consistent with that found by Hähnel et al. /5/.
Our results confirm those of other authors reporting that
the ERn occurrence frequency is greater in ERc+ than in ERc-
tumours.

Our finding of correlation between ERnf and PRc, and a
lack of correlation between ERnb and PRc, is in agreement

Table 1. Frequency of occurrence of "free" /ERnf/, estrogen-bound /ERnb/ and "total" /ERnt/ nuclear estrogen
receptor in human breast cancer
Patients' age: 34 - 83 years; total number of cases: 78

Receptor	% of total	ERn,	fmol/mg of DNA	
		range	mean value	median value
ERnf+	49	10-1220	184	97
ERnb+	67	10-744	132	71
ERnt+	73	12-1830	246	141

ERn+ $\geqslant$ 10 fmol/mg of DNA

Table 2. Simultaneity of occurrence of cytoplasmic estrogen
/ERc/ and progesterone /PRc/ receptors and "total" nuclear
estrogen receptor /ERnt/ in human breast cancer
Patients' age: 34 - 83 years; total number of cases: 78

ERc	+	+	+	+	−	−	−	−
ERnt	+	+	−	−	+	+	−	−
PRc	+	−	−	+	+	−	−	+
% of total	28.2	23.1	3.8	10.3	10.2	12.8	10.3	1.3

ERc+ and PRc+ > 5 fmol/mg of cytoplasmic protein
ERnt+ $\geqslant$ 10 fmol/mg of DNA

with the results of Hähnel et al./5/. In contrast with the
finding of Romić-Stojković and Gamulin /4/, in our material
the frequency of PRc occurrence in ERc- ERn- tumours was
extremely low / 1%/; this testifies against the possibility
of ER-independent PRc synthesis.

The occurrence of ERn, in the absence of ERc, may point
to ERc translocation in the presence of endogenous estrogens.
However, the fact that many ERc+ /58%/ and ERc- /37%/ of
breast cancers contained - in addition to ERnb - also ERnf
suggests the presence of estrogen-independent translocation;
the frequency of occurrence of ERnb, as compared with that
of ERnf, in ERc+ tumours was only slightly higher /71% and
57%, respectively/. It is well known that about 10% of ERc-
breast cancers regress in response to endocrine therapy.
The difference between this value and the frequency of ERn
occurrence in ERc- tumours /37%/ may testify to disturbances
in the receptor mechanism at the posttranslocation stage.
These disturbances seem to also be suggested by the fact that
36% of the investigated breast cancers contained no PRc,
despite the presence of ERn /"free" or estrogen-bound/.

REFERENCES

1. Garola RE, McGuire WL: An improved assay for nuclear
   estrogen receptor in experimental and human breast cancer.
   Cancer Res /37/: 3333-3337, 1977.
2. Paszko Z, Padzik H, Pieńkowska F, Chrapusta S, Konopka B,
   Peczko D, Wąsowska B, Kwiatkowska E: Receptory hormonów
   stereoidowych: występowanie w rakach sutka kobiet, przydat-
   ność do doboru chorych do endokrynnej terapii i prognozo-
   wania rozwoju choroby. Pol Tyg Lek /38/: 676-683, 1983.
3. Thorsen T: Occupied and unoccupied nuclear oestradiol
   receptor in human breast cancer: relation to oestradiol
   and progesterone cytosol receptors. J Steroid Biochem
   /10/; 661-668, 1979.
4. Romić-Stojković R, Gamulin S: Relationship of cytoplasmic
   and nuclear estrogen receptors in human breast cancer.
   Cancer Res /40/: 4821-4825, 1980.
5. Hähnel R, Partridge RK, Gavet L, Twaddle E, Ratajczak T:
   Nuclear and cytoplasmic estrogen receptors and progesterone
   receptors in breast cancer. Europ J Cancer /16/: 1027-1033
   1980.

ACTIVATION AND TRANSLOCATION OF ESTRADIOL RECEPTORS IN NITROSOMETHYLUREA-
INDUCED MAMMARY CARCINOMAS OF RATS

E. HEISE AND W. DIETRICH

Many controlled clinical trials have shown that only about 50-60% of estradiol receptor-positive mammary carcinomas responded favourably to endocrine therapy (1). The results of molecular biological research have indicated that the cytoplasmic receptor, after steroid binding, becomes translocated into the nucleus, where an interaction between the translocated receptor-steroid complex and the genome of the cell takes place. Before becoming translocated, the hormone receptor complex has to be activated by a mechanism which is not fully understood. It is easily conceivable that this chain of events may be disturbed after the formation of the cytoplasmic estradiol-receptor complex in hormone-unresponsive mammary carcinomas, even though a cytoplasmic receptor complex may be detected. It is reasonable, therefore, to investigate the process of receptor activation and translocation in more detail. We performed the experiments with the nitrosomethyl-urea (NMU)-induced mammary carcinomas of rats, described first by Gullino (2). To study the process of receptor activation and translocation, it was necessary to isolate cytosol and nuclei from tumour tissue and to measure the estradiol receptor activity in both components separately. Firstly we determined the estradiol receptor activity in the cytosol of the tumours by the charcoal assay using 7 different concentrations of ^3H-estradiol in a range from $10^{-10}M$ to $5 \times 10^{-9}M$. The incubation of the cytosol with the different ligand concentrations was performed at 2^oC for 18hr. To eliminate non-specific estradiol binding, aliquots of the cytosol were incubated with the several estradiol concentrations, with addition of a 100-fold excess of diethylstilboestrol (DES). More than 30 tumours were investigated and a very high degree of reproducibility in relation to maximal binding capacity ($n=40\pm10fm/mg$ protein) and affinity constant ($Kd = 22 \pm 1.1 \times 10^{-10}M$) was found. Because activation of the cytoplasmic estradiol-receptor complex requires elevated temperature it was necessary at first to study the influence of temperature on the stability of the receptor complex. For this, cytosols were charged with ^3H-estradiol at 2^oC for 18hr and thereafter aliquots

503

incubated at 30 or 37°C for 30 or 60min. Then the cytosols were cooled to 0°C for 30min, and the unbound estradiol removed by charcoal treatment. Fig. 1 shows the results. It can be seen that an incubation at 30°C has only a small influence on the receptor activity whereas an increase of temperature to 37°C induced a remarkable loss of receptor activity.

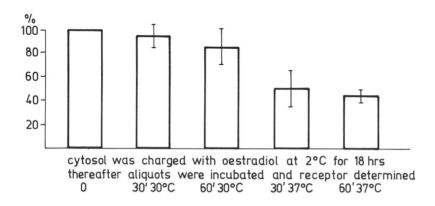

FIGURE 1. Influence of temperature on receptor stability.

Most authors demonstrate an activation of the receptor complex by measuring its ability to translocate. This can be done by incubation of cytosol after activation with purified nuclei and determination of nuclear bound estradiol-receptor complex. Aurichio et al (3) could show that a combined incubation of cytosol and purified nuclei from mouse and calf uteri at elevated temperature induced a very rapid inactivation of the cytoplasmic receptor complex. Therefore it seemed to be reasonable to study in the NMU-tumour system the influence of nuclei on the activity of the cytoplasmic estradiol receptor in more detail at first before performing activation and translocation experiments. Firstly cytosol was charged with ^{3}H-estradiol and incubated thereafter with purified nuclei in a ratio of 1:1. Figure 2 shows the results obtained under the various conditions used.

source	expt. conditions	source	expt. conditions	receptor activity %
cytosol	2°C 18 hrs ÷		÷	100
cytosol	2°C 18 hrs ÷	+ nuclei	2°C 3 hrs + DCC[1]	84 ± 5 (5)
cytosol	2°C 18 hrs + DCC[1]	+ nuclei	2°C 3 hrs ÷	94 ± 5 (5)

[1] dextran coated charcoal

FIGURE 2. Influence of nuclei on cytoplasmatic receptor activity at 2°C.

The first incubation of cytosol with ^{3}H-estradiol was carried out at 2°C for 18hr; the second incubation with nuclei was for 3hr at 2°C. Thereafter the unbound ligand was removed by charcoal treatment. Under these conditions about 15% of the cytoplasmac estradiol receptor activity disappeared. However, it was not possible to decide whether the receptor activity lost was due to a translocation process or to a nuclei-incuded degradation of the receptor. Therefore the experiment was repeated, but with the unbound estradiol being removed before incubation of cytosol with nuclei. The results obtained are shown in the last line of figure 2. It can be seen that under these conditions apparently only a very small part of the receptor activity disappeared. We assume that this small loss of receptor activity from cytosol was due to a translocation of cytoplasm into nuclei or to an attachment of receptor to nuclei, because radioactivity could be extracted from the centrifuged nuclei by ethanol, the amount of which corresponded to the receptor activity lost from cytosol. From these two sets of experiments we concluded that the difference of the receptor activities which disappeared under the two different experimental conditions of charcoal treatment reflected that part of receptor activity which was degradated under the influence of nuclei. This degradative influence of nuclei became pronounced if charged cytosol and nuclei were incubated together at elevated temperature. As can be seen from figure 3, even a short combined incubation of cytosol and nuclei at 30°C induced a remarkable disappearance of receptor activity from cytosol.

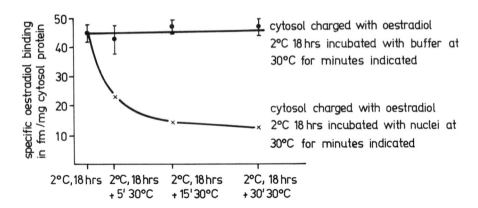

FIGURE 3. Influence of nuclei on receptor activity at elevated temperature.

In this case too, only a small amount of radioactivity could be extracted from the separated nuclei, which did not correspond to the receptor activity lost. Therefore we assumed that the lost receptor activity was not translocated but degraded under the influence of nuclei. To demonstrate activation and translocation, cytosol was charged with ^3H-estradiol at 2°C for 18hr and incubated at elevated temperature to activate the receptor complex. Then the receptor activity was determined in an aliquot of the cytosol in the usual way using dextran-coated charcoal. Thereafter the cytosol was cooled and, after mixing with purified suspended nuclei, incubated again. After separation of cytosol and nuclei the receptor activities were determined in the cytosol and in the nuclei. We found that the inactivating properties of nuclei were dependent on Mg-ions and could be suppressed using phosphate buffer instead of Tris-buffer. Therefore the experiments were performed using Tris-buffer and EDTA for tissue homogenisation and preparation of cytosol and nuclei. The results obtained are seen in figure 4.

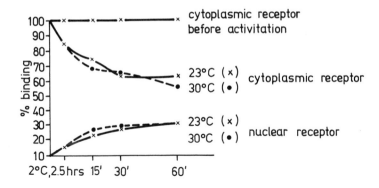

FIGURE 4.   Activation and translocation of the receptor.

The upper part of the figure shows the disappearnce of the estradiol receptor from the cytosol which amounted to more than 30% of the receptor activity originally found in the cytosol.   The lower part of the figure shows the protein-bound radioactivity found in the nuclei after activation of the cytosol and incubation with nuclei which corresponded to that lost from cytosol.   These findings show that the experimental conditions used (phosphate-buffer + EDTA, without Mg-ions) induced a complete inhibition of the inactivating effect of nuclei on the cytoplasmic receptor-complex and enabled the activation and translocation process to be measured with high accuracy.   Further experiments have to be done to optimise this system and to test the possibility of using purified nuclei from NMU-induced mammary carcinomas as a standard system to measure activation and translocation of cytoplasmic estradiol receptor complexes from other biological sources, such as human mammary tumours.

REFERENCES

1.   Jensen EV: Some newer endocrine aspects of breast cancer.   New Eng J Med
     (291): 1252-1254, 1974.
2.   Gullino PM, Pettigrew HM, Grantham FH: N-Nitromethylurea as mammary gland
     carcinogen in rats.   J Natl Cancer Inst (54): 401, 1975.
3.   Aurichio F, Migliacco A, Rotondi A: Inactivation of estrogen receptor in
     vitro by nuclear dephosphorylation.   Biochem J (194): 569-574, 1981.

HORMONE RECEPTORS IN GYNECOLOGICAL TUMOURS AND THEIR RELEVANCE FOR THERAPEUTIC MANAGEMENT

G. TRAMS AND W.E. SIMON

INTRODUCTION

The effect of steroid hormones is mediated by the interaction with specific hormone receptors of the target cell. It was obvious, that this concept should be applied to the management of so-called hormone responsive tumours. Steroid-hormone receptors - mostly oestrogen receptors - have been detected in the following neoplasias of the female reproductive system: cervical cancer, endometrial cancer, ovarian cancer, breast cancer. Our information on the implication and function of receptor protein in these tumours is still incomplete and their presence does not necessarily indicate responsiveness to endocrine manipulation. Although there is a reasonable chance of successful hormonal treatment of carcinomas of the endometrium and the breast, the same does not hold true for cervical and ovarian cancers. The present paper deals with the practical value of receptor measurements in patients with endometrial, ovarian or breast cancer.

Endometrial Cancer

Both oestrogen (ER) and progesterone (PgR) receptors have been determined in malignant lesions of the endometrium, and most investigations indicate that more differentiated tumours have a greater proportion of receptor-positive tissues than less differentiated ones; this holds true especially for the progresterone receptor. Some clinical data seem to suggest that receptor-positive tumours have a significantly higher chance to respond to endocrine therapy. In a cumulative series of 85 patients with advance of recurrent endometrial carcinomas, who received progestin therapy, 90% of tumours were progesterone-receptor positive, in the group of responders. Whilst in 91% of non-responders receptors were lacking. A prospective receptor-orientated trial would be required to evaluate the benefit of an adjuvant treatment with high doses of gestagenic compounds for endometrial carcinomas.

509

Ovarian Cancer

Independent from receptor assay some efforts were made to treat advanced ovarian cancer with hormones (e.g. progesterone) or anti-hormones (e.g. danazol, tamoxifen) alone or in combination with other chemotherapy. Results obtained were not convincing that this kind of endocrine treatment was of significant benefit for the patient. Nevertheless, some investigators have determined steroid-hormone receptors in carcinomas of the ovary. We have assayed 83 ovarian tumours for steroid receptors. Excluding benign tumours and ovarian metastases, 57 primary ovarian carcinomas were evaluated. In 33%, both receptor types were present, in 42% there were only oestrogen, and in 1.6%, only progesterone-receptors. 22.8% of tumours were completely receptor-negative. The total of 75% of oestrogen receptor-positive tumours was comparable to results obtained in breast cancer tissues. Androgen-receptor assay was positive in 25.5% of tumours, and corticosteroid-receptor assay in 20.4%. The attempt to correlate histological type with receptor level of the tumour, showed no clear correlation beween these two parameters, but there was a tendency for the endometrial lesions to show a higher percentage of progesterone-receptor positive tumours than the other forms.

In a limited number of tumours we were able to compare receptor level with histological grading of the tumours and their proliferative behaviour in long term tissue cultures.

Breast Cancer

It is well-established that receptor status can be used as a guide to therapy in breast cancer patients with advanced disease, but the question remains, whether receptor distribution in the primary tumour is an indicator for later development of metastases. We have, therefore, carried out retrospective analyses of multiple receptor measurements. Tissue specimens were taken simultaneously or at different time intervals in the same patient.

Simultaneous ER-determination - performed in specimens from primary tumours and lymph node metastases - were concordant in nearly 90% of cases. Serial biopsies at different time intervals were taken in 151 patients for ER analysis and in 83 patients for both ET and PgR analysis. The percentage of consistent results decreased to about 65% both for ER and PgR. Levels for the complete receptor pattern changed in more than half of all cases. This could be due to intervening endocrine therapy. In the ER-positive group, 64 patients received a systemic therapy between biopsies and 37 patients were assayed for PgR. The rate of discordant receptor levels - both ER and PgR - was found to be significantly higher in the subgroups of patients receiving intervening endocrine treatment. Similar observations have been made by other groups. The change from receptor-positive to receptor-negative would be consistent with the view that intervening endocrine therapy may lead to a selection of receptor-negative or receptor-deficient cells. Results from various centres indicate that the steroid-receptor level offers an additional prognostic tool to evaluate the necessity of adjuvant therapy. Since 1976, 515 primary breast carcinomas (stage I-III) were treated in our hospital with a modified radical mastectomy. Patients with histologically evident tumour in one or more axillary lymph nodes received 6 or 12 cycles of adjuvant CMF-treatment. Patients with negative lymph nodes were followed up without further therapy. Assays in 236 patients were carried out for ER and PgR, and in 221, for DHT-R. After a follow-up of 3-4 years, the clinical data of these groups were analysed with respect to relapse-free survival. In node-negative patients, a non-significant tendency to a better course of disease in receptor-positive patients, was seen for all three receptor types. In the CMF-treated, node-positive patients survival was increased where ER was present, but there was no difference at all for PgR and DHT-R.

ABSTRACTS OF PROFFERED PAPERS AND POSTERS

1. NEW AGENTS: EXPERIMENTAL STUDIES

PRETHERAPEUTIC IN VITRO PREDICTION OF HUMAN TUMOUR DRUG RESPONSE.
St. Tanneberger, E. Nissen, H. Lenk, W. Arnold, Akademie der Wissenschaften
der DDR, Berlin, East Germany.

Cell biological systems for prediction of individual human tumour drug
sensitivity have been recommended for more than 20 years (Tanneberger et al,
Cancer Treat. Rev., 1983 in press).

1981/82 a new assay basing on organ cultures on viable tumour slices have
been elaborated by us (Nissen et al, Period. Biolog. 84, 371-373, 1982). The
advantages of cultivation of viable tumour slices are: less time is required
for preparation of the cultures, mechanical trauma is reduced, the slices can
be examined under the microscope after air fixation and staining, the slices
are very uniform in shape and dimension. The evaluation of drug sensitivity
is easier, because slices have a higher ^{3}H-thymidine uptake.

The results of drug sensitivity in vitro (microsome activated
cyclophosphamide 12; 6μg/ml) and data of in vivo treatment (cyclophosphamide
120; 60mg/kg) correlated very well in different experimental systems (Lewis
lung carcinoma, 2 human lung cancer nude mouse xenografts). In
contradistinction to these findings up to now only in 5/11 patients were
found a correlation between results in vitro and success of treatment in vivo
after 3 months observation time.

****

CONTINUOUS CELL LINES AS AN EXPERIMENTAL MODEL FOR BLADDER CANCER
CHEMOTHERAPY. J.R.W. Masters, P.H. Hepburn and R.T.D. Oliver, Dept Pathology,
Institute of Urology, St. Paul's Hospital, London, England.

Numerous systems are used in experimental cancer chemotherapy, including
induced and transplantable animal tumours, human tumour xenografts and a
variety of tissue culture methods. Each of these models has limitations.
Continuous cell lines are unique in providing a pure, reproducible and
relatively homogeneous population of human tumours cells. Their in vitro
drug sensitivities may be of particular relevance to intravesical
chemotherapy, because in contrast to systemic administration the duration and
drug concentration to which the tumour cells will be exposed are known.
Therefore, the biological and growth characteristics of twelve continuous
cell lines derived from transitional cell cancers of the human bladder were
determined, including tumorigenicity in "nude" mice and isozyme patterns.
Population doubling times ranged from 17-93hr and colony forming efficiency
from 3-87%. In vitro sensitivities to adriamycin and methotrexate were
determined using clonogenic assays. Profound differences in sensitivity were
observed, the proportion of surviving clonogenic cells following exposure to
30ng/ml adriamycin ranging from 0.7-42.0% and to 100ng/ml methotrexate from
1.5-89.5%. It is concluded that this panel of cell lines shows a wide range
of biological characteristics and drug sensitivities, perhaps comparable to
those encountered clinically in this disease, and may provide a model system
with which to conduct in vitro phase II trials.

517

CHEMICAL AND BIOLOGICAL PROPERTIES AND MODE OF ACTION OF 8-CARBAMOYL-3-(2-CHLOROETHYL)IMIDAZO[5,1-d]-1,2,3,5-TETRAZIN-4(3H)-ONE, A NOVEL BROAD SPECTRUM ANTITUMOUR AGENT.

M.F.G. Stevens, R. Stone and G.U. Baig, Cancer Research Campaign Experimental Chemotherapy Group, Dept of Pharmacy, University of Aston in Birmingham, Birmingham, England.
E. Lunt and C.G. Newton, May & Baker Ltd., Dagenham, Essex, England.

The title compound is synthesised by interaction of 5-diazoimidazole-4-carboxamide with 2-chloroethyl isocyanate in a variety of solvents at 20-60ºC in the dark. It has curative activity against L1210 and P-388 leukaemia and also shows marked activity against a variety of other tumours, including LL, C88, B16 M5076, ADJ/PC6A and TLX/5 lymphoma. It also markedly inhibits metastasis observed with the LL tumour. Biochemical studies carried out recently at the University of Aston suggest a relation to the triazene type of antitumour agent, and chemical degradation studies to be described indicate that the compound may unusually be a pro-drug of the active but unstable 5[3-(2-chloroethyl)triazen-1-yl]imidazole-4-carboxamide (MCTIC).

****

LYCURIM IN COMBINATION CHEMOTHERAPY WITH 3,4,5-TRIHYDROXYBENZO HYDROXAMIC ACID IN VITRO. <u>J. Ban and G. Weber</u>, Central Inst. for Tumors & Allied Diseases, Zagreb, Yugoslavia and Lab. for Exp. Oncology, Indiana Univ. School of Medicine, Indianapolis, Indiana, U.S.A.

The purpose of this study was to test for possible synergism in the cytotoxic activity of the alkylating agent, lycurim (LY) in the combination with 3,4,5-trihydroxybenzohydroxamic acid (VF 122), an inhibitor of ribonucleotide reductase. Experiments were performed on proliferating rat hepatoma 3924A cells in tissue culture. Lycurim also inhibited the activity of transaldolase. In tissue culture LY killed both exponentially growing and plateau phase cells. VF 122 inhibited ribonucleotide reductase activity <u>in vitro</u> with IC_{50} = 10µM and proved to be a better inhibitor of this enzyme than hydroxyurea. In tissue culture VF 122 was a cycle-specific agent. LY together with VF 122 gave synergistic killing in hepatoma 3924A cells treated for 7 days as determined by colony-forming ability. It was concluded that synergism was time-dependent because only summation was observed when the cells were treated with both drugs for 1hr.

Supported by NIH Grants CA-13526 and CA-05034.

PHENOTYPIC AND GENOTYPIC CHANGES INDUCED BY THIOPROLINE IN CANCER CELLS IN TISSUE CULTURE. GUIDELINES FOR CLINICAL STUDIES OF THE DRUG. M. Gosalvez, Dept Experimental Biochem, Clinica Puerta de Hierro, National Center of Medical Research, Madrid 35, Spain.

Studies with thioproline in HeLa cells and fibroblastic cell lines at different saturation densities suggest that the phenotypic reversion obtained in most cells, in optimal conditions, with very low concentrations of thioproline plus diazepam, at low calcium levels, using a six-day treatment schedule started 24 hours after subcultivation, seems to be accompanied by several genotypic changes in part of the cells. All our experimental and theoretical studies with thioproline and the Zipper Mechanism strongly suggest that thioproline could again reverse cancer in humans, given at low doses either alone or with its cooperators, if tumours with the adequate thioproline-sensitivity hallmarks are gathered and proper and precise conditions for thioproline administration are followed. The following guidelines are suggested for thioproline given alone in lung cancers. Pathology: very well differentiated epidermoid lung cancers. Stage: as early as possible after diagnosis; if possible, prior to chemotherapy with cytotoxic drugs. Immunological hallmarks: 1) presence of lymphocyte HLA-A28 locus histocompatibility antigen; 2) high titer of the C1q constituent of complement; 3) presence of blood group antigen Ii; 4) high titer of anti-erythrocyte antibodies. Biochemical hallmarks: 1) high circulating levels of cyclic AMP; 2) high prostacycline levels; 3) high circulating levels of putrescine; 4) high circulating levels of low molecular weight mitochondrial polyribonucleotides. Dosage: 100mg thioproline daily in the first half hour after awakening (i.v. or i.m.). (Supported by the Spanish N.I.H. and Assessorial Commission of the Presidency).
****

USE OF MESNA IN REDUCING BLADDER TOXICITY. D. Schmähl, German Cancer Research Center, Heidelberg, F.R.G.

Acute and chronic toxicity in the urinary bladder is a severe complication in cancer chemotherapy with oxazaphosphorines. The former is expressed as hemorrhagic cystitis, the latter results in papillomas and carcinomas of the urinary bladder. Experimental studies by Brock and coworkers and by our own working group demonstrated that concomitant administration of mesna (sodium 2-mercaptoethane sulfonate) can significantly reduce the toxic and carcinogenic effects of oxazaphosphorines in the urinary bladder, without interfering with their therapeutic efficacy. The mechanism of action is suggested to consist in interception of the toxic activity of acrolein, a metabolite of oxazaphosphorines. To our knowledge, mesna has to be considered the first rationally developed antidote against the carcinogenic effect of alkylating compounds in a specific organ. The results of the above mentioned experimental investigations are at present being confirmed in clinical trials.

NORMAL TISSUE PROTECTION DURING HIGH-DOSE CHEMO/RADIOTHERAPY BY A "PRIMING DOSE" OF CYCLOPHOSPHAMIDE. A.C.M. Martens and A. Hagenbeek, Radiobiological Institute TNO, Rijswijk, The Netherlands.

With respect to cancer treatment it has been reported, that after "priming" with small doses of cyclophosphamide a subsequent high-dose treatment is far better tolerated (Millar and Hudspith, Cancer Treat. Rep. 60: 409, 1976). This principle was investigated in a rat leukaemia model (BNML) that shows a striking resemblance with human acute myelocytic leukaemia. Priming doses were given at a dose of 10mg.kg^{-1} i.p. 48 hours preceeding a second high-dose treatment with either cyclophosphamide or whole body X-irradiation. Both normal and leukaemic rats were treated. Firstly, in normal rats there was a protection against radiation-induced bone marrow failure (6.0 Gy X-rays), although no drastic increase in the irradiation dose was tolerated. Following a priming dose, CFU-S numbers were increased 2 to 3 days thereafter. Secondly, normal rats received a priming dose, followed by a supralethal dose of whole body X-irradiation (12.0 - 16.0 Gy). Bone marrow transplantation prevented death due to aplasia. No consistently convincing protection of the intestinal epithelial against the radiation damage was observed. In leukaemic animals, however, we observed an improvement in the tolerance towards the high-dose treatment. Protection against the early toxicity death within 24 hours) could be achieved by priming 48 hours prior to a high-dose of cyclophosphamide or irriadation were administered. A second observation induced by "priming" was the d day-delay in the numerical decrease of CFU-S in the bone marrow. As a result this led to an improved survival. Most data on the optimal time scheduling of the priming dose will be presented.

****

5-ACETOXY-2-(4-ACETOXYPHENYL)-1-ETHYL-3-METHYLINDOLE (D 16726): PRECLINICAL EVALUATION OF A NEW MAMMARY TUMOUR INHIBITING DRUG. E. Von Angerer and J. Prekajac, Inst. Pharmacy, Univ. Regensburg, Regensburg, F.R.G.
M. Berger, DKFZ, Heidelberg, F.R.G.

Derivatives of 2-phenylindole inhibit the growth of estrogen-dependent mammary tumours (Von Angerer and Prekajac, J. Med. Chem. 26: 113, 1983). The title compound was selected for further studies because of the high affinity of its free hydroxy derivative for the calf uterine receptor (RBA = 9.5; estradiol = 100) and its antiuterotrophic properties in the immature mouse. It proved to be active against experimental hormone-dependent mammary tumours. The average size of DMBA-induced tumours in the rat was reduced after 4 weeks treatment with 6 x 4mg/kg/week s.c. The growth of MNU-induced tumours in the rat was inhibited by administration of 5.7mg/kg/week (tumour volume 19.7; control 39.7, after 5 weeks). In the human MCF-7 tissue culture, cell number and thymidine incorporation decreased with increasing concentrations of D 16726 (ED_{50} ca. 100nM).

ROLIN ENHANCING EFFECT UPON IN VITRO PHA-PROLIFERATION OF NORMAL HUMAN PERIPHERAL BLOOD LYMPHOCYTES. S. Perez-Cuadrado, L Llorente, M.C. Moreno and V. Bellido, Department of Immunopathology, Nat. Inst. of Oncology, Madrid, Spain.

Rolin is a modulating agent obtained from Siccacel (Cybila) that can enhance the PHA-proliferation index of PBL from normal individuals. A 42% rise of the PHA-index above the physiological level has been shown by us in normal rabbits, following the i.v. injection of a suitable dose (1st Can. Res. Cong., Madrid, 1982). In this study, 650 in vitro cultures were done to assess the Rolin-effect upon the PHA-index of PBL from 151 normal volunteers, 13 male and 138 female. In every case several tests were done, each of which contained the same amount of PBL enriched plasma, PHA and TC (Difco); escalated doses of Rolin were also added except to test-tubes which represented the PHA-index. After 72hr of incubation at 37°C, the blastoid-cells of each test were assessed. Data showed a significative dose-dependent enhancing effect of Rolin upon the PHA-index of PBL from normal persons (P < 0.001). The set of tests having a full-dose of Rolin got the highest activity (119% of normal PHA-index); doses above and below this had less effect. Taking the individual highest reponse, regardless of the dose, the Rolin-induced enhancement got up to 136%, 142% and 159% of the normal PHA-index in the sub-sets with 2, 3 and 6 Rolin doses, respectively. A positive activity, at least for one of the doses, was observed in 82% of the cases; in the set of 81 cases which had three doses of Rolin, 40% of them showed a positive effect to all three doses. Probably, Rolin induces the differentiation from pre-T to T-cells, sensitive to PHA. Partially supported by the Spanish F.C. de la AECC.

****

DTIC: TOWARDS AN APPROPRIATE ALTERNATIVE. D.E.V. Wilman, Inst. Cancer Res., Sutton, Surrey, England.

As a result of relatively poor patient tolerance, considerable effort has been made over the past decade in the search for a suitable second-generation clinical alternative to 5-(3,3-dimethyl-1-triazeno)imidazole-4-carboxamide (DTIC, Dacarbazine). Our own investigations have produced an extensive structure-activity series of photostable aryltriazenes. From this study we have concluded that the necessary requirements for antitumour activity in this class of compounds are a carrying group (aryl or heterocyclic) at N^1 and a methyl group at N^3, together with a readily metabolisable group also at N^3. Triazenes of this type undergo hepatic oxidative metabolism to produce a cytotoxic monomethyltriazene. Selected examples of these compounds have been tested against a number of human tumour xenografts. In the U.S.A., the National Cancer Institute has demonostrated that compounds such as 1-(4-carbamoylphenyl)-3-ethyl-3-methyltriazene (CB 10-335) have marked activity against colon and lung tumour xenografts. Perhaps of more interest is the activity towards Grade IV astrocytoma xenografts. Subcutaneous implants of such tumours are sensitive to both DTIC and 1-(4-carbamoylphenyl)-3-methyl-3-pentyltriazene (CB 10-350) but an intracerebral implant is sensitive only to CB 10-350. Experimental antitumour activity is not the sole criterion in selecting a drug for Phase I clinical trial. Highly lipophilic molecules such as the 4-carbamoylphenyltriazenes, whilst necessary for penetration of the blood brain barrier, are difficult to formulate. Recent studies with DTIC suggest that human liver may be incapable of sufficient activation of the dialkyltriazenes by oxidative metabolism. Rather an alternative prodrug may be required.

DRUG RESISTANCE OF HUMAN GLIOMA CELL LINES IN CULTURE - THE ROLE OF MEMBRANE TRANSPORT. S Merry and S.B. Kaye, Dept. Clin. Oncology, University of Glasgow, Glasgow, Scotland.

In animal tumour models resistance to adriamycin (ADR) and vincristine (VCR) has been shown to be associated with an energy-dependent cellular drug efflux mechanism which can be inhibited by calcium antagonists such as verapamil. The aim of this study is to establish the relevance of these data to human tumours. Our previous studies with human glioma cell lines have identified one cell line (MCF) sensitive to both ADR and VCR, and another (UVW) resistant to both drugs. Cell monolayers in soda glass tubes were exposed to radioactively labelled drug, cooled rapidly (0-5°C) and washed. Drug-free medium was added, the cells were incubated and intracellular drug determined by measuring label released into the medium. The plateau level of drug was determined for each cell line in the presence (6mM glucose) and absence (no glucose, 10mM NaN$_3$) of an energy source. For ADR the removal of the energy source made no apparent difference to the plateau drug level of MCF, however for UVW plateau drug level rose by at least 300%. A similar increase in plateau drug level was observed in UVW when cells were exposed to verapamil in the presence of energy. For VCR, a 100% increase in plateau drug level of UVW cells was noted when the energy source was removed. These preliminary data suggest that for certain drugs resistant human tumour cells may possess a similar energy-dependent drug efflux mechanism to that seen in animal tumour models and this may be reversed with verapamil. Studies with other cell lines, including lung carcinoma, are now in progress.

****

LETHAL AND KINETIC EFFECTS OF AMSA IN A RANGE OF HUMAN TUMOUR CELL LINES AND ITS VALUE IN OVERCOMING INDUCED DRUG RESISTANCE IN A SERIES OF MURINE L5178Y LYMPHOMA SUBLINES IN VITRO. R.D.H. Whelan and B.T. Hill, Cellular Chemotherapy Laboratory, Imperial Cancer Research Fund, London, England.

4'-(9-acridinylamino)methanesulfon-m-anisidide (AMSA), currently undergoing Phase II clinical trials, shows activity in childhood leukaemia. The drug's lethal and kinetic effects were investigated in Syrian hamster ovary cells (NIL8) and a human neuroblastoma line (CHP100). Cytotoxicity increased exponentially with drug concentration and duration of exposure. Plateau-phase cells were significantly more resistant to AMSA than log-growing cells. Lethal effects of AMSA on synchronised cells showed no cell cycle specificity in contrast to adriamycin which kills cells predominantly in late S and G$_2$. Flow microfluorimetric analyses of asynchronous cells provided no evidence of delay or arrest in cell cycle progression by AMSA. To identify any value for AMSA in overcoming resistance to other antitumour drugs we screened (i) a range of in vitro selected resistant sublines of the murine L5178Y lymphoma and (ii) a series of human neuroblastoma, prostate, colon and breast tumour cell lines. AMSA proved effective against murine cells resistant to methotrexate, 5-fluorouracil, vincristine and cis-platinum but showed complete cross resistance with adriamycin. In contrast, no positive correlations were found with the human tumour cell lines where IC50 values varied 12-fold for a 24 hour exposure to AMSA. These studies provide evidence of differing responses to AMSA depending on the model system adopted for screening and caution against general extrapolation of data from a single test system.

A NOVEL HPLC PROCEDURE FOR MEASUREMENT OF 6-MERCAPTOPURINE IN PLASMA.
N.K. Burton, G.W. Aherne and V. Marks, Dept. Biochemistry, University of
Surrey, Guildford, England.

Although 6-mercaptopurine (6MP) is a well established cytotoxic drug, little
information about its clinical pharmacology is available. Existing HPLC
methods have not proved entirely satisfactory due to plasma interference. A
novel procedure has been developed which exploits the specific reaction of
bimanes with thiol groups to produce a stable fluorescent adduct (Newton et
al, Anal. Biochem. 114: 383, 1981). Following ethanol protein precipitation
of plasma and treatment with chloroform, an aliquot of the aqueous layer is
dried in air at 40°C, reconstituted in reaction buffer (50mM ammonium hydrogen
carbonate and 1mM EDTA, pH 7.3) and allowed to react with bimane (5μg/ml
final concentration) at room temperature for 2-18 hours. The reaction is
stopped by acidification and 20μl injected onto a 25cm 5μm Hypersil ODS
column and eluted with 20% acetone : water at a flow rate of 1ml/min.
Detection of the 6MP-bimane adduct was carried out using an excitation
wavelength of 392nm : emission wavelength of 465nm. The sensitivity of this
method is at least 10ng/ml in plasma with an overall assay CV of 2%. The
retention time of 6MP is 7.7min which allows good resolution from any plasma
interference.

****

POTENTIATION OF THE CYTOTOXICITY OF ANTIBODY-TOXIN A CHAIN CONJUGATES.
D. McIntosh, Chester Beatty Laboratories, Inst. Cancer Res., London, England.

As part of a research programme on the in vitro eradication of malignant
cells from bone marrow, conjugates of monoclonal antibody and A chains of
plant toxins have been prepared and tested. Fib75 is a monoclonal antibody
recognising a 19000 molecular weight glycoprotein on all differentiated human
cells with the exception of those of the lymphoid series (Edwards et al,
Transplant. Proc. 12:398, 1980). Two conjugates were prepared by covalently
linking Fib75 to the A chains of abrin or ricin. Both were tested in tissue
culture against EJ, a cell line derived from a human bladder carcinoma.
Cytotoxic activity was assayed by measurement of the inhibition of ^{3}H-leucine
incorporation into cellular protein, and both conjugates gave ID50 values in
the region of 10^{-11}M. It has been reported (Cassellas et al, Protides of the
Biological Fluids, 1982; Neville & Youle, Immunol. Rev. 62, 1982) that
lysosomotropic amines and toxin B chains can enhance toxic and conjugate
cytotoxicity. In the present system methylamine and ammonium chloride, both
previously described as having potentiating activity were without effect.
However chloroquine at appropriate concentrations gave significant promotion
of the cytotoxic action of both conjugates. At 0.1mM chloroquine, the ID50
of Fib75-SS-ricin A was enhanced by one order of magnitude and that of the
analagous abrin A chain conjugate by two. Preliminary results indicate that
isolated B chains of abrin and ricin also possess the capacity to enhance
toxin A chain-conjugate activity.

THE EFFECT OF INHIBITORS OF POLY(ADP-RIBOSE)POLYMERASE ACTIVITY ON THE CYTOTOXIC ACTION OF BIFUNCTIONAL ALKYLATING AGENTS AND RADIATION. J. Walling, I.J. Stratford and P.W. Sheldon, MRC Radiobiology Unit, Harwell, Oxon, England and Institute of Cancer Research, Sutton, Surrey, England.

Analogues of benzamide and nicotinamide are known to inhibit the action of poly(ADP-ribose)polymerase in mammalian cells. It has been proposed that this enzyme is important in the repair of DNA single strand breaks and inhibition of its activity is known to increase damage caused by radiation and monofunctional alkylating agents.

The electron affinic compound CB 1954 (2,4-dinitro-5-aziridinyl benzamide) has previously been shown to increase the radiation sensitivity of hypoxic mammalian cells when the agent is present only shortly before and during irradiation. The increase in radiation sensitivity caused by this and other benzamide analogues is far greater than would be predicted from electron affinity considerations. This report shows that these increases in activity may be associated with effects on poly(ADP-ribose) synthesis.

Further, we also show that CB 1954 can increase the cytotoxic action of the bifunctional alkylating agent melphalan, both in vitro and in vivo. For example, the surviving fraction of V79 cells treated with $1\mu g/ml$ melphalan for 1hr at 37°C is 0.4. In contrast, cells given a non-toxic concentration of CB 1954 (0.2mM) prior to, during and for a few hours after treatment with melphalan have their survival reduced to 0.04. Similarly, the effect of melphalan on the Lewis lung tumour in mice is considerably enhanced by addition of CB 1954. Data showing enhancement ratios greater than 2 will be presented.

****

CHARACTERISATION OF A MURINE RENAL CELL CARCINOMA MODEL POTENTIALLY USEFUL IN SELECTING NEW CHEMOTHERAPEUTIC AGENTS. M. Vandendris, P. Dumont, R. Heimann and G. Atassi, Bordet Inst., Brussels, Belgium.

A murine renal cell carcinoma transplantable in CDF1 mice, the RC tumour was characterised and used for the evaluation of chemotherapeutic agents. Survival time as well as tumour growth were consistent and reproducible. Median survival time (MST) of mice inoculated intraperitoneally with 10^6 tumour cells was 16.6 days and 21.4 days after subcutaneous transplant. The percent increase in lifespan (ILS) and long-term survivors (LTS) on Day 60 were used to assess the effectiveness of the drugs. Sixteen drugs with known clinical activity and 4 new drugs were evaluated. Three different doses per drug were given intraperitoneally on Days 1, 5, 9, 13 and 17 (schedule q4D x 5). The most effective agents against the RC tumour were cyclophosphamide (ILS > 387%; LTS = 100%), methyl-CCNU (ILS > 209%; LTS = 50%) and cisplatin (ILS > 200%; LTS = 60%). A new epoxide derivative : the triglycidyl urazole (TGU) showed a high effectiveness (ILS > 185%; LTS = 90%). Methotrexate, bleomycin, 5-fluorouracil, vindesine and vinblastine revealed a satisfactory activity (ILS > 50%). In these experiments, the RC tumour revealed as responsive to alkylating agents and antimetabolites as P388 leukaemia and almost as responsive to antimitotics as L1210 leukaemia. These results would suggest that the RC tumour is more sensitive to chemotherapeutic agents than P388 and L1210 leukaemias and may be used in selecting new anticancer drugs in a primary screen.

PERTURBATION OF S-ADENOSYLHOMOCYSTEINE (SAH) AND S-ADENOSYLMETHIONINE (SAM) LEVELS FOLLOWING 2'-DEOXYCOFORMYCIN (dCf) AND 2'-DEOXYADENOSINE (AdR) ADMINISTRATION. J. Renshaw and K.R. Harrap, Inst. Cancer Res., Sutton, Surrey, England.

In mice treated with the adenosine deaminase inhibitor dCf (0.27mg/kg daily x 5) in combination with AdR (267mg/kg daily x 5), death was attributable to acute hepatic dysfunction (Paine et al, Cancer Treat. Rep. 65: 259, 1981). The dose of AdR was the primary determinant of hepatotoxicity. Preliminary investigations demonstrated dramatic increases in liver SAH levels suggesting that inhibition of SAH hydrolase by AdR may be the primary biochemical lesion (Renshaw et al, J. Clin. Chem. Clin. Biochem. 20: 409, 1982). Elevated SAH levels with depressed SAM:SAH ratios will result in inhibition of transmethylation reactions essential to normal tissue function and survival. Further investigations have revealed that while SAH and SAM levels and their ratios normalise by 24 hours after each days' treatment for the first 2 days no such recovery is demonstrated thereafter. Elevations of liver SAH levels are such that efflux of SAH from the liver into the plasma occurs with subsequent excretion of substantial quantities of SAH in the urine. The "trapping" of adenosine in SAH may contribute to the reduced levels of ATP demonstrated in vivo following dCf treatment which in conjunction with elevated dATP levels may result in compromised energy metabolism (Siaw et al, Proc. Natl. Acad. Sci. USA 77: 6157, 1980). It is suggested that the monitoring of plasma and/or urinary SAH levels during dCf treatment of patients may prove useful for the prediction of systemic toxicity.

****

THE DEVELOPMENT OF RESISTANCE TO METHOTREXATE IN A HUMAN LEUKAEMIA (AML) GROWING IN NUDE MICE. M. Jones, S.J. Harland and S. Sparrow, Inst. Cancer Res. & Royal Marsden Hospital, Sutton, and MRC Toxicology Unit, Woodmansterne, Surrey, England.

The line was derived by s.c. implantation of 2.4×10^6 leukaemic cells. The resultant solid tumour was shown to be sensitive to methotrexate at its third passage. Development of the resistant line commenced at passage 5. Treated animals received 2 courses of 5 daily injections at each passage and donors were taken from the treated groups. At passage 7 of the resistant tumour (passage 11 of the parent line) identical treatment produced 53% inhibition and 95% inhibition respectively. Histologically both lines are very similar. The parent line has been found to be a rich source of human DHFR.

INHIBITORS OF THYMIDINE (TdR) SALVAGE. S.E. Barrie, J.A. Stock, L.C. Davies and K.R. Harrap, Inst. Cancer Res., Sutton, Surrey, England.

Inhibition of the de novo TMP biosynthetic pathway by the quinazoline antifolate, CB 3717, or methotrexate (MTX) can be circumvented by the salvage of exogenous TdR (Jones et al, Eur. J. Cancer 17: 11, 1981; Taylor et al, Molec. Pharmacol. 21: 204, 1981). The enzyme responsible for this is thymidine kinase (TdRK), and inhibition of this enzyme should potentiate the effects of the above antitumour agents. For a compound to be a specific TdRK inhibitor suitable for use in vivo, certain criteria should be met: (1) The compound must inhibit both TdRK, and ^{3}H-TdR incorporation by whole cells, (2) The compound must not inhibit TdR phosphorylase, otherwise TdR degradation would be reduced and the circulating levels of TdR elevated, (3) The compound must be non-toxic when administered alone.
Many potential inhibitors have been synthesised and tested but only 3 have fulfilled these criteria - 5'-NH$_2$,5'-deoxy-TdR, 3'-benzyl-TdR and 3'-propargyl-TdR. These compounds were competitive inhibitors of TdRK (Ki 6, 35, 20μM respectively) and inhibited the incorporation of 1μM ^{3}H-TdR into cells in vitro (I$_{50}$ 10^{-5}, 6 x 10^{-5}, 5 x 10^{-5}M respectively). They did not significantly inhibit TdR phosphorylase activity from either gut or liver (Ki >5mM). They were not toxic to L1210 cells in vitro (ID$_{50}$ >1mM, 0.8mM, >1mM respectively).
These compounds inhibited the rescue by TdR of L1210 cells treated with a cytotoxic concentration of CB 3717 in vitro. It is expected, therefore, that the combination of these specific TdRK inhibitors with either CB 3717 or MTX will give increased antitumour activity in vivo.
****

STUDIES ON THE MECHANISM OF CB 3717 INDUCED HEPATOTOXICITY. D.R. Newell, M. Manteuffel Cymborowska, A.H.Calvert and K.R. Harrap, Inst. Cancer Res., Sutton, Surrey, England.

CB 3717 is a folate-based inhibitor of thymidylate synthetase currently undergoing clinical evaluation. However, its assessment has been hindered by the frequent occurrence of hepatotoxicity. In an attempt to elucidate the mechanism of this toxicity, studies have been performed in mice using a therapeutic but non-toxic dose (100mg/kg i.p.). Experiments with ^{14}C-CB 3717 demonstrated that hepatic uptake of CB 3717 is rapid and extensive (at t = 1.33hr, hepatic ^{14}C-CB 3717 = 2.2mM). In view of the known ability of organic anions to bind to and inhibit hepatic glutathione-s-transferases (EC 2.5.1.18, GSH-T) (Kaplowitz, Am. J. Physiol. 239: G439-G444, 1980) the inhibition of GSH-T by CB 3717 was examined in vitro and weak non-competitive inhibition demonstrated (Ki = 400 μM). In vivo, pretreatment (2hr) with CB 3717 slightly reduced the paracetamol induced depletion of liver GSH, suggesting that inhibition of GSH-T by CB 3717 may have pathological significance. Indeed, pretreatment (2hr) of mice with CB 3717 increased the whole animal toxicity of paracetamol (LD50: paracetamol alone 476mg/kg; CB 3717 + paracetamol 283mg/kg). However, a more interesting observation is that CB 3717 alone induces a moderate (30-40%) and sustained (0.5 - >4hr) depletion of liver GSH. This effect of CB 3717, plus its weak inhibition of GSH-T may make patients more susceptible to hepatotoxic insults. If this is so, the concurrent administration of a nucleophile should reduce the hepatotoxicity of CB 3717 in man.

This work was supported in part by a grant from the Federation of European Biochemical Societies.

STUDIES RELATING TO THE REVERSAL OF THE CYTOTOXICITY OF THE THYMIDYLATE SYNTHETASE INHIBITOR CB 3717. G.A. Taylor, A.L. Jackman, S.E. Barrie and K.R.Harrap, Inst. Cancer Res., Sutton, Surrey, England.

The quinazoline based folate analogue CB 3717 is an antitumour agent, at present under clinical study, which has thymidylate synthetase (TS) as its sole cytotoxic locus. Unlike other antimetabolites affecting TMP synthesis the effects of the drug can be totally reversed by thymidine (TdR) alone both in vivo and in vitro. Our in vitro studies to define the requirements for the reversal of the cytotoxicity of CB 3717 have demonstrated that the methods generally used for this type of study are inaccurate and misleading. Cell counts (48hr) of L1210 suspension cultures (initial cell density 10^4/ml) indicate that high levels (>2μM TdR) are required whereas colony assays suggest that low levels (>0.2μ M TdR) are sufficient. By monitoring the metabolism of TdR in suspension cultures this apparent anomaly has been resolved. Cytotoxicity was apparent when the concentration of TdR in the medium decreased to <0.05 M. Depletion of TdR occurred by (i) incorporation into DNA, which is dependent upon the cell concentration (for example 10^4cells/ml supplemented with 0.5 moles/litre TdR incorporated 50% of this within 24 hours), (ii) catabolism to thymine by TdR phosphorylase. The nucleoside transport inhibitor dipyridamole (10μM) effectively blocked both the incorporation of TdR into DNA and the circumvention of CB 3717 inhibition of TS but did not affect the TdR phosphorylase activity present in the serum. We have shown that the level of TdR required to overcome CB 3717 toxicity to L1210 cells in vitro is within the range 0.05 - 0.17μ M. Deoxyuridine (100μM) which is metabolised by TdR kinase and TdR phosphorylase did not affect the metabolism of TdR (1μM) nor its ability to overcome CB 3717 cytotoxicity.

****

STUDIES WITH MUTANT L1210 CELL LINES THAT HAVE ACQUIRED RESISTANCE TO CB 3717. A.L. Jackman, D.L. Alison, A.H. Calvert, S.E. Barrie and K.R. Harrap, Inst. Cancer Res., Sutton, Surrey, England.

The development of resistance to antimetabolites is often associated with either overproduction of the target enzyme or deletion of the enzymes responsible for activation of the drug. Cell lines possessing such defects may be useful for the elucidation of metabolic pathways and the effects of inhibitors. In addition, cells that overproduce enzyme can be a useful source of large quantities of enzyme for primary structure analysis and associated studies. CB 3717 is a quinazoline analogue of folic acid that competitively inhibits thymidylate synthetase (TS) (Ki = 4nM). Its single locus of action and lack of requirement for metabolic activation made it useful in raising several monoclonal cell lines which overproduce the target enzyme TS (>30 fold). Thymidine kinase is not elevated. This acquired resistance to CB 3717 (>100-fold) is stable in the absence of the drug (>9 months). Studies with TS purified from one of these cell lines suggest that it is identical to that of the sensitive line and future work will determine whether gene amplification is the cause of resistance. Two cell lines also have a small increase in DHFR (>5-fold), and are slightly cross-resistant to MTX. 5-fluorouracil (FU) and 5-fluorodeoxyuridine (FUdR) may inhibit TS through their active metabolite, 5-fluorodeoxyuridylate, but can also be incorporated into nucleic acids. Unexpectedly no cross-resistance was observed to either compound. However 10μ M thymidine failed to give protection from the cytotoxicity of FU and FUdR in contrast to the sensitive L1210 line. Current work should determine which factors influence the cytotoxic loci of these fluorinated pyrimidines in sensitive and resistant cell lines.

2. NEW AGENTS/COMBINATIONS: CLINICAL STUDIES

PAC POLYCHEMOTHERAPY OF STAGE III + IV OVARIAN CARCINOMA. B.O. Schulz, B. Weppelmann, H.-J. Friedrich, K. Hof and D. Krebs, Dept. of Obstet. & Gynec., Medical School of Luebeck, F.R.G.

During the past 25 years 730 patients with ovarian carcinoma were registered at the Medical School Luebeck. Therapy and development of all cases were documented by codification sheets.

62 patients were treated by PAC: platinum $50mg/m^2$ d1, adriamycin $50mg/m^2$ d2, cyclophosphamide $500mg/m^2$ d2; mannitol hydration programme.

Medium survival 20 months.
Response rate 41/62 (65%; CR = 14, PR = 12, NED = 15).

Retrospective comparisons of selected groups show improved survival rates (1, 2, 3 years) after PAC polychemotherapy (n = 50) versus cyclophosphamide monotherapy (n = 93) in cases of undifferentiated epithelial ovarian carcinoma.

After initially BSOHO and extensive tumor debulking with tumor rests <2cm ⌀ in epithelial stage III + IV ovarian carcinoma (n = 47) the two years survival rate was 65%.

BSOHO followed by PAC (n = 24)   70%
BSOHO followed by cyclophosphamide (n = 23) 58%

Updated data of subgroups will be presented.
****

WEEKLY LOW DOSE 4 EPI-ADRIAMYCIN-EFFECTIVE SINGLE AGENT CHEMOTHERAPY FOR ADVANCED BREAST CANCER WITH LOW TOXICITY.
W. Mattsson, Dept. Oncology, Centralsjukhuset, Karlstad, Sweden, and W.G. Jones, University Dept, Cookridge Hospital, Leeds, England.

This study is based on the experience of Mattsson et al (Clin. Therap. 2: 193-203, 1982) with low dose weekly adriamycin therapy. 4 epi-adriamycin is reported more effective (Casazza et al, 1978) and less toxic (Bonfante et al, 1979) than adriamycin. 39 patients with bi-dimensionally measurable lesions were given 4 epi-adriamycin 20mg intravenously weekly. The majority (34/39) had received previous therapy to which they were resistant. All had advanced disease. Age range 42-89 (mean 64) performance status (WHO, 1978) range 0-3 (mean 2). The lesions were assessed by direct measurement or radiologically. The WHO criteria of response were used. 2 (5%) patients achieved Complete Response (duration: 52, 48 + weeks), 18 (46%) a Partial Response (duration: range 4-56, mean 30+ weeks). A No Change was seen in 11 (28%) patients (duration: 4-40+, mean 14+ weeks) and 8 (21%) showed Progression after (a minimum of) 4 weeks treatment. This gives an objective response rate of 51%, which is better than previously reported for any single agent. No significant toxicity was observed. No myelosuppression was seen. Nausea and vomiting (graded very slight and not occurring with every course) was seen in 3/39 (8%), occasional slight nausea in 8/39 (21%), and slight alopecia (similar to that with oral cyclophosphamide) in 8/39 (21%). All possible effects were recorded, the majority were negligible - 23 (59%) patients had no complaints. This therapy represents effective treatment without toxicity of clinical importance for patients with advanced breast cancer.

531

COMBINATION TREATMENT OF MALIGNANT GLIOMAS WITH DIBROMODULCITOL (DBD).
D. Afra, S. Eckhardt and L. Institoris, National Institute of Neurosurgery, National Institute of Oncology, CHINOIN Pharm. Work, Budapest, Hungary.

DBD-based combined chemotherapy of malignant gliomas (Grade 3 and 4) has been performed in two different trials. In a Phase 3 trial all patients got a uniformly high voltage radiotherapy. In Group 1 no other treatment was administered. In Group 2 DBD was applied during and after irradiation in a single dose of 400mg/sq.m, every fifth day. Patients designated to the third arm of the protocol (Group 3) received the same dose of DBD during irradiation. Treatment was continued with a combination of CCNU (80mg/sq.m) and DBD (200mg/sq.m) in courses lasting a month. Patients who had radiotherapy alone had a median survival time of 40 weeks. The median survival times in Groups 2 and 3 were 57 and 60 weeks which proved to be statistically significant: $p < 0.0025$ and 0.0001, respectively. In a subsequent Phase 2 study DBD has been applied in daily doses of 130-160mg/sq.m during irradiation in a total dose of 6-7500mg. After a rest of 4-6 weeks a combination of CCNU + PCB and CCNU + DBD was given in alternating courses. In this study a median survival time of 55-58 weeks is to be expected. It can be assumed that the main factor in improving survivals was the concurrent use of DBD during irradiation.

****

INITIAL CLINICAL SUDIES WITH IPROPLATIN (CHIP, JM9). P.J. Creaven, S. Madajewicz, L. Pendyala, Z. Wajsman, E. Pontes and A. Mittelman, Roswell Park Memorial Institute, Buffalo, New York, U.S.A.

Iproplatin (CHIP, JM9) was given to 21 patients (pts) with advanced solid tumors at doses of 20-350mg/m^2 preceded by 2L of 0.5N saline and to 16 pts at doses of 270-350mg/m^2 without pretreatment hydration (PH) in a phase I trial. Toxicity was N&V in all pts at doses >20mg/m^2, myelosuppression [after first dose median nadir of WBC 4,200/cu.mm, platelets 82,000/cu.mm at 270mg/m^2 (n=12); WBC 3,200/cu.mm, platelets 41,000/cu.mm at 350mg/m^2 (n=14)], diarrhoea in 4, skin rash in 3, hypersensitivity in 2. In pts treated with 350mg/m^2 without PH, creatinine clearance (CrCl) was 102 $\pm$ 23ml/min before and 115 $\pm$ 33ml/min 3-4 weeks after therapy (n=12). Subsequently, 6 end stage pts with non-seminomatous germ cell tumors failing on third line therapy which included cisplatin were treated, 3 with iproplatin alone and 3 with combination therapy in which iproplatin replaced cisplatin. There were 1 CR, 2 PR and 2 MR in this group. One pt developed severe N&V, dehydration, hyperuricemia and acute renal failure which resolved with rehydration. One pt with renal failure from cisplatin therapy, on hemodialysis, received 3 courses of iproplatin. Recovery of total platinum was 10% in the urine in 72hr and 23.9% in the dialysate over 4hr when the drug was given immediately prior to hemodialysis. In this pt total platinum had a $t_{\frac{1}{2}\beta}$ of 69.3hr and a Cl_β of 9.73L.h^{-1}. Unchanged iproplatin had a $t_{\frac{1}{2}}$ of 1.23h and a Cl_β of 11.5L.h^{-1}. These values were within 1 S.D. of the mean for all pts. One pt with bladder carcinoma with renal failure (CrCl 10ml/min) had a CR but died from drug related myelosuppression. Iproplatin is myelosuppressive and active in cisplatin resistant germ cell tumours. Supported in part by USPHS CA-21071 and Bristol Laboratories.

TAMOXIFEN INDUCED FLUORESCENCE: SPECTROFLUORIMETRIC STUDY AND CLINICAL APPLICATIONS OF THE ION-PAIR EOSIN TAMOXIFEN. J. Mouriquand, M.H. Bartoli, J. Rochat, H. Beriel and J. Louis, Faculte de Medecine et de Pharmacie de Grenoble, La Tronche, France.

In acid solution, Tamoxifen molecule is protonized and forms with Eosin a fluorescent ionic association (λexc. 480nm, λ em 565nm). This reaction is quantitatively linked to the concentration of Tamoxifen. Similar studies are applied to metabolites of Tamoxifen (N-Desmethyl-Tamoxifen and 4-Hydroxy-Tamoxifen). These fluorescent properties are used on Papanicolaou stained smears of 66 human breast carcinomas. A short pretreatment before surgery allows to detect on imprints of tissue sections Tamoxifen-induced fluorescent intracytoplasmic granules. 29 patients out of 66 cases present with such a fluorescence and compares well with the average 50 per cent clinical response to such an antiestrogen treatment. This predictive test as to therapeutical responsiveness is correlated with ultrastructural aspect and Progesterone receptor content of such treated tissues. The correlation is highly significant.

****

EB-VIRUS ANTIBODY TITERS IN TWO SISTERS WITH NASOPHARYNGEAL CARCINOMA AND IN SEVERAL MEMBERS OF THEIR FAMILY. G.P. Stathopoulos and S. Kottaridis, Hippokration Hospital, Athens, Greece.

Two sisters presented with nasopharyngeal carcinoma within a time of four months the one from the other. They were both initially treated with RT. EB-virus antibody titer for MA, VCA, EA (R+D) and EBvA were studied and all found elevated, except of VCA IgA in patient one. In this patient the disease soon recurred and despite the treatment she died within a few months. Patient two survived for three more years during which the disease recurred and partly responded to chemotherapy and radiotherapy. At the end of the third year the patient deteriorated and died three months later. Two months before death EB-virus antibodies were all found elevated apart from VCA IgA which was negative. It is concluded that EB-virus antibodies particuarly VCA IgG and EA (D) increase with advancing tumour but VCA IgA turns to negative, possibly representing a bad prognostic sign. Twelve healthy members of the two sisters' family were also studied and are discussed.

LOCO-REGIONAL CHEMOTHERAPY WITH ADRIAMYCIN - INTRAVESICAL, INTRAPLEURAL, AND INTRAHEPATIC ADMINISTRATION. S. Eksborg, B.J. Cedermark, F. Edsmyr and A. Larsson, Karolinska Pharmacy and Karolinska Hospital, Stockholm and Uppsala University Hospital, Uppsala, Sweden.

By loco-regional chemotherapy it is possible to increase the therapeutic efficiency of many cytostatic drugs by an enhanced local concentration compared to intravenous administration. Sometimes a reduction of side effects is also obtained as a result of a decreased systemic concentration. Superficial bladder tumours have been successfully treated according to a standardized procedure (Eksborg et al, Europ. Urol. 6:218, 1980), with negligible plasma concentrations of the drug (<2ng/ml). Intravesical instillation of adriamycin after transurethral resection (TUR) resulted in plasma concentrations not exceeding 100ng/ml. Malignant pleural effusions are efficiently treated by intrapleural instillation therapy with adriamycin. Only mild side effects including nausea and vomiting were recorded following such therapy. Maximum plasma concentration found after intrapleural instillation of 50mg adriamycin was <100ng/ml, the elimination half-life being 2.5 hours. Comparison of area under plasma concentration time curves (AUC) after intravenous and intrapleural administration revealed that large amounts of adriamycin are adsorbed from the pleura. Plasma pharmacokinetics of adriamycin after intravenous and intrahepatic administration to patients with malignant liver tumour showed a large interindividual variation. On the average the AUC values after intravenous administration were 1.5 times higher and the maximum plasma concentration 1.7 times higher than after intrahepatic administration.

****

ETOPOSIDE (VP 16-213) AS A FOURTH DRUG IN COMBINATION WITH BVP FOR TREATING METASTATIC GERM CELL TUMOURS. P.M. Wilkinson, R.T.D. Oliver, C. Williams, T.J. McElwain and M.J. Peckham, Holt Radium Institute, Christie Hospital; St. Peter's Hospital, London, Southampton General Hospital, Royal Marsden Hospital, Sutton.

The demonstration that Etoposide could induce durable complete response in patients who had failed cis-Platinum therapy led to a collaborative attempt to develop a combination incorporating this drug as a fourth drug with Bleomycin, Vinblastine and cis-Platinum for patients whose initial staging investigations suggested a poor prognosis. For the initial phase 1 study Etoposide was used at the dose of $100/m^2$ x 5 days every 3 weeks, the other drugs being continued at the same dose as in the modified Einhorn regime. Twenty patients were entered on this initial study. There were 3 treatment related deaths (15%) and in 10 patients it was necessary to stop the Etoposide because of dangerous infectious episodes. Because of this unacceptable toxicity subsequent patients received Etoposide $100/m^2$ for three days. An additional 37 patients were treated. Three patients died on treatment (myocardial infarct: bleeding duodenal ulcer: uncontrolled infection). The remaining patients tolerated the treatment without major dosage reduction. 28 (76%) became long term disease free survivors (82% if deaths on treatment are excluded). No patient becoming disease free has relapsed.

INVESTIGATIONS ON LEUCOVORIN RESCUE AFTER METHOTREXATE TREATMENT OF HUMAN OSTEOSARCOMA CELLS IN VITRO. H. Diddens and D. Niethammer, Div. of Paed. Haematology, Dept. of Paediatrics, Univ. of Tübingen, Germany.

High-dose methotrexate (MTX) therapy with subsequent Leucovorin (LV) rescue in the treatment of osteosarcoma is based on the assumption that the cells of this tumour have a highly impaired active membrane transport system for folates. In normal cells this system is shared by MTX. It is assumed, that in contrast to normal tissues the tumour cells cannot be rescued by the MTX-antidote folinic acid (LV) from the cytotoxicity of this drug. Based on therapeutic regimens used in the clinic 3 osteosarcoma lines and 1 fibroblast line were exposed to MTX and/or LV in various dosages and time schedules. The cells were grown in monolayers and the effect on the cell growth was evaluated. It turned out that the cytotoxic effect of MTX (10^{-7}-10^{-4}M) can be overcome by relatively low doses of LV (10^{-8}-10^{-5}M). Studies on MTX transport showed that MTX uptake in osteosarcoma cells is saturable and highly temperature dependent thus indicating a carrier mediated active transport system. These results are not consistent with the above concept and they should be taken into consideration when designing new therapeutic regimens.

****

EARLY CLINICAL STUDIES WITH CB 3717 (N-(4-(N-((2-AMINO-4-HYDROXY-6-QUINAZOLINYL)METHYL)PROP-2-YNYLAMINO)BENZOYL)-L-GLUTAMIC ACID) AT THE ROYAL MARSDEN HOSPITAL. D.L. Alison and A.H. Calvert, Inst. Cancer Res., Sutton, Surrey, England.

The folate analogue CB 3717, a potent inhibitor of thymidylate synthetase, was used to treat 77 patients with a wide variety of tumours at the Royal Marsden Hospital. The starting dose of 100mg/m^2 was escalated to 500mg/m^2 and was given by a 1 hour infusion every 3 weeks. Transient reversible rises in serum liver transaminase levels associated with malaise occurred in 50% of patients. Other toxicities observed included occasional skin rashes and, rarely, myelosuppression. None of these side effects showed a dose relationship and the severity of malaise and rashes was ameliorated by administering prednisolone for 1 week after treatment. Renal toxicity was not evident at doses up to 450mg/m^2 and pharmacokinetic studies showed the 24 hour renal excretion of CB 3717 to be fairly constant at 25%. At higher doses, the renal excretion was considerably reduced. Out of 21 heavily pretreated patients with ovarian carcinoma, 1 complete, 1 partial and 3 minor responses were seen, while out of 11 breast carcinoma patients, 3 partial and 1 minor responses occurred. In addition 1 out of 2 patients with mesothelioma had a partial response. We believe that this is the first clinical evaluation of a cytotoxic agent whose antitumour locus is exclusively thymidylate synthetase (Jackman et al, Brit. J. Cancer 46:505, 1982; Jackman et al, In "Advances in Tumour Prevention, Detection and Characterisation", Volume 7, 1982). The antitumour responses observed suggest that further evaluation of the therapeutic effects of this biochemical lesion is justified.

3. NEW AGENTS: CYTOTOXIC MECHANISMS

DNA REPAIR ENZYMES AND CROSSLINKS: PREVENTION OF BCNU INTER-STRAND CROSSLINKING IN VITRO BY O6-METHYLTRANSFERASE. A.L. Harris, P. Robins and T. Lindahl, CRC Unit, Royal Victoria Infirmary, Newcastle upon Tyne & Imperial Cancer Research Fund, Mill Hill, London, England.

Human cell lines differ in their rate of removal of a specific alkylation lesion from DNA O6-methylguanine (O6MeG) (Sklar and Strauss, Nature 289, 1981). Mex⁻ cell lines (slow removal rate) are more sensitive to methylnitrosourea (MNU), and also the clinically used nitrosoureas (CCNU, BCNU, streptozotocin and chlorozotocin) than Mex⁺ cell lines. We have shown an enzyme in human Mex⁺ cell lines that acts only once and removes the methyl group from O6MeG leaving the base intact (O6MeG transferase, O6MeGT). We now show that purified O6MeGT can prevent cross-linking produced by BCNU. BCNU initially forms mono-adducts with DNA which then form cross-links slowly over several hours. Phage M13 double-stranded covalently closed circular DNA (DSCCC) was incubated at 37°C in Tris-HCl,DTT buffer with 500μm BCNU. At various times DNA was alkali-denatured and renatured and electrophoresed on 0.8% agarose gels to separate DSCCC from irreversibly denatured form IV DNA. One crosslink per DSCCC prevents irreversible alkali-denaturation. 500μm BCNU for 3 hrs was sufficient to crosslink 60% of DSCCC. Incubation with 4μg of purified O6MeGT prevented crosslink formation and allowed irreversible alkali denaturation. Equivalent amounts of BSA or buffer alone did not affect the reactivity of BCNU with DNA. Thus BCNU crosslinks can be prevented by O6MeGT. Results suggest that initial mono-adduct is at the O6 position of guanine. As O6MeGT is a suicide enzyme current modes of utilising nitrosoureas may not be optimal.

****

CIS-DIAMMINEDICHLOROPLATINUM TOXICITY AND DNA CROSSLINKING IN HUMAN MELANOMA AND LYMPHOBLAST CELLS. J. Hansson, U. Ringborg and R. Lewensohn, Department of Oncology, Radiumhemmet, Karolinska Hospital, Stockholm, Sweden.

Treatment of human malignant melanoma with cis-platinum has resulted in less than 20% responses (Friedman, Cisplatin 33: 462, Academic Press, 1980). Among the dose limiting toxicities exerted by cis-platinum in clinical practice is myelosuppression. Whether the clinical resistance of melanoma to cis-platinum is cellular or still not understood. We have now investigated the in vitro-sensitivity of human melanoma cell line (RPMI 8322) and phytohemagglutinin stimulated human lymphocytes to cis-platinum. When trypan blue exclusion was measured the concentration of cis-platinum needed for equal toxicity was more than 4 times higher in the melanoma cell line as compared to the human lymphoblasts. DNA crosslinks in the two cell populations were measured by Kohn's alkaline elution technique. After exposure of the cells for 30 min to different concentrations of cis-platinum and 5.5hr further incubation the amount of total crosslinks in the lymphoblasts was twice that registered in the melanoma cells. At this time the interstrand crosslinking effect in the melanoma cells was 3-4 times that in the lymphoblasts. Longer drugfree incubation times resulted in a further build-up of interstrand crosslinks in the lymphoblasts but not in the melanoma cells. At 24hr, when maximum crosslinking was noted in the lymphoblasts, the crosslinking difference was 10 times. At even longer incubation times less crosslinking was noted, presumably representing a DNA-repair process. Whether the lower crosslinking in the DNA of melanoma cells is due to less drug available at target site or to less binding sites may as yet not be concluded.

539

EXPERIMENTAL TRIAL OF NEW ALKYLATING HEXITOLS. J. Sugar, S. Somfai-Relle, I. Palyi, E. Institoris, E. Olah and O. Csuka, Research Institute of Oncopathology, Budapest, Hungary.

The second generation drugs of alkylating hexitol derivatives are 1,2:5,6-dianhydro-3,4-diacetyl-galactitol (diac-DAG) and 3,4-disuccinyl-dianhydro-galactitol (disu-DAG). Diac-DAG was found to have the best therapeutic index in the i.m. inoculated Walker carcinoma. Disu-DAG contains free acidic groups at the ends of the substituent, it has 3 times higher therapeutic index in the Walker model and is more favourable on P388 i.p., S180 s.c., Colon 26 s.c., Yoshida i.p., Guerin s.c., Lewis lung tumours and B16 melanoma. K562 human tumour cells were about four times more resistant against both drugs than the P388 mouse lymphoma cells with plating efficiency. 3924A hepatoma cells were more sensitive to disu-DAG in plateau than in log phase. In synchronised cultures cells were most sensitive to diac-DAG at the G1/S transition. Both DAG and diac-DAG formed interstrand cross-linking in DNA of Yoshida sarcoma tumour cells after in vivo treatment. The alkylation proceeded at the nitrogen 7 atom of guanine base forming 1,6-di-(guanin-7-yl)-1,6-dideoxygalactitol moieties in tumour cell DNA. Some correlation was found between the number of cross-linking induced by the two agents and their antitumour effects.

****

SITES AND EXTENTS OF ALKYLATION IN TUMOUR CELL DNA AND THEIR RELATION TO ANTITUMOUR EFFECTS OF DIBROMODULCITOL AND DIANHYDROGALACTITOL. E. Institoris*, J. Tamas** and L. Institoris***, *Nat. Oncol. Inst., **Central Res. Inst. Chem. Hung. Acad. Sci., ***Chinoin Pharm. Work., Budapest, Hungary.

It has been revealed that dibromodulcitol (DBD) and one of its conversion products dianhydrogalactitol (DAG) alkylate DNA in vivo yielding 3-alkyladenine, 7-alkylguanine and di(guanin-7-yl)-galactitol. The doses of the two drugs which produced nearly equal tumour inhibitory effects on Yoshida sarcoma cells resulted in the same amount of diguaninyl moieties in the tumour cell DNA but DBD produced six times as much monoalkylpurines as the DAG did. The persistence of monoalkylguanine and diguaninyl-galactitol in DNA was followed as a function of time. There was no significant loss of either monoalkylguanine or diguaninyl derivatives during the observation period i.e. 7-36hr, whereas the physical measurements of the amount of renaturable DNA showed a rapid opening of cross-links in the same period. The removal of cross-linking is proceeded by a two-step mechanism. In the first step, one arm of the cross-links is removed, leaving the DNA non-renaturable. While the other arm of cross-link is still attached covalently to the DNA molecule rendering possible the detection of the diguaninyl moiety in DNA. In the second step the other arm of the cross-link will be excised more later, probably at the same rate as it is in the case of monoalkylguanine.

HEXAMETHYLMELAMINE: METABOLIC ACTIVATION AND CYTOTOXICITY. <u>M.M. Ames</u> and <u>M.E. Sanders</u>, Mayo Clinic, Rochester, Minnesota, U.S.A.

Hexamethylmelamine (HMM) is an investigational s-triazine antitumour agent with established antitumour activity against human malignancies. We have shown that HMM is metabolically activated by hepatic monooxygenases to reactive species which covalently bind to microsomal protein and to calf thymus DNA. The N-methylol intermediate in HMM demethylation covalently binds to protein and calf thymus DNA in the absence of activating systems (Ames <u>et al</u>, Cancer Res. 43: 500, 1983). When HMM is incubated for 1hr with continuous human tumour cell lines in culture, no inhibition of colony formation is observed at concentrations as high as 200µg/ml. In this same system, mitomycin C totally abolishes colony formation at concentrations of 0.4µg/ml. When HMM is similarly incubated in the presence of 9,000 x g rat liver supernatant activating system, colony formation is inhibited only when NADPH is added to incubation mixtures. Cyclophosphamide was used as a positive control for these studies. We have also determined that HMM is significantly metabolised in an NADPH dependent manner by rat kidney, lung and brain microsomal preparations, but not by tumour cells under identical conditions. Cytotoxicity appears to be dependent on conversion of HMM to alkylating metabolites by hepatic and possibly extrahepatic tissues rather than formation of such metabolites by tumour cells. Supported in part by RCDA CA0755 (MMA), and CA30250, DHHS.

****

MELANOGENESIS IN HUMAN MALIGNANT MELANOMA XENOGRAFTS. <u>S. Sparrow,</u> <u>S. Billington and J. Rickard</u>, Toxicology Unit, Medical Research Council Laboratories, Carshalton, Surrey, England.

Chemotherapy can increase the pigment production of human malignant melanomas when grown as xenografts in athymic nude mice. Of five largely amelanotic human melanomas treated with a phenyltriazene (CB 10-286) three showed some response in terms of growth rate. These three tumours also exhibited an increase in melanin production when examined histologically. Homogenates of these tumours which had not been subjected to chemotherapy showed a marked inhibition of the conversion of DOPA to melanin. In one case there was an increase in the rate of melanin production when the tumour had been subjected to chemotherapy. Using HPLC to study the conversion of 5,6-dihydroxyindole to melanin it was found that the inhibition could occur at this stage of the metabolic pathway and that a non-responding tumour had a conversion factor that increased the rate of melanin production from 5,6-dihydroxyindole.

DNA CROSS-LINKING AND CYTOTOXICITY IN NORMAL AND TRANSFORMED HUMAN CELLS
TREATED IN VITRO WITH M&B 39565. N.W. Gibson, J.A. Hickman* and L.C.
Erickson, Lab. Molec. Pharm., NCI, Bethesda, Maryland, U.S.A. and *CRC
Experimental Chemotherapy Group, Univ. Aston, Birmingham, England.

Normal (IMR-90) and SV-40 transformed (VA-13) human embryo cells were treated
with M&B 39565 (8-carbamoyl-3-(2-chloroethyl)imidazo[5,1-d][1,2,3,5]-
tetrazin-4(3H)-one) and the effects on cell viability and cellular DNA
integrity were studied. M&B 38565 was compared to one of its potential
decomposition products 5-(3-(2-chloroethyl)triazen-1-yl)imidazo-4-carboxamide
(MCTIC). M&B 39565 and MCTIC were 5-6 fold more toxic to VA-13 cells than to
IMR-90 cells for drug concentrations which produced a 2 log cell kill, as
measured by colony forming assays. Using alkaline elution analysis VA-13
cells exhibited concentration dependent DNA interstrand cross-link formation.
However, in IMR-90 cells little or no interstrand cross-link formation was
detected. The DNA interstrand cross-link formation in VA-13 cells was found
to peak 12 hours after drug removal. A linear correlation between DNA
interstrand cross-link formation and log cell kill was observed in VA-13
cells, but not in IMR-90 cells. DNA-protein cross-link formation was found
to be comparable in both cell lines for each drug, suggesting that drug
penetration and intracellular drug reactivity was similar. Initial chemical
decomposition studies suggest that both M&B 39565 and MCTIC may produce a
chloroethyldiazo species. This species has been implicated in the formation
of chloroethyl-DNA adducts which convert to DNA interstrand cross-links in
mammalian cells treated with chloroethyl nitrosoureas (Erickson et al, Nature
288: 727, 1980). These data suggest that DNA interstrand cross-link
formation may be a common mechanism for the in vitro cytoxicity of M&B 39565
and MCTIC.

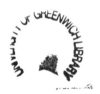

4. NEW AGENTS: METABOLISM AND PHARMACOKINETICS

IN VIVO PHARMACOKINETICS OF DAUNORUBICIN IN BONE MARROW IN ADULT ACUTE NONLYMPHOCYTIC LEUKAEMIA. P. Sonneveld*, H.A. Wassenaar**, K. Nooter* and B. Löwenberg**, *Radiobiological Institute TNO, Rijswijk; **Rotterdam Radiotherapeutic Institute, Rotterdam, The Netherlands.

Remission-induction chemotherapy of adult acute nonlymphocytic leukaemia (ANLL) with the new EORTC protocol LAM-6 includes Daunorubicin (DNR) as the anthracycline instead of Adriamycin, which was included in previous protocols. This choice was made in order to reduce bone marrow toxicity while maintaining the antileukaemic effect. In this study, the tissue concentrations of DNR and its metabolites in nucleated bone marrow and peripheral blood cells were investigated, together with the plasma pharmacokinetics, as measured with High Pressure Liquid Chromatography (HPLC). In 5 ANLL patients studied, during 3 repetitive injections of DNR, accumulation of DNR and its major metabolite was observed in plasma and blood leukocytes. In bone marrow, a considerable variation of DNR concentrations was found (tissue levels of DNR: $0.44 \times 10^{-5}M - 6.36 \times 10^{-5}M$ and of Daunomycinol: $1.33 \times 10^{-5}M - 10.0 \times 10^{-5}M$). In one patient no drug was detectable in bone marrow. Evidently, no correlation could be observed between bone marrow concentrations and plasma concentrations of DNR. Also, in patients studied during a second induction course, the cellular concentrations of DNR in hypoplastic bone marrow were different, when compared with the initial treatment. This study demonstrates that bone marrow concentrations of DNR have large individual variation, which may be indicative for the outcome of therapy.

****

PHARMACOLOGIC CHARACTERIZATION OF TEROXIRONE (HENKEL COMPOUND) IN ANIMALS AND HUMANS. M.M. Ames, J.S. Kovach, J. Rubin and D. Moertel, Mayo Clinic, Rochester, Minnesota, U.S.A.

Teroxirone (T, Henkel compound) is a triepoxide antitumour agent first studied in Europe. A more soluble preparation is being evaluated in the U.S. We have studied the disposition and metabolism of T in rabbits, rats and humans. We have developed an hplc assay based on derivatisation of T with diethyldithiocarbamate (DDC). T was analysed following extraction from biological fluids, derivatization with DDC, and normal phase hplc analysis. Following rapid i.v. infusion to patients, plasma disappearance is characterized by a one-compartment open model with mean values for $t\frac{1}{2}$, total body clearance and volume of distribution of 1.4min, 5.7ℓ/min, and 13ℓ, respectively. When T is administered by i.v. infusion (60-240min), plateau plasma concentrations are rapidly achieved, followed by rapid disappearance at the end of infusion. T is rapidly metabolised by hepatic, but not lung, microsomal preparations. Metabolism is NADPH independent and is inhibited by cyclohexene oxide. Epoxide hydrolysis products were detected in microsomal preparations and rabbit urine following administration of T. T cytotoxicity to human tumour cell lines in culture is abolished in the presence of 9,000 x g rat liver preparations, and is restored by the addition of cyclohexene oxide to incubation mixtures.

Supported in part by RCDA CA0755, DHHS (MMA), Contract CM27548, DHHS, and American Cancer Society Grant CH-143.

545

PHARMACOKINETICS AND TOXICITY OF VP 16 (ETOPOSIDE) IN PATIENTS WITH GESTATIONAL CHORIOCARCINOMA AND MALIGNANT TERATOMA. C.J. Brindley, P. Antoniw, E.S. Newlands and K.D. Bagshawe, Dept. Medical Oncology, Charing Cross Hospital, London, England.

18 patients with malignant teratoma each received VP16 in combination with cyclophosphamide and actinomycin D, and 7 patients with gestational choriocarcinoma recieved VP16 alone. VP16 (100mg/m^2) was administered on 5 consecutive days as an i.v. infusion of 30 minutes. Blood samples were taken immediately before and after infusion. Serum concentrations of the drug were measured by HPLC and are shown below.

Mean (+ S.D.) VP16 Concentration (μg/ml)

	Choriocarcinoma	Teratoma
5-20 mins after infusion	20.54 $\pm$ 2.59	20.04 $\pm$ 2.70
24hr after infusion	0.40 $\pm$ 0.27	0.56 $\pm$ 0.21

The major dose-limiting toxicity of VP16 is myelosuppression and there appears to be a linear correlation ($p < 0.001$) between WBC nadir and mean VP16 serum concentrations in those patients with malignant teratoma. However, when given as a single agent in gestational choriocarcinoma this relationship was not observed. The effect of altering the dose and schedule of VP16 on the pharmacokinetics and toxicity of the drug is being investigated.

****

TISSUE DISTRIBUTION AND MYELOTOXICITY OF DAUNOMYCIN IN NORMAL AND LEUKEMIC RATS: RAPID BOLUS INJECTION VERSUS CONTINUOUS INFUSION. K. Nooter, P. Sonneveld, J. Deurloo, R. Oostrum, F. Schultz, A. Martens and A. Hagenbeek, Radiobiological Institute TNO, Rijswijk, The Netherlands.

The present study was designed to compare the pharmacokinetic and cytotoxic behaviour of daunomycin (DAU), administered either as a rapid bolus inj. or as a 3-hour infusion in normal and leukemic rats. DAU and its metabolite duanomycinol (DAUNOL) were determined by HPLC (Baurain et al, Cancer Chem. Pharm. 2: 37, 1979) in plasma, urine, bile and tissues. After an i.v. bolus inj. of 7.5mg/kg in BN rats the plasma level decreased biphasically (t$\frac{1}{2}$ = 18.4min and 472min). The organs showed 2 types of time/conc. curves. One type, found in lungs, liver, kidneys and heart, had an initial high drug conc. followed by a relatively rapid elimination. In the other type, found in hemopoietic tissues, the drug uptake phase lasted longer (about 1.5hr) and the elimination phase was slower. After DAU infusion a plasma steady-state level is reached in 1.5hr and high peak levels are absent. DAU infusion led to substantially lower tissue levels, including heart tissue. The experiments in which the myelotoxicity was estimated by CFU-S (colony forming units-spleen) survival (Sonneveld et al, Cancer Chem. Pharm. 5: 167, 1981) showed that bolus inj. killed twice as much CFU-S than did infusion (18% versus 34%). DAU bolus inj. or infusion in rats made leukemic by transplantable leukemia cells, led only to a slight increase in drug content in those tissues that were infiltrated by leukemic cells. About 90% of the leukemic CFU-S survived after infusion, while by bolus inj. 50% of the LCFU-S were killed. In conclusion, DAU infusion is less toxic for heart and bone marrow but DAU bolus inj. has a better therapeutic effect.

METABOLISM OF 4-HYDROXYANDROSTENE-3,17-DIONE BY RAT LIVER. I.B. Parr and M.G. Rowlands, Inst. Cancer Res., Sutton, Surrey, England.

4-Hydroxy-4-androstene-3,17-dione (4OHA) is an effective inhibitor of aromatase in vitro whilst in vivo it acts as an anti-estrogen (Brodie et al, Endocrinol. 100: 1684, 1977). The metabolism of (^{14}C) 4-OHA was studied using rat hepatocytes (prepared by perfusion technique). After incubation at 37°C for 1hr, 70% of the total radioactivity added was in the aqueous residue remaining after extraction with ethyl acetate. Steroid constituents of the aqueous phase were absorbed on to amberlite X AD-2 resin, eluted with MeOH and separated by TLC. The only area of radioactivity on the TLC plate was associated with a band which stained strongly positive with a naphthoresorcinol spray reagent specific for glucuronide.

****

ENZYME INHIBITION STUDIES WITH DERIVATIVES OF AMINOGLUTETHIMIDE. M.G. Rowlands and M. Bunnett Inst. Cancer Res., Sutton, Surrey, and M.J. Daly, P.J. Nicholls and H.J. Smith, Welsh School of Pharmacy, UWIST, Cardiff, Wales.

Aminoglutethimide, 3-(4-aminophenyl)-3-ethylpiperidine-2,6-dione, (AG) in combination with replacement glucocorticoid is an effective endocrine therapy in advanced postmenopausal breast cancer (Santen, Breast Cancer Res. and Treat. 1: 183, 1981). AG blocks oestrogen biosynthesis via inhibition of peripheral aromatase and adrenal desmolase enzyme complexes. The aromatase blockage appears to be the clinically relevant site of action and the development of a potent, specific aromatase inhibitor would be of therapeutic advantage. 3-(4-aminophenyl)-1-ethylpyrrolodine-2,5-dione (I) and its N-methylated analogue (II) have been synthesised and assayed in vitro for activity against bovine adrenal desmolase and human placental aromatase. Comparison was made with AG and its N-methylated analogue (III). Compound I was as potent as AG against aromatase, with little activity against desmolase indicating that for these 4-aminophenyl derivatives the pyrrolidinedione ring confers greater selectivity of action than the piperidinedione ring system of AG. The methylated analogues displayed weak, non-selective inhibition. Analogues of AG and compound I lacking the amino group or substituted with a nitro group were weakly active against both enzymes, indicating the importance of the amino moiety for inhibitory activity. Further analogues of AG and compound I are being synthesised to explore the structure activity relationships.

THE SPECIES DEPENDENT PHARMACOKINETICS OF DTIC. R.B. Vincent, C.J. Rutty and G. Abel, Inst. of Cancer Res., Sutton, Surrey, England.

5-(3-Dimethyl-1-triazeno)imidazole-4-carboxamide (DTIC) is an antitumour agent which has limited use in the treatment of malignant melanoma. DTIC is known to undergo oxidative N-demethylation to give 5-(3-monomethyl-1-triazeno)imidazole-4-carboxamide (MIC) via an intermediate carbinolamine 5-(3-hydroxymethyl, 3-monomethyl-1-triazeno)imidazole-4-carboxamide (HMIC). MIC undergoes rapid chemical decomposition yielding a methyl carbonium ion which can methylate DNA. Thus the antitumour activity of DTIC is dependent upon metabolism of the drug. In view of the marked species differences in the N-demethylation of pentamethylmelamine (PMM) described earlier (Rutty et al, Cancer Chemother. Pharmacol. 8, 105, 1982), the metabolism of DTIC in mouse, rat and man was examined. The plasma half life ($t\frac{1}{2}\beta$) of DTIC in the rat (29.6mins) was significantly greater than in the mouse (8.6mins), and greater still in 4 patients studied to date (57-100mins). Of greater significance were the peak levels of the cytotoxic metabolites HMIC and MIC found in the plasma of mice (33.8µM) which were very much higher than in either rat (2.0µM) or man (6.7µM). Correspondingly, DTIC shows marked activity versus a mouse plasmacytoma, but is without activity against the Walker 256 tumour grown in the rat. These findings suggest that the poor clinical activity of DTIC is at least in part due to the low level of metabolism of the drug in man.

****

PRELIMINARY STUDIES ON THE METABOLISM AND PHARMACOKINETICS OF THE DIALKYLPHENYLTRIAZENES. C.J. Rutty, G. Abel, R.B. Vincent, P.M. Goddard and K.R. Harrap, Inst. Cancer Res., Sutton, Surrey, England.

The metabolism and pharmacokinetics of a series of dialkylphenyltriazenes have been examined with a view to selecting an appropriate clinical alternative to DTIC. A number of these compounds have shown activity against a mouse PC6 plasmacytoma. However, it has previously been demonstrated for pentamethylmelamine (PMM) and DTIC, agents which, like the dialkylphenyltriazenes, are believed to require metabolic activation, that such antitumour activity does not adequately reflect the clinical situation because of marked species differences in oxidative N-demethylation. In an examination of the pharmacokinetics of 1-p-carboxamidophenyl-3,3-dimethyltriazene (CB 10-286) this compound was found to be more rapidly metabolised in the mouse (plasma $t\frac{1}{2}\beta$ = 3.7mins) than in the rat ($t\frac{1}{2}\beta$ = 16.9mins), and resulted in the generation of some four-fold higher levels of the monomethyltriazene, which is the putative active metabolite. However, by pretreating rats with oral sodium phenobarbitone it was possible to mimic the mouse pharmacokinetics in the rat. Despite marked antitumour activity of 1-p-carboxyphenyl-3,3-dimethyltriazene (CB 10-277) this compound failed to undergo any N-demethylation in vitro, in contrast to the carboxyamido derivative. Furthermore, there was no apparent formation of a monomethyl metabolite in vivo. The apparent lack of oxidative N-demethylation of this particular triazene brings into question the hypothesis that such metabolism is a prerequisite of antitumour activity for this class of compounds.

THE ROLE OF GLUTATHIONE AND GLUTATHIONE S-TRANSFERASES IN ACQUIRED DRUG RESISTANCE. A.L. Wang and K.D. Tew, Lab of Molecular Pharmacology, Div of Medical Oncology and Dept of Biochemistry, Lombardi Cancer Center, Georgetown University, Washington, DC, U.S.A.

A selected population from a wild type (WS) Walker 256 rat mammary carcinoma has been demonstrated to have a 20-fold resistance to nitrogen mustards. However, these resistant cells (WR) have no collateral resistance to nitrosoureas. A direct correlation between the carbamoylating activity and cytotoxicity has been found in this cell line. A one-hour incubation with N,N'-bis-(trans-4-hydroxycyclohexyl)-N'-nitrosourea (BCyNU) (which decomposes to produce carbamoylating isocyanate species, but no alkylating species) at a concentration of $5 \times 10^{-3}M$ resulted in a 50% inhibition of glutathione reductase (GR) activity in WS and 100% in WR. Similar nitrogen mustard concentrations had no effect on GR activity. The basal levels of this enzyme showed that the GR activity in the WR cells was approximately half of the WS (3.98 vs 8.67 nmoles NADPH oxidised/mg protein/min). Glutathione S-transferases have been shown to protect cells against alkylating species. Basal activity in WR is twice that of WS (28.3 vs 14.1 nmoles/mg/min with CDNB as substrate). ID_{50} concentrations of alkylating and carbamoylating agents did not deplete transferase activity. The reduced efficiency of GR in WR cells may account for their relative sensitivity to carbamoylation. The presence of double minutes, a marker for gene amplification, and the increased glutathione S-transferase activity in the WR may be commensurate with an increased capacity of the resistant cells to deal with the electrophilic alkylating species and express resistance.

****

DISPOSITION OF TRICYCLIC NUCLEOSIDE 5'-PHOSPHATE (TCN-P, NSC 280594) IN MAN AND RAT. P.J. Basseches, G. Powis, J.S. Kovach and R.L. Richardson, Dept. Oncology, Mayo Clinic, Rochester, Minnesota, U.S.A.

TCN-P is the monophosphate ester of an unusual tricyclic nucleoside (TCN). TCN-P and TCN were assayed by reverse phase HPLC (Basseches et al, J. Chromatogr. 233: 227, 1982). TCN-P is converted to TCN by human plasma in vitro at 37° with a $t_\frac{1}{2}$ of 23min. TCN-P was administered to patients in phase I trial as a daily 10min infusion of 5 to 44mg/m², for 5 days. TCN-P is rapidly accumulated by rbc and could not be consistently detected in plasma at doses <36mg/m². Peak TCN-P concentrations in whole blood occurred within 5min of administration and were >10μg/ml at a dose of 44mg/m². TCN-P was slowly eliminated from blood with an initial $t_\frac{1}{2}$ of 6hr and a slower second phase of elimination which was not accurately defined. Blood concentrations of TCN-P 24hr later were 4μg/ml. These concentrations were maintained over 5 day administration with no accumulation of the drug. TCN in plasma was around 0.2 g/ml at a dose of 44mg/m² and was maintained over 5 days. No other metabolites were detected in blood or plasma. TCN is metabolised by rat liver microsomes with loss of in vitro cytotoxicity, to the bicyclic open ring metabolite. The metabolite was detected in rat bile as 13% of a dose of TCN 6.9mg/kg, in 12hr. Over the same time 46% of dose was excreted as unchanged TCN in bile. The metabolite could not be detected in rat blood. (Supported by NCI Contract CM27548 and ACS CH143).

CIRCADIAN VARIATION IN THE PHARMACOKINETICS OF SOME CYTOTOXIC DRUGS AND SYNTHETIC STEROIDS. J. English, G.W. Aherne and V. Marks, Dept. Biochemistry, University of Surrey, Guildford, Surrey.

Circadian variations in the toxicity and efficacy of a number of cytotoxic drugs and synthetic steroids have been found in rodents (Scheving et al, Chronobiologia 7: 33, 1980), but the possibility of these changes being due to variations in the pharmacokinetics has seldom been investigated. This study reports changes in T$\frac{1}{2}$ and AUC which depend on the time of day of drug administration. Drugs were injected into male Norwegian hooded rats (250-300g) maintained on a light dark schedule of 0630-1830hr light : 1830-0630hr dark, via surgically exposed femoral veins and blood samples were obtained from the tail veins. Drug concentrations were measured by RIA.

Time of Dose (GMT)	Bleomycin 500 µg/kg		AraC 1mg/kg		VCR 100µg/kg		Prednisolone 1mg/kg	
	T$\frac{1}{2}$	AUC	T$\frac{1}{2}$	AUC	T$\frac{1}{2}$	AUC	T$\frac{1}{2}$	AUC
0600	53+10	290+21	54+3	17+2	56+3	67+7	20+2	178+17
1200	23+2	215+19	33+1	8+1	39+4	41+6	15+2	79+6
1800	31+2	175+34	37+2	11+1	42+6	42+3	21+1	84+7
2400	23+1	263+22	16+1	9+1	37+2	35+4	16+1	79+3

Each value for T$\frac{1}{2}$ (min) and AUC (ng/ml.hr; µg/ml.hr for AraC) represents the mean + SEM (n = 6). The clinical relevance and mechanisms behind these variations remain to be investigated.

****

ANTITUMOUR AND PHARMACOKINETIC STUDIES WITH PLATINUM COORDINATION COMPLEXES FOLLOWING ORAL ADMINISTRATION. Z.H. Siddik, P.M. Goddard, F.E. Boxall, *C.F.J. Barnard and K.R. Harrap, Inst. Cancer Res., Sutton, Surrey and *Johnson Matthey Res. Centre, Sonning Common, Reading, England.

Cisplatin and its analogues, cis-diammine(1,1-cyclobutanedicarboxy lato)platinum II (CBDCA, JM8) and cis-dichloro-trans-dihydroxy-bis(isopropylamine)platinum IV (CHIP, JM9), are active against a number of experimental rodent neoplasms when administered parenterally. This is the first report to describe the antitumour activity of this class of compounds following oral administration via a stomach tube. The complexes were tested against the ADJ/PC6A plasmacytoma grown s.c. in female Balb C⁻ mice, and the Walker 256 carcinosarcoma grown i.m. in male Wistar rats. Cisplatin had a TI (therapeutic index; LD_{50}/ED_{90}) of 4-5 against the ADJ/PC6A and a TI of 2 against the Walker 256. Comparable or lower activity against the ADJ/PC6A has also been demonstrated for CBDCA and CHIP. Following an oral dose of 50mg/kg in mice of the three complexes, maximum platinum levels in blood (1.5-2.4µg/ml) are achieved 1-4 hours after drug administration. Urinary excretion is greatest for cisplatin (15% of dose in 48 hours), followed by CHIP (13%) and CBDCA (9%). The major part (60-80%) of the dose, however, is excreted in the faeces. These results indicate that the orally administered cisplatin and the two analogues are absorbed to an appreciable extent into the systemic circulation. This is probably important in producing the observed antitumour activities of the complexes when given by this route of administration.

AUTHOR INDEX

Abel, G. 548
Adams, G.E. 241
Afra, D. 532
Aherne, G.W. 523, 550
Alexander, P. 43
Alison, D.L. 527, 535
Allen, J.M. 469
Ames, M.M. 541, 545
Antoniw, P. 546
Arnold, W. 517
Atassi, G. 524
Bagshawe, K.D. 546
Baig, G.U. 518
Baines, M.J. 182
Baker,M.H. 485
Ban, J. 518
Barnard, C.F.J. 550
Barrie, S.E. 526, 527
Bartoli, M.H. 533
Basseches, P.J. 549
Bedford, P. 383
Belanger, A. 475
Bellido, V. 521
Berger, M. 520
Beriel, H. 533
Besserer, J. 315
Beunner, K.W. 95
Billiaert, P. 153
Billington, S. 541
Black, L.J. 457
Bloch, A 251
Bloom, S.R. 469
Bogden, A.E. 215
Boggust, W.A. 301
Bondy, P.K. 295
Booth, R.J. 289
Boritzki, T.J. 315
Boxall, F.E. 550
Brindley, C.J. 546
Brodie, A. 451
Bunnett, M. 547
Burton, N.K. 523
Calman, K.C. 153
Calvert, A.H. 526, 527, 535
Canellakis, Z.N. 295
Carter, S.K. 49

Casazza, A.M. 345
Cavalli, F. 95
Cedermark, B.J. 534
Chrapusta, S. 497
Cleare, M.J. 357
Clemens, J.A. 457
Clink, H. 33
Cobb, W.R. 215
Cole, V.M. 257
Cook, P.D. 13
Coombes, R.C. 451, 485
Courtenay, V.D. 221
Creaven, P.J. 532
Crofts, M. 33
Csuka, O. 540
Daly, M.J. 547
Davies, L.C. 526
de Haan, H.A. 445
de Marco, A. 345
Deurloo, J. 546
Devleeschouwer, N. 463
Dhaliwal, H.S. 117
Diddens, H. 535
Dietrich, W. 503
Diver, J. 445
Drumm, A. 301
Duch, D.S. 333
Dumonde, D.C. 283
Dumont, P. 524
Dupont, A. 475
Eckhardt, S. 77, 532
Edsmyr, F. 534
Einhorn, L.H. 135
Eisenbrand, G. 351
Eksborg, S. 534
English, J. 550
Eppenberger, U. 491
Erickson, L.C. 371, 542
Evans, B.D. 395
Facchinetti, T. 345
Foster, A.B. 485
Fox, B.W. 227, 383
Fox, K.R. 377
Friedlos, F. 389
Friedrich, H.-J. 531
Fry, D.W. 315

583

To Zoe who
died age 15 of
cancer.
I miss you x x